Blood Safety

Hua Shan • Roger Y. Dodd
Editors

Blood Safety

A Guide to Monitoring and Responding to Potential New Threats

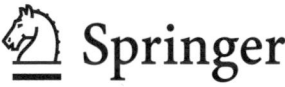
Springer

Editors
Hua Shan, MD, PhD
Department of Pathology
Stanford University
Stanford, CA
USA

Roger Y. Dodd, PhD
American Red Cross
Medical Office
Rockville, MD
USA

Department of Pathology
Johns Hopkins University
Baltimore, MD
USA

ISBN 978-3-030-06851-6   ISBN 978-3-319-94436-4   (eBook)
https://doi.org/10.1007/978-3-319-94436-4

© Springer International Publishing AG, part of Springer Nature 2019
Softcover re-print of the Hardcover 1st edition 2019
This work is subject to copyright. All rights are reserved by the Publisher, whether the whole or part of the material is concerned, specifically the rights of translation, reprinting, reuse of illustrations, recitation, broadcasting, reproduction on microfilms or in any other physical way, and transmission or information storage and retrieval, electronic adaptation, computer software, or by similar or dissimilar methodology now known or hereafter developed.
The use of general descriptive names, registered names, trademarks, service marks, etc. in this publication does not imply, even in the absence of a specific statement, that such names are exempt from the relevant protective laws and regulations and therefore free for general use.
The publisher, the authors, and the editors are safe to assume that the advice and information in this book are believed to be true and accurate at the date of publication. Neither the publisher nor the authors or the editors give a warranty, express or implied, with respect to the material contained herein or for any errors or omissions that may have been made. The publisher remains neutral with regard to jurisdictional claims in published maps and institutional affiliations.

This Springer imprint is published by the registered company Springer Nature Switzerland AG
The registered company address is: Gewerbestrasse 11, 6330 Cham, Switzerland

Foreword

Assuring the safety of blood transfusions has been a fundamental and ongoing challenge from the earliest days of human experimentation with transfusion in the late seventeenth century. Introduction of cross matching at the dawn of the twentieth century based on Karl Landsteiner's landmark discovery of blood groups ushered in the modern era of transfusion medicine by dramatically reducing deaths from blood incompatibility. Rapid advances in anticoagulation permitted blood storage, replacing direct donor to patient transfusions with the use of banked blood, enabling the widespread practice of transfusion.

With expanded use, infectious disease risks of transfusion soon became apparent. First were reports of syphilis transmissions in 1911 and 1915, leading to universal donation testing, ongoing since 1938. Posttransfusion hepatitis was discovered in 1943, and a remarkably high incidence was documented in the early 1960s. Universal donation testing for HBsAg was implemented in 1971 based on the serendipitous discovery of the "Australia antigen" in 1962 and its subsequent linkage to some, but not most posttransfusion hepatitis. Association of posttransfusion hepatitis with paid donation led to the adoption of volunteer (unpaid) collections also in the 1970s. Continued transmission of non-A, non-B hepatitis unfortunately was considered benign for lack of a clear disease association. This misperception delayed an aggressive response until epidemiologic studies established morbidity of the condition, and the discovery of hepatitis C virus as the etiologic agent of non-A, non-B hepatitis allowed development of specific donor screening tests, implemented in 1990.

In the cases of syphilis and hepatitis B, the public health authorities and blood banking community reacted over time with appropriate scientific studies, technological innovations, and safety interventions without major public pressure or apparent concern. Conversely, the crisis of confidence and demand for accountability which followed the revelation in 1982 that the emerging epidemic of AIDS, a fatal and sexually transmissible infection, had severely compromised blood product safety, especially for clotting factor recipients, began a new era of blood safety decisionmaking under intense congressional and public scrutiny, mainly focused on product manufacturers and Food and Drug Administration (FDA). Underlying the controversy whether public health authorities had acted appropriately to address blood safety in the face of the HIV/AIDS epidemic was a deeper question whether the US system had the leadership, organization, and mind-set necessary to cope with a novel, rapidly evolving, and uncertain epidemic threat. These issues were addressed in the 1995 report of the Institute of Medicine (IOM) on *HIV and the Blood Supply: An Analysis of Crisis Decisionmaking* which called for more coordinated institutional leadership, transparent risk communications, and timely and proportionate responses in periods of scientific uncertainty. In 1996, echoing similar concerns, a congressional committee faulted governmental agencies for a "mute public health response" to the silent epidemic of hepatitis C virus (HCV), including inadequate efforts to notify transfusion recipients of possible exposure to HCV prior to effective testing of blood donations. FDA responded in 2000 with rulemaking to establish HCV "lookback" procedures like those in place for HIV.

In the immediate wake of the HIV epidemic, regulatory efforts centered on risk reduction for human T-lymphotropic retrovirus (HTLV) and hepatitis C and on improving compliance of the blood industry with current good manufacturing practices. However, responding to epidemic diseases became a dramatic, recurrent, and disruptive theme as nature tested us repeatedly with threats from novel and emerging agents. Epidemics affecting blood safety unfolded, while progress was ongoing to address slower evolving threats from Chagas disease, malaria, babesiosis, and bacterially contaminated platelet collections. Human outbreaks of zoonotic infections emerged as particular concerns. The 1996 report of presumptively food acquired cases of variant Creutzfeldt-Jakob disease in the United Kingdom, a fatal condition, caused FDA in 1999 to recommend for the first time preventive measures against a potentially serious but uncertain threat to blood safety based just on a theoretical likelihood of transfusion transmission. West Nile virus (WNV), which became widespread in the United States in 2002, represented the first instance of a vector-borne epidemic disease that threatened blood safety only during acute environmental outbreaks and only for a brief period of asymptomatic infection in the donor. Prior to WNV, blood safety threats were recognized only for diseases transmitted during chronic, asymptomatic infections. Another mosquito-borne flavivirus, Zika virus (ZIKV), reached Puerto Rico in December 2015 after massive spread in southern countries of the Americas. While the course of the ZIKV epidemic in the Continental United States could not be predicted, urgent and universal interventions to protect blood safety were mandated in 2016 based on the severe neurological risks to a fetus from an infected mother, difficulties in identifying areas with active mosquito-borne transmission, impacts of donor deferrals on local blood supplies, and the possibility of a secondary epidemic spread by sexual transmission. Again, decisionmakers were challenged to act in the face of scientific uncertainty.

Over time, the introduction of validated virus reduction steps in manufacturing processes eliminated nearly all known infectious risks from clotting factors and other plasma derivatives. These measures further obviated the need to introduce new safeguards for subsequently emerging viral epidemics. This demonstrated their presumptive value as precautions against unknown agents of future concern. Similarly, pathogen reduction technology for blood components, currently approved only for plasma and some types of platelets, holds the promise of a more precautionary approach to emerging infectious diseases (EIDs) affecting transfusion safety. However, pending the availability of pathogen reduction methods for all blood components, donor screening for risk factors and laboratory testing of donations remain the principal safety interventions for EIDs.

The chapters of this book summarize the scientific state of the art on assessing and responding to potential new threats to blood safety. No less important is the question whether the lessons of the HIV/AIDS epidemic, summarized in the 1995 IOM report, will remain in the forefront of the minds of decisionmakers as time goes on. I suggest that readers of this book reflect on the history of the spread of HIV as they enjoy a highly edifying account of the strategies that have been developed in the last several decades to predict, monitor, assess, and respond to potential new infectious threats to blood safety.

May 2018

Jay S. Epstein, MD
Senior Advisor for International Blood Regulatory Affairs
Center for Biologics Evaluation and Research
US Food and Drug Administration
Silver Spring, MD, USA

Contents

Part I Recent Progress

1. **Prediction and Prevention: Interventions to Enhance Blood Safety**.................................. 3
   Roger Y. Dodd

2. **Assessing the Threat: Public Health** 17
   Hans L. Zaaijer

3. **Assessing the Threat: Public Concern** 35
   Anne Wiles, Judie Leach Bennett, and Dana Devine

4. **Health Economics in Blood Safety**............................ 53
   Brian Custer

5. **Decision Systems** 83
   Philip Kiely

Part II Case Studies

6. **HIV and Blood Safety**.. 125
   Mrigender Virk and Hua Shan

7. **vCJD Case Studies** 143
   Patricia Hewitt and Robert Will

8. **Case Study: West Nile Virus**................................. 157
   Roger Y. Dodd

9. **Zika Virus** 163
   Luiz Amorim

Part III Current Concerns

10 The Emergence of Zoonotic Pathogens as Agents of Concern in Transfusion Medicine..................................... 189
Louis M. Katz

11 Tick-Borne Infections: Beware the Tortoises Among Us........... 207
David A. Leiby

Part IV International Collaboration

12 International Collaboration for Improving Global Blood Safety and for Monitoring and Responding to Potential Microbial Threats... 225
Jose Ramiro Cruz, Rene Berrios Cruz, Jorge Duque Rodríguez, and Silvina Kuperman

Index.. 251

Contributors

Luiz Amorim, MD Hemorio Blood Center, Rio de Janeiro, Brazil

Judie Leach Bennett, LL.B, LL.M Canadian Blood Services, Ottawa, ON, Canada

Rene Berrios Cruz, MD Ministry of Health, National Blood Service, Managua, Nicaragua

Jose Ramiro Cruz, MSc, DSc International Affairs Committee, Grupo Cooperativo Iberoamericano de Medicina Transfusional, Ashburn, VA, USA

Brian Custer, MPH, PhD Epidemiology and Health Policy Science, VP Research and Scientific Programs, Blood Systems Research Institute, San Francisco, CA, USA

Department of Laboratory Medicine, University of California San Francisco, San Francisco, CA, USA

Dana Devine, PhD University of British Columbia Centre for Blood Research and Canadian Blood Services, Vancouver, BC, Canada

Roger Y. Dodd, PhD American Red Cross, Medical Office, Rockville, MD, USA

Department of Pathology, Johns Hopkins University, Baltimore, MD, USA

Patricia Hewitt, FRCP, FRCPath Department of Microbiology Services, NHS Blood and Transplant, London, UK

Louis M. Katz, MD America's Blood Centers, Washington, DC, USA

Philip Kiely, BSc (Hons) Australian Red Cross Blood Service, Melbourne, Australia

Department of Epidemiology and Preventive Medicine, Monash University, Melbourne, Australia

Silvina Kuperman, MD Centro Regional de Hemoterapia, Hospital de Pediatria Garrahan, Buenos Aires, Argentina

David A. Leiby, PhD Division of Emerging and Transfusion-Transmitted Diseases, OBRR/CBER, U.S. Food and Drug Administration, Silver Spring, MD, USA

Jorge Duque Rodríguez, MD, MC Facultad de Medicina, Area de Investigacion, Universidad Autonoma de Chihuahua, Chihuahua, Mexico

Hua Shan, MD, PhD Department of Pathology, Stanford University, Stanford, CA, USA

Mrigender Virk, MD Department of Pathology, Stanford Hospital, Stanford, CA, USA

Anne Wiles, PhD Risk Sciences International, Ottawa, ON, Canada

Robert Will, MA, MD, FRCP National CJD Research and Surveillance Unit, Western General Hospital, Edinburgh, UK

Hans L. Zaaijer, MD, PhD Department of Blood-borne Infections, Sanquin Blood Supply Foundation, Amsterdam, The Netherlands

Department of Clinical Virology, Academic Medical Center, Amsterdam, The Netherlands

Part I
Recent Progress

Chapter 1
Prediction and Prevention: Interventions to Enhance Blood Safety

Roger Y. Dodd

Introduction

The safety of the blood supply has been a matter of concern from the outset with the successive recognition of transfusion-transmitted syphilis, closely followed by hepatitis outbreaks. Indeed, hepatitis was, for many years, regarded as an accepted and intractable outcome of transfusion, particularly in the United States. In the late 1950s and the 1960s, there were concerted efforts to understand and to minimize this problem, culminating in the recognition of causative agents and implementation of specific donor tests. However, it was not until the AIDS crisis in the 1980s that safety became an overriding priority. In retrospect, AIDS was a harbinger of the global dissemination of a transfusion-transmissible, epidemic infection. This set the scene for aggressive attention to blood safety but also established the expectation that there might be other transfusion-transmissible disease outbreaks in the future, but the fear was focused on chronic, parenterally transmitted agents. Agents with the potential for transfusion transmission must have an asymptomatic phase with circulation in the blood, must survive the processes inherent in collection and storage of blood, and must be infectious by the intravenous route. The advent of West Nile fever in the United Sates was yet another unexpected threat to blood safety, but it has been followed by a cascade of other global outbreaks of tropical arboviruses with actual or theoretical implications to the blood supply. The issue is whether or not there are means to foresee and defend against such events.

R. Y. Dodd
American Red Cross, Medical Office, Rockville, MD, USA

Department of Pathology, Johns Hopkins University, Baltimore, MD, USA
e-mail: Roger.Dodd@redcross.org

Emerging Infectious Diseases

Over that past 30 years or so, emerging infectious diseases have become an intense focus of attention. The simplest definition is that these are diseases whose frequency has increased over the prior 20 years [1]. There are many drivers for emergence, but some of the most important are environmental change, rapid transportation, urbanization, conflict, and failure of control measures. In addition, the agents themselves may mutate and acquire different properties.

Some emerging infections clearly impact blood safety. The first of these was AIDS. HIV, the causative agent, originated in primates in Africa and was likely transmitted to humans as a result of preparation of meat from such primates. Subsequent human to human transmission probably occurred horizontally via the sexual route and perhaps vertically to infants. Large-scale emergence of the disease was attributable to travel and extensive sexual networks, particularly among men having sex with other men. Infection is almost invariably chronic, and there is a very long asymptomatic period during which the virus is present in the circulation. This long incubation period was not appreciated at first and resulted in the silent spread of the virus including its transmission by blood transfusion. Ultimately, although HIV/AIDS had a serious negative impact on blood safety and on public confidence, it did stimulate a proactive response to recipient protection.

A second emerging infection with potentially severe implications to transfusion was variant Creutzfeldt-Jakob disease (vCJD), another zoonosis, caused by ingestion of the infectious prion responsible for bovine spongiform encephalopathy (BSE, mad cow disease) [2]. In this case, the potential for transfusion transmission was predicted before any cases were seen, an important step, because this disease also has a very lengthy latency. It is important to note that, although the BSE and vCJD outbreak emerged in the United Kingdom, concern and prevention were global. Indeed, globalization and transportation were definitively involved in the spread of BSE and vCJD.

In 1999, West Nile virus (WNV) was identified for the first time in North America, with a few cases in New York City. In the next few years, it expanded across the continent. In 2002, a total of 23 cases of transfusion transmission were reported in the United States, and there were estimates that hundreds of thousands of individuals had been naturally infected by mosquitoes [3]. Universal blood donor testing for WNV RNA was in place by mid-2003. WNV is an arbovirus, transmitted by culicine mosquitoes, and the primary amplifying hosts are birds. Human-to-human transmission does not occur (other than by transfusion), and the human is an accidental, dead-end host. The appearance and scope of the outbreak were completely unexpected. Initially, there was little concern about blood safety, as the previous focus had been on chronic infections. In the case of WNV, the size of the outbreak was such that there was a significant chance of collecting blood from an individual during the short (7–10 day) viremic phase of early infection. The virus now appears to be endemic in the United States with annual periods of human infection and disease.

The early twenty-first century in the Americas has been characterized by continuing waves of epidemics of tropical arboviruses, essentially all of which are transmitted by *Aedes* mosquitoes. Unlike WNV, the relevant viruses are transmissible by the human-mosquito-human route. They are actually or potentially transmissible by transfusion. They include dengue, chikungunya, and Zika viruses. Most recently, Zika virus has received particular attention, largely because it is responsible for a very serious fetal disease syndrome, which includes microcephaly [4]. In the United States, universal, individual donation NAT has been required since late 2016, although only a few tens of positive donations were found nationwide during the first year and a half of testing.

A critical question is whether or not these outbreaks could have been predicted as a first step toward control or prevention of adverse outcomes. The purpose of the remainder of this chapter is to discuss the extent to which this may be achieved and the available interventions to manage the risk.

Horizon Scanning

Early recognition of a potential threat is a critical step toward establishing readiness for the impact of an emerging infection. Fortunately, general awareness of emerging infections has led to a great deal of interest in this area, and tools are readily available [5].

Probably the best source of primary information is ProMed-mail, a simple list server that provides frequent bulletins about infectious disease events worldwide (http://www.promedmail.org). It is possible to receive documented alerts on human, animal, and plant diseases or to select one or two of these categories. The information is carefully curated for reliability, and, in many cases, brief commentary is appended to the news item. All postings are also maintained in a web-based searchable database. In normal use, one or two posts are received each day via e-mail and each report may have up to four or five different items. High profile outbreaks may be followed, as updates are posted as appropriate.

The websites of national and supranational health organizations are also rich sources of information about disease outbreaks. Globally, the World Health Organization (WHO) is most comprehensive, but each WHO region also has a website. In the case of the Americas, the PAHO site is most informative. The US Centers for Disease Control and Prevention (CDC) has an excellent site which also covers outbreaks outside the United States. Similarly, the European Center for Disease Control (ECDC) has a topical and informative site. Most countries also have similar sites.

Another very useful primary source is HealthMap (http://www.healthmap.org/en/), which reports on and tracks infectious diseases through a mapping interface, which may be used interactively. There are many additional components, including topical reports on events, and the website deserves careful exploration. Additionally, social media should not be overlooked, as many of these, and similar programs have Twitter feeds that are reliable pointers to important information.

Horizon scanning using these tools, however, only identifies and perhaps describes the extent of an outbreak but does not usually provide any information about its implications for blood safety. As a broad generalization, to be transfusion-transmissible, an infectious agent must have an asymptomatic phase during which the agent is present in the blood. This requirement reduces concern about many respiratory and enteric infections. Even so, precautions may be appropriate if the transmission route is not clearly known, and the epidemiology of the infection involves rapid and extensive spread, as was the case for SARS. In this case, WHO rapidly recommended precautions to protect blood safety.

Thus, if the outbreak is of a known disease, it is reasonable to consider the likelihood of transfusion transmission before preparing to develop interventions [6].

An interesting, but rare event would be the recognition of a transfusion-transmitted infection before an outbreak of the disease had been established. It could be argued that this is possible in special circumstances, and, indeed, some viruses have been identified in the context of searches for otherwise unknown hepatitis viruses. However, the viruses identified this way do not appear to be pathogenic. On the other hand, it is true that astute physicians reported the earliest (unexpected) evidence of transfusion transmission of some known agents. West Nile virus is good example of this situation.

Prediction

Given the available information, is it possible to predict an outbreak of a transfusion-transmitted infection and thus be fully prepared when the outbreak occurs? The simple answer is "sometimes," but the inherent problem is that emerging infections are themselves not predictable. The situation is made more complex by the fact that, currently, in most cases the best intervention is to develop and implement a sensitive test for donated blood. Industry is understandably not usually willing to commit to test development until the market need is apparent, a situation usually linked to demonstrated transfusion transmissions of the emerging agent. However, it is clear that the extent and urgency of the eventual intervention are associated with the severity of the disease.

Recently, tropical arboviruses have been a matter of particular concern in the Americas, and they illustrate different circumstances. The appearance of West Nile virus in the United States in 1999 could not have been predicted. In contrast, the appearance of Zika virus in the United States led to rapid and perhaps overzealous implementation of universal testing [7]. In this case, however, there was an immediate history of the rapid spread of other tropical arboviruses (most notably chikungunya virus) throughout the Caribbean and South America and subsequently into Puerto Rico and to other mainland areas in the United States with a high density of vector competent mosquitoes. This, in addition to the association of the virus with the severe impact of Zika virus on the fetus, encouraged manufacturers to research the development of appropriate test systems, and testing was in place at essentially the same time as the appearance of autochthonous infections on the US mainland.

This latter experience suggests that, in some circumstances, it may be possible to predict outbreaks of certain diseases. Indeed, there have been organized efforts to do exactly this for some arboviral diseases in Europe. More specifically, careful analysis of environmental, meteorological, and human movement parameters can identify likely areas for the presence of particular mosquito vectors. Evaluation of population travel patterns can be used to indicate the risk of introduction of a given agent into these areas and thus to target areas of potential risk for an outbreak. These methods have been successfully implemented for malaria, WNV, and dengue [8]. Additionally, in some cases, the dynamics of the outbreak can be predicted.

Although it apparently did not offer a real risk to blood safety, the explosive outbreak of SARS in 2003 is a counterexample, in which a local epidemic of a zoonosis spread around the world in a few months. This was totally unpredictable, and it provoked the hasty implementation of donor deferral policies as a precautionary response, as the pathogenesis of the disease was initially unclear.

Interventions: Donor Suitability

The safety of the blood supply is a matter of considerable medical, political, and public concern. Accordingly, a great deal of effort is exerted to prevent transfusion transmission of agents known or thought to be transmissible by transfusion [9]. The remainder of this chapter will review available measures used to achieve this outcome. These measures vary by country in some cases because the threat is local and in other cases because resources are limited or public health priorities differ.

Donor Information-Based Strategies

It is not always recognized that the process for identifying donor populations has a significant impact on the infectious risk profile, as demonstrated by the decreased prevalence of infection markers among first-time donors compared to the population at large; however, this issue will not be discussed here. Neither will routine donor evaluations of self-reported health and vital signs be discussed, although some of these measures undoubtedly eliminate a number of donors in the early acute phase of infections. Of more relevance to this chapter are strategies that are implemented in order to reduce the risk of specific infections. These generally reflect specific questioning of potential donors in order to determine medical history, exposure risk, or behavioral risk for given infections.

Medical History

This approach is frequently used when a novel infection occurs but prior to the recognition of its cause and the development of appropriate tests. Perhaps the most obvious example of this approach was questioning presenting donors about a history of viral hepatitis, which was implemented long before the etiology of transfusion-transmitted hepatitis was understood. Arguably, the question likely did prevent some transmissions because of the chronic nature of infection by at least some hepatitis viruses, but would have been ineffective in the face of asymptomatic infection. This intervention has mostly been abandoned in the face of effective testing protocols. Asking prospective donors about symptoms of given infections has continued and was an important component of early efforts to impact the risk of transmission of HIV. More recently, questions about the symptoms of tropical arbovirus infections have also been introduced, at least pending the availability of suitable screening tests. In general, however, this approach is neither sensitive nor specific. There have been some instances where such questioning has been eliminated when shown to be ineffective.

Another aspect of this approach is the use of post-donation information, often called PDI. In most blood systems, donors are encouraged, after donation, to inform the blood center of any illness or symptoms occurring during the few days following their donation. This implies that an infectious agent could have been circulating in the donor's blood and allows the blood center to recover the donation prior to its release or use. This approach is known as passive PDI. However, in situations where there is a known risk, such as the presence of an ongoing outbreak, an active form of PDI has, on occasion, been used [10]. In this case, the blood product is quarantined, and its donor is contacted within a few days, and the product is released only after the donor has affirmed that there were no symptoms post-donation. This approach is difficult to employ for platelets, because of their short shelf life.

Risk Exposure

Donors may be asked questions about circumstances that are known, or thought, to offer increased risk of infection with specific agents. This is again a long-standing practice, which should be open to review and change as more effective and accurate measures become available. The risks that are generally considered relate to contact with known cases of a specific disease, exposure to environments where transmission risk is increased (such as a prison) or travel from an area known or thought to offer risk. Most recently, this approach has been invoked in the United States for travel to areas affected by outbreaks of Zika virus, although the questioning stopped once universal donor testing was put in place. Residence in areas with ongoing risk of vCJD is another example. Conversely, a number of countries ask questions designed to avoid collecting blood from people who have recently traveled from the

United States, as a measure to reduce risk of West Nile virus infection. This approach is potentially sensitive but has very poor specificity. It has the advantage that it can be implemented (and abandoned) relatively quickly. This type of questioning can have a significant effect on blood supplies, as a broadly based travel question, for example, can impact 3% or more of all donors.

Risk Behaviors

The third class of questions ask the presenting donor whether or not he or she has engaged in activities or behaviors known to be associated with infection, usually by a specific known agent or group of agents. These questions tend to be intrusive and may, in many cases, require self-reporting of behaviors that may be socially challenging, such as improper injecting drug use. In other cases, the donor may well feel that the questions are discriminatory to a given lifestyle or sexual affinity; this is particularly the case with questions intended to elicit risk for HIV infection. This situation is not readily ameliorated, particularly when specific questions are required by the regulator. There have been attempts to avoid this situation through educational activities designed to encourage self-deferral prior to interview or to give donors the opportunity to indicate that his or her donation should not be used for transfusion (confidential unit exclusion, or CUE). In the United States, CUE has been essentially abandoned as evaluative studies suggested that it was of little benefit. There is published evidence that donors do not always respond accurately to some of these risk behavior questions. A number of studies indicate that around 2% of accepted donors will acknowledge in post-donation studies that they had risk behaviors that should have disqualified them from donation [11]. There is interest and discussion about development of risk questions that do not lead to a sense of discrimination among some donors, but this is not necessarily easy. However, as we develop increasingly sensitive tests and pathogen inactivation, it is to be hoped that such donor questioning could be eliminated.

Interventions: Testing

Although the interventions noted above likely eliminate the majority of donors and donations offering the risk of infection, those methods are neither sensitive nor specific and may be unreliable. There is little question that testing methods are currently perceived as the most significant blood safety intervention. Conceptually, this approach was initiated at some level as a result of cases of transmission of syphilis by transfusion, but the origins of current technology came from attempts to manage the transmission of viral hepatitis by transfusion. These efforts started before the causative agents of hepatitis were characterized or isolated, so the original focus was on the use of liver function tests – an approach known as surrogate testing. The recognition the association of what we now know as hepatitis B surface antigen with one form of transfusion-transmissible hepatitis in the late 1960s led directly to testing that is still in place. Posttransfusion hepatitis continued to occur, however, and it took another 20 years to isolate the hepatitis C virus. In the interim, AIDS and its agent HIV appeared, and testing started in 1985 in the United States. It became apparent that these early tests were not able to identify all infectious donations, and, staring in 1999, additional testing for viral nucleic acids was initiated.

Surrogate Testing

A definition of surrogate is "substitute," and this is a useful definition: in the absence of a specific test for the infectious agent itself, a different analyte or characteristic is used. In the case of surrogate tests for viral hepatitis, tests that are commonly used to detect liver damage (most often blood tests for alanine aminotransferase [ALT]) were used. Clearly, there is a rationale behind this approach, but it was eventually shown to be neither sensitive nor specific. It was, however, in general use until the implementation of a specific test for hepatitis C antibodies. More controversial was the use of a test for antibodies to the hepatitis B core antigen (anti-HBc) in order to reduce the risk of transmission of HIV, prior to the actual recognition of that virus. This approach was based upon epidemiologic data showing that many AIDS patients also had anti-HBc. This was because the hepatitis B virus shared some of the same transmission routes as HIV, although this was, of course, not clear until the virus had been characterized. Ironically, testing for anti-HBc was eventually mandated in the United States, as an additional measure to reduce the transmission of hepatitis B virus by transfusion. A number of other surrogate tests have been used, but generally only on a small scale, and mostly in the context of AIDS, prior to the availability of tests for antibodies to HIV. As noted above, surrogate tests usually lack both specificity and sensitivity, and it is difficult to explain the meaning of an abnormal test result to the donor.

Specific Tests for Pathogens

The presence of pathogens in blood can be identified by a number of different methods. Conceptually, direct observation of the pathogen is simplest but generally insensitive and dependent on the nature of the agent itself. For many years, testing has been based upon serologic approaches. The apparent prototype was testing for HBV, based upon detection of a viral antigen circulating in the blood, but subsequent to this, almost all chronic transfusion-transmissible infections were detected by tests for antibodies to the agents. Subsequently, in a return to testing directly for the pathogen, nucleic acid testing was implemented for HBV, HCV, and HIV. This approach has proved effective for acute infections such as West Nile fever and Zika.

Direct Tests

The most obvious direct testing method is by microscopic observation, as performed, for example, for malaria. However, this approach is very insensitive, and it is confined to agents that are visible by light microscopy. Thus it is restricted to parasites and bacteria and cannot be used for viral infections. Because only a very small volume of sample can be observed, there is also a serious constraint in the sensitivity of testing: for malaria, for example, 50 to 100 parasites per microliter are routinely identified although a highly skilled operator may be able to recognize as few as 5 per microliter.

In many countries, platelet concentrates are routinely evaluated for the presence of bacteria, which may readily proliferate during room-temperature storage of the component. In most cases, a sample of the platelet product is used to inoculate a culture bottle, which is then incubated in an automated device, routinely used for diagnostic blood cultures in the hospital environment [12, 13]. The device monitors the products of bacterial growth in the bottles. If the platelet sample contains viable bacteria, then growth is detected, in most cases, within 24 h, a time at which the parent product is released. Mounting evidence, however, indicates that this method may detect only about 50% of contaminated platelets, most often because the relatively small sample taken for testing did not capture one or more of the contaminating bacteria, which are initially at very low concentration in the component. Despite these issues, bacterial culture has resulted in a measureable decrease in the incidence of patient septic reactions attributable to bacterial contamination in platelets.

Serologic Tests

At least until the end of the twentieth century, transfusion-transmissible agents of most concern were all responsible for chronic infections: syphilis, hepatitis B and C, HIV, HTLV, and malaria. A common feature of all of these infections is the ability of the infectious agent to persist in the face of the immune response. Consequently, the presence of circulating antibodies is frequently an indication that the infectious agent is present. Because antibody is usually present at much greater level than the agent itself, serologic testing is more sensitive than direct detection. Of the pathogens listed immediately above, all but HBV were detected in donations (at least initially) solely by tests for the corresponding antibodies.

The test for HBV was based upon an unusual characteristic of the virus, that is, the production of excess viral coat material (HBsAg), which circulates in the blood stream. The levels of HBsAg are often enough to be detected by simple test methods, such as agar gel diffusion. Indeed, when routine testing was introduced in the early 1970s, tests were based upon some form of passive or active gel diffusion. Those tests were soon supplanted by radioimmunoassay, which was itself replaced by enzyme immunoassays. Subsequently, other detector systems, such as chemiluminescence, have been introduced, but the principle is the same. In some countries, including the United States and Japan, additional testing is now performed for the HBV antibody to core antigen (anti-HBc), in order to identify donors with occult HBV infection (OBI), which is defined as HBV infection without detectable HBsAg.

In 1985, tests for antibodies to HIV were licensed and rapidly implemented. This testing achieved a major decline in the incidence of transfusion-transmitted HIV infection, although earlier efforts based upon donor education and questioning also contributed [14]. Serologic tests were subject to continuing improvement, particularly for sensitivity, but it became apparent that the early stages of infection resulted in circulating virus prior to the development of detectable levels of antibody. This was named the window period and was as long as 45 days with the earliest tests and 22 days after some levels of improvement [15].

Concern about retroviruses led to the initiation of antibody testing for HTLV (1 and 2) in a number of countries and subsequently, the identification of HCV, the virus causing non-A, non-B hepatitis, led to the development of antibody tests for this infection. Subsequently, testing for antibodies to *Trypanosoma cruzi*, the agent of Chagas disease, was implemented in the United States, although it has been in place for many years in South and Central America and parts of Mexico.

A further development for HCV and HIV testing has been the development of the so-called fourth-generation serologic tests. These tests detect antibodies but also simultaneously may detect viral antigens, which are detectable during the latter part of the window period. The level of viral antigens is low and not comparable to the high levels of HBsAg. Nevertheless, this approach adds some additional level of safety in circumstances where NAT is not available.

Rapid Tests

A number of rapid tests for key markers for HBV, HCV, and HIV are available. They are usually based upon lateral flow technology and generate a result in around 15 min. Although logistically attractive, they are not generally recommended for blood donor testing as they are less sensitive than standard tests. However, they are definitely better than not testing at all and may be of value in locations without available resources for full-scale testing. In China and some other locations, rapid tests for HBsAg are used for first-pass testing to avoid collection of blood from donors with positive findings, thus saving resources [16]. In these instances, however, accepted donors are also tested with regular tests.

Nucleic Acid Testing

As pointed out above, even the most sensitive serologic tests demonstrably fail to detect donor infectivity during the window period. This failure led directly to the adoption of tests for viral nucleic acids as a further supplement to serologic tests. It is of some interest to note that the practice actually originated in parts of Europe and that the initial objective was to reduce the prolonged window period for HCV. In the United States, however, the major driver for adoption was the further reduction of risk of transmission of HIV. Many blood systems now routinely test all donations for HBV, HCV, and HIV using multiplex NAT, either singly or in mini pools [17]. The analytic sensitivity of these methods is in the range of a few copies per mL, and their use has reduced the residual risk of transfusion transmission to less than one per million in the United States. Additionally, NAT is used as the sole approach to detection of WNV and Zika virus, both of which are arboviruses causing acute infection. For these (and similar viruses), serologic tests are of little use, as infectivity appears to be absent once antibodies are detectable.

In addition to its sensitivity, NAT has the advantage that new tests can be developed relatively rapidly, as it is not necessary to develop and qualify antibodies or other rare reagents. Once testing platforms are available, they can readily accept newly developed tests. These factors contributed to the rapid adoption of tests for WNV and Zika virus in the United States. However, they are not necessarily appropriate for many parts of the developing world.

Interventions: Pathogen Inactivation

Pathogen reduction, based upon pathogen inactivation technology, offers considerable promise in the context of blood safety. At the time of writing, methods to treat plasma and platelet concentrates are commercially available and in use in a number of countries. Methods for treatment of whole blood and red cell concentrates are in development, and some are in clinical trials. The most promising methods have been shown to inactivate 5 or more $\log_{10}$ of infectivity of many viruses and bacteria, in the absence of significant impact on blood components. There is documented evidence that a method used on platelet concentrates has essentially eliminated the risk of bacterial sepsis after implementation in France, Belgium, and Switzerland [18]. Methods for plasma and platelets have been approved in the United States as an alternative to NAT for Zika virus. This system has also been approved in place of bacterial culture. Currently, however, it is unclear whether use of pathogen reduction will entirely supplant all other tests in current use.

Global Implications of Interventions

The WHO considers that the minimum requirement for blood safety is to test for syphilis, HBV, HCV, and HIV. This expectation has largely been met, but this is an incomplete approach to minimizing transfusion-transmitted infections, particularly if only a single test is used. However, not every country or blood system has the resources to go beyond the minimum requirement. It is unrealistic to expect that all countries should meet the same standard, no matter how desirable that is. Another issue is that risks do vary geographically, as exemplified by Chagas disease and HTLV, so additional local measures may be appropriate. An obvious question is the role of pathogen reduction in the developing world. Clearly, it would be desirable to use this technology to displace the need for other interventions, but this is offset by concerns about costs and appropriate infrastructure. Some methods have been evaluated in this environment, but it is probably too early to assess their true potential and benefit.

References

1. Lederberg J, Shope RE, Oakes SC. Emerging Infections. Microbial Threats to Health in the United States. Wahington D.C.: National Academies Press; 1992. p. 1–294.
2. Seed CR, Hewitt PE, Dodd RY, Houston F, Cevenakova L. Creutzfeldt-Jakob disease and blood safety. Vox Sanguinis, Published early on-line 22nd January. 2018;113:220. https://doi.org/10.1111/vox.12631.
3. Pealer LN, Marfin AA, Petersen LR, Lanciotti RS, Page PL, Stramer SL, et al. Transmission of West Nile virus through blood transfusion in the United States in 2002. N Engl J Med. 2003;349:1236–45.
4. Fauci AS, Morens DM. Zika virus in the Americas – yet another arbovirus threat. N Engl J Med. 2016;374:601–4.
5. Christaki E. New technologies in predicting, preventing and controlling emerging infectious diseases. Virulence. 2015;6:558–65.
6. Stramer SL, Hollinger FB, Katz LM, Kleinman S, Metzel PS, Gregory KR, Dodd RY. Emerging infectious disease agents and their potential threat to transfusion safety. Transfusion. 2009;49(Suppl 2):1S–29S.
7. US Food and Drug Administration. Revised recommendations for reducing the risk of Zika virus transmission by blood and blood products. Guidance for Industry, August 2016. https://www.fda.gov/downloads/BiologicsBloodVaccines/GuidanceComplianceRegulatoryInformation/Guidances/Blood/UCM518213.pdf.
8. Semenza JC. Prototype early warning systems for vector-borne diseases in Europe. Int J Environ Res. 2015;12:6333–51.
9. Perkins HA, Busch MP. Transfusion-associated infections: 50 years of relentless challenges and remarkable progress. Transfusion. 2010;50:2080–99.
10. Appassakij H, Promwong C, Rujirujindakul P, Wutthanarungsan R, Silpapojakul K. The risk of blood transfusion-associated Chikunguya fever during the 2009 epidemic in Songkhla Province, Thailand. Transfusion. 2014;54:19454–2.
11. Custer B, Kessler D, Vahidnia F, Leparc G, Krysztof D, Shaz B, et al. Risk factors for retrovirus and hepatitis virus infections in accepted blood donors. Transfusion. 2015;55:1098–107.

12. Eder AF, Kennedy JM, Dy BA, Notari EP, Weiss JW, Fang CT, Wagner S, Dodd RY, Benjamin RJ, Blood Centers ARC. Bacterial screening of apheresis platelets and the residual risk of septic transfusion reactions: the American red Cross experience (2004-2006). Transfusion. 2007;47:1134–42.
13. McDonald C, Allen J, Brailsford s RA, Ball J, Moule R, et al. Bacterial screening of platelet components by National Health Service Blood and transplant, an effective risk reduction measure. Transfusion. 2017;57:1122–31.
14. Busch MP, Young MJ, Samson SM, Mosley JW, Ward JW, Perkins HA. and The Transfusion Safety Study Group. Risk of human immunodeficiency virus (HIV) transmission by blood transfusions before the implementation of HIV-1 antibody screening. Transfusion. 1991;31:4–11.
15. Petersen LR, Satten GA, Dodd RY, Busch M, Kleinman S, Grindon A, Lenes B. HIV seroconversion study group. Duration of time from onset of human immunodeficiency virus type 1 infectiousness to development of detectable antibody. Transfusion. 1994;34:283–9.
16. Weng Z, Zeng J, Li T, Xu X, Ye X, et al. Prevalence of hepatitis B surface antigen (HBsAg) in a blood donor population born prior to and after implementation of universal HBV vaccination in Shenzhen, China. BMC Infect Dis. 2016;16:498.
17. Roth WK, Busch MP, Schuller A, Ismay S, Seed CR. Jungbauer, et al. international forum: international survey on NAT testing of blood donations: expanding implementation and yield from 1999 to 2009. Vox Sang. 2012;102:82–90.
18. Benjamin RJ, Braschler T, Weingand T, Corash LM. Hemovigilance monitoring of platelet septic reactions with effective bacterial protection systems. Transfusion. 2017;57:2946–57.

Chapter 2
Assessing the Threat: Public Health

Hans L. Zaaijer

Introduction

A threat to the safety of blood components and blood products may arise because a new outbreak occurs. Recent examples are outbreaks caused by arboviruses (dengue, West Nile fever, chikungunya, and Zika), coronaviruses (MERS and SARS), and zoonotic outbreaks caused by the BSE/variant Creutzfeldt-Jakob disease (vCJD) agent from cattle, by the *Coxiella burnetii* bacterium from goats, and by hepatitis E virus genotype 3 (HEV-3) from pigs. Theoretically, threats may come from agents that always have been around; a "new" threat may arise because we realize that an "old" agent is less innocent for certain recipients than assumed.

Other chapters describe the prediction and monitoring of threats. In this chapter, it is described how the consequences for public health of a transfusion-transmitted agent can be estimated. A checklist is provided for a structured inventory of the relevant properties of an emerging transfusion-transmitted agent. Once completed, this inventory gives an indication of the transfusion-associated morbidity and mortality that can be expected and of mitigating interventions that can be considered. The inventory is based on the approach as designed by the author in 1998 for the Dutch blood transfusion service. It has been found to be useful in real-life blood banking, but it has not been validated or acknowledged officially; other approaches may be as good or better. Subsequently two models are described for a more quantitative analysis of the impact of a transfusion-transmitted infection; both models are available in the public domain. Finally, some examples are given of advanced, agent-specific studies which were performed to assess the impact of an emerging

---

H. L. Zaaijer
Department of Blood-borne Infections, Sanquin Blood Supply Foundation,
Amsterdam, The Netherlands

Department of Clinical Virology, Academic Medical Center, Amsterdam, The Netherlands
e-mail: h.zaaijer@sanquin.nl

blood-borne threat. In a wider context the Alliance of Blood Operators developed the Risk-Based Decision Making framework for risk mitigation in blood safety, as yet it is beyond the scope of this chapter.

Assessing the Threat: A Structured Approach

The emergence of a (potential) blood-transmitted agent necessitates the evaluation of the threat it poses to the safety of blood components and blood products. This assessment serves several goals: (1) possibly short-term measures must be taken to limit blood-borne spread of the agent; (2) relevant gaps in our knowledge of the agent must be identified and addressed; (3) health authorities and the general public must be provided with relevant information regarding the safety of the blood supply; (4) parameters must be provided to modelers enabling cost-benefit analysis of potential interventions; and (5) a long-term safety policy must be defined. Assessing the threat of a transfusion-transmitted pathogen includes two steps:

Step 1: Collect Facts and Uncertainties

The properties of the agent that are relevant for blood banking must be collected. To complete this inventory, the checklist as presented in Table 2.1 of this chapter can be used. The inventory may seem to contain some redundancies, but it must be realized that, for example, the detection of a viral genome by PCR in blood components does not equate with infectivity. Concurrent antibodies may neutralize the agent, or only noninfectious RNA or DNA remnants of the agent may be present. Proven transmission of the agent by blood components does not equate with disease in the recipient. For example, so far, disease caused by transfusion-transmitted dengue, chikungunya, or Zika virus infection seems an exception.

Using the data as obtained in step 1, additional calculations and modeling may be performed to provide detailed figures for the expected morbidity and mortality and for the efficacy of interventions. The costs and benefits of preventive interventions, such as the introduction of donor deferral and donor screening, must be estimated. Unfortunately, detailed numerical analysis may take considerable time. Often safety measures must be considered in absence of a detailed cost-benefit analysis. The exact methodology for modeling and cost-benefit analysis is beyond the scope of this chapter but is partly covered by a following paragraph of this chapter.

Step 2: Report and Conclude

The inventory of Step 1 must be reported and summarized in a format that is understandable for blood bank directors, physicians, safety boards, and government officials. A practical format for the report is provided in Table 2.2. The report not only must present the relevant properties of the agent in a readable way, the data as obtained in step 1 must be interpreted, and three conclusions must be presented:

Table 2.1 Fact finding

To obtain an inventory of the relevant properties of an emerging agent, data can be collected using the following checklist:

A. General Issues

A.1 In what way did the agent emerge? ....
(e.g., Was the agent recently introduced among humans? Or was the agent recently discovered while being present for a longer period?)

A.2 Nature of the agent:

(a) Virus	Enveloped/non-enveloped			
	RNA virus/DNA virus			
	Taxonomy:			
(b) Bacterium	Gram positive/Gram negative			
	Coccus/bacillus/.........			
	Taxonomy:			
(c) Protozoan	Taxonomy:			
(d) Others	....			

B. Epidemiology

B.1 Prevalence and incidence

	Prevalence	Incidence	Ref.
(a) Among blood donors in region/country:			
....	....	....	...
....	....	....	...
(b) In other groups:			
....	....	....	...
....	....	....	...
(c) In endemic areas:			
....	....	....	...

(continued)

Table 2.1 (continued)

To obtain an inventory of the relevant properties of an emerging agent, data can be collected using the following checklist:			
....	....	....	...
....	....	....	...
B.2 Risk factors for infection			
	Yes/no/unknown	Useful for donor exclusion?	
		Yes/no	Ref.
Age	....	....	...
Diet	....	....	...
IV drug abuse	....	....	...
Ethnicity	....	....	...
Travel	....	....	...
Others:	....	....	...
B.3 Transmission routes of the agent			
	Proven/probable/possible/unlikely/no/unknown		Ref.
Transplacental	....		...
Perinatal	....		...
(Feco-)oral, dietary	....		...
Inhalation	....		...
Intra-familial	....		...
Parenteral (ivd)	....		...
Iatrogenic, via:			
RBCs	....		...
Platelets	....		...
FFP	....		...
SD-plasma	....		...
Clotting factor	....		...

Ig	....	...
Leukocytes	....	...
Stem cells	....	...
Solid organs	....	...
Others:	....	...
B.4 Course of infection in healthy donors		
Incubation period:	.... (average, min, max)	Ref.
duration of viremia/bacteremia:	.... (average, min, max)	...
	%/majority/minority/unknown	Ref.
		...
Asymptomatic infection in	.... of cases	...
Symptoms occur in	.... of cases	...
Infection resolves in	.... of cases	...
Chronic infection develops in	.... of cases	...
Fatal outcome in	.... of cases	...
Immunity after resolved infection?	Proven/probable/possible/unlikely/no/unknown/not applicable	
In healthy donors	....	...
In immunosuppressed patients	....	...
B.5 Course of infection in subsets of the population (*not* acquired via blood components/products)		
Are certain persons at increased risk for (consequences of) infection?		
	Yes/no/unknown	Ref.
Fetus	....	...
Neonate	....	...

(continued)

Table 2.1 (continued)

To obtain an inventory of the relevant properties of an emerging agent, data can be collected using the following checklist:

Child	….
Pregnant woman	….
Adults	….
Elderly	….
Others: …………	….
Immune suppressed recipients:	
Hematological patients	….
Solid organ transplant	….
Others: …………	….

B.6 Course of infection in recipients of infectious blood components/products

Has blood-borne transmission been documented?
If so what were the consequences for the recipient?

	Documented		
	Yes/no	Outcome of infection	Ref.
Neonate	…	…	…
Child	…	…	…
Pregnant woman	…	…	…
Adults	…	…	…
Elderly	…	…	…
Others: …………	…	…	…
Immunosuppressed recipients			
Hematological patients	…	…	…
Solid organ transplant	…	…	…
Others	…	…	…

Are infected recipients infectious for others? ………………………

B.7 Treatment and prophylaxis

		Available		
Pre-exposure prophylaxis		Yes/no	(e.g., vaccination)	
Post-exposure prophylaxis		Yes/no	(e.g., immunoglobulins)	
Treatment of infection		Yes/no	(e.g., antibiotics, antivirals)	

C. Transmission and Infectivity

C.1 Tropism

Tissue and/or cell tropism(s) of the agent: ....

C.2 Presence of the agent in blood components or products

	Presence/absence is proven/probable/possible/unknown	Ref.
Whole blood	....	...
RBCs	....	...
Platelets	....	...
FFP	....	...
Leukocytes	....	...
....	....	...

("proven": as demonstrated by transmission, detection [PCR, culture], etc.)

("probable/possible": as suggested by biological or epidemiological properties of the agent)

C.3 Presence of infectivity in donated blood:

(a) Before symptoms appear:	Proven/probable/possible/unlikely/no/unknown	
Duration of infectivity:	....	Ref.: ...
(b) During clinical stage:	Proven/probable/possible/unlikely/no/unknown	
Duration of infectivity:	....	Ref.: ...
(c) After clinical cure:	Proven/probable/possible/unlikely/no/unknown	
Duration of infectivity:	....	Ref.: ...

(continued)

Table 2.1 (continued)

To obtain an inventory of the relevant properties of an emerging agent, data can be collected using the following checklist:		
(d) In asymptomatic cases:	Proven/probable/possible/unlikely/no/unknown	
Duration of infectivity:	……………..	Ref.: ….
C.4 Minimum infective dose		
What is known of (the course of) the *level* of viremia/bacteremia/parasitemia?		
What is known of the minimum infective dose for humans?		
D. Mitigating Interventions		
D.1 Which selection criteria could be suitable for deferral of at-risk donors?		
D.2 Which laboratory markers (serology, NAT) could be suitable for detection of infectious donors?		
D.3 Which selection criterial or laboratory markers could be suitable to identify "safe" donors? (e.g., immune donors after resolved infection, non-traveling donors, etc.)		
D.4 Is quarantine of material and follow-up testing of the donor applicable?		
D.5 Sensitivity of the agent for inactivation or removal:		
	Proven/probable/possible/ unlikely/no/unknown	Ref.
Effect of storage at room temperature	………………	…
Effect of storage at +4° C	………………	…
Effect of storage at −20° C	………………	…
Leukodepletion	………………	…
Pasteurization	………………	…
Solvent-detergent	………………	…
Dry heat	………………	…
Nanofiltration	………………	… (Pore size: ………………)
Presence of neutralizing antibodies	………………	…
Commercial pathogen reduction	………………	…
……………….	………………	…

Table 2.2 Reporting key data and recommendations for an emerging transfusion-transmitted agent

This table provides an example for the layout of a report providing relevant properties of an emerging transfusion-transmitted agent, targeted at blood bank and public health officials. (This "quick scan" document layout is used by the committee for emerging infections of Sanquin Blood Supply Foundation, for reporting to the Medical Advisory Board.)
Quick scan for agent X
Paragraphs:
1. Short summary, presented as a limited number of bullets
2. Background information: reference to the relevant pages in "Control of Communicable Diseases Manual" or another high-quality text book
3. To what extent can infection X be expected among blood donors?
4. Has transmission via blood been documented?
5. Presence of X in the blood
During symptomatic infections (incubation period, symptomatic phase, reconvalescence)
During asymptomatic infections
Are these resolving and/or chronic infections?
6. Severity of infection
Course and outcome in children, adults, and immunosuppressed persons
7. Short description of global epidemiology of X
8. Short description of local epidemiology of X
9. Potential blood safety measures
10. Blood policies elsewhere (USA, Canada, EU, Australia, etc.)
11. Conclusion and recommendations
12. Knowledge gaps to be addressed
13. Authors and revisors
14. Sources of information

1. An estimate must be provided of the expected morbidity and mortality, caused by the emerging agent via blood transfusion and blood products. Often, in the absence of hard data, only a carefully phrased educated guess is possible.
2. Safety measures must be described that (may) reduce the expected transmission via blood components and blood products.
3. Gaps in the knowledge of the agent must be identified that must be addressed.

Quantitative Analysis of the Impact of a Transfusion-Transmitted Infection and of Countermeasures

Tools for Quantitative Assessment of Transfusion-Transmitted Infections

The previous paragraph offers an approach to quickly obtain a thorough, but qualitative assessment of the threat to blood safety, caused by an emerging agent. Based on this approach, some excerpts from previous real-life situations and reports are:

- "Given the efficacy of our inactivation procedures for enveloped viruses, it is unlikely that our plasma products transmit GB-virus-C."
- "Last spring, up to 1 in 5000 donors was silently highly viremic for parvovirus-B19." (It was found that approximately every 4 years, parvovirus-B19 infections show a considerable seasonal peak, with many donors being silently infected).
- "In the years following the outbreak of Q-fever, 1 in 100 infected persons may silently harbor chronic Coxiella infection, which amounts to 1 in 1000 blood donors in the affected area." (According to literature, roughly one in one hundred persons who acquire *Coxiella burnetii* infection will develop chronic infection, while in a specific affected area, one in ten citizens became infected via air-borne transmission).
- "Zika virus especially is a threat for pregnant women. An estimated 0.1% of our RBC transfusions concern pregnant women." (Gynecologists and transfusion specialists were asked about the number of transfusions among pregnant women; and detailed transfusion data were available from a comparable country).

Such remarks are useful because they highlight the problem, but they provide insufficient quantitative information about the impact of the threat on public health. To facilitate a more quantitative analysis of the consequences of an emerging infection for the safety of blood components and blood products, two models are available in the public domain. The models are compared in a review by Kiely et al. [1]. In response to the West Nile virus outbreak in the USA, Biggerstaff and Petersen (CDC, Fort Collins, USA) designed a model for the estimation of the number of silently viremic blood donors, based on a combination of deterministic calculations and a Monte Carlo simulation [2, 3]. Others used the Biggerstaff-Petersen model to assess chikungunya outbreaks in La Reunion [4], Thailand [5], and Italy [6], a dengue outbreak in Australia [7], a Ross River virus outbreak in Australia [8], and a hepatitis A outbreak in Latvia [9].

Van der Poel (Sanquin Blood Supply Foundation, Amsterdam), Janssen (Transfusion Technology Assessment, University of Utrecht), and Domanovic (ECDC, Stockholm) initiated the computer-based, interactive "European Up-Front Risk Assessment Tool" (EUFRAT), for the quantitative estimation of transfusion transmission risks as posed by emerging infections [10]. The tool is freely accessible via http://eufrattool.ecdc.europa.eu. EUFRAT supports local outbreaks, and threats that are introduced by traveling donors, returning from affected areas abroad. After data have been entered, EUFRAT calculates the number of infected and diseased recipients. Entering the data includes five steps:

- In step 1 predefined parameters for 18 infectious agents can be selected, or a new, still undefined agent can be chosen. Subsequently it must be indicated whether donors are involved who visited an outbreak-affected region, whether data on infected donors are available, whether the infection has a chronic phase, and whether donor deferral or donor screening is available.

- Dependent on the choices entered in step 1, in steps 2 to 5, specific parameters must be entered concerning "disease and outbreak," "donor screening and donation testing," "blood component production and donor exposure," and "recipient population."

EUFRAT has been used to assess the impact of chikungunya in Italy [11], Q-fever in the Netherlands [11, 12], Ross River fever in Australia [8], and dengue in donors returning from affected areas [13].

Advanced Quantitative Assessment

As a rule, in the early phase of an emerging infection, insufficient data are available to determine precisely the impact of the threat and the costs and benefits of mitigating interventions such as the deferral of at-risk donors and the introduction of molecular or serological screening of donors. Sometimes the true costs and benefits of a safety measure only become clear years after its introduction. For example, universal leukodepletion of blood donations was hoped to reduce the risk of transmission of the vCJD agent. The filters involved were expensive. The efficacy of prion protein removal by leukodepletion is based on indirect evidence, obtained using laboratory animals which only partially reflect human blood donors incubating vCJD. Years later, leukodepletion filters have become very cheap; they virtually remove the risk of CMV, EBV, and HTLV transmission; they reduce transfusion reactions and alloimmunization; and it still is expected that they reduce the risk of vCJD transmission. All in all, leukodepletion turned out to be very effective but in unexpected ways. On the other side of the spectrum is the donor screening for HIV RNA in countries with a low incidence of HIV infection. Introduction of universal HIV RNA donor screening was considered to be indispensable for the societal trust in blood transfusion. However, in countries with a low incidence of HIV infection, "HIV NAT only" donations may not be encountered. Based on carefully collected data and using advanced modeling, Borkent and colleagues calculated that triplex-NAT donor screening for HIV, HCV, and HBV, on pools of six donations, costs Euro 5,200,000 per quality-adjusted life year (QALY) gained in the Netherlands [14]. For this exercise, detailed characteristics of blood transfusion, recipients, and local HBV, HCV, and HIV epidemiology were taken into account.

A more recent example of advanced modeling, performed to estimate the consequences of an emerging infection for public health, concerns the analysis of transfusion-transmitted HEV genotype 3 infection:

- Of all HEV infections nationwide one in 700 is estimated to be due to blood transfusion, while for chronic HEV infections this is one in 3.5. HEV screening of Dutch whole blood donations in pools of 24 would prevent 4.52 of the 4.94 transfusion associated chronic HEV infections expected annually, at approximately Euro 310,000 per prevented chronic case [15].

These seemingly simple findings could not be generated using the Biggerstaff-Petersen model or the EUFRAT tool; they were obtained by dedicated modeling, after several studies generated essential data:

- During 2013–2016 the monthly screening of 2000 plasma donations for HEV RNA provided detailed data on the incidence of HEV infection, the duration of viremia, and the distribution of viremia levels.
- A British study provided data on the infectivity of HEV via transfusion [16].
- In academic hospitals the course of HEV infection in vulnerable subsets of patients was elucidated.

It became clear that especially solid organ- and stem cell transplant patients are at risk for developing chronic hepatitis E, sometimes with rapid onset of cirrhosis.

- For these groups of patients, the exposure to blood components and other sources of HEV was determined.
- The effect of timely diagnosis of hepatitis E and subsequent antiviral treatment was studied.
- The costs and the yield of donor screening for HEV RNA using different pool sizes were calculated.

These examples of quantitative analysis point to a sobering conclusion. Reliable and detailed quantitative analysis of the impact of a transfusion-transmitted infection, including the costs and yield of mitigating measures, needs a team of specialists and considerable time. Figure 2.1 illustrates the complexity of only one aspect of this matter. Considering the impact of a transfusion-transmitted infection in terms of lost years of life and chronic sequelae, the a priori life expectancy of the exposed recipients varies considerably [17]. Figure 2.1 shows that platelets often are transfused to persons with (potential) long life expectancy, including young adults, children, and neonates at the far left of the graph, while Fig. 2.1 shows that the majority of fresh frozen plasma units was administered to patients with short life expectancies. Considering an emerging transfusion-transmitted threat, it appears that especially the administration of infectious platelets may have considerable consequences.

An Unresolved Issue: Presence of DNA or RNA of a Pathogen Does Not Equate with Infectivity

No matter how detailed the knowledge of the course of viremia and the occurrence of antibodies for an emerging agent in donors with asymptomatic infection, the infectivity of blood donors in different phases of infection cannot be fully predicted. Only targeted studies provide clarity, as illustrated by the following three examples.

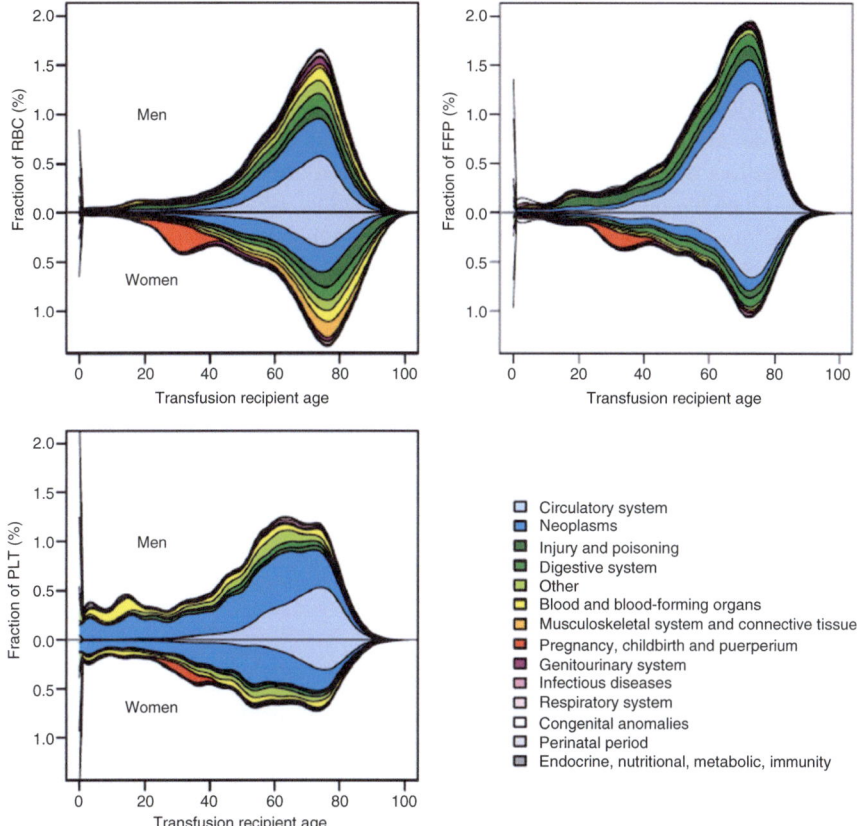

Fig. 2.1 Characteristics of recipients of red blood cells, platelets, and fresh frozen plasma. (Reproduced with permission from John Wiley and Sons, from Borkent-Raven et al. [17])

The donor-recipient HEV transmission study by Hewitt and colleagues showed that only 18 of 43 recipients (42%) of a blood component from an HEV-viremic donor acquired infection [16]. Absence of HEV antibodies and a high viral load in the donor made transmission more likely. The results of this study helped to estimate the minimum infectious dose of HEV and the infectivity of units of red blood cells, platelets, and plasma, given the levels of viremia in donors [15].

Remarkable details have been reported about the complex relation between infectivity of donated material and the detection of West Nile virus RNA in blood and organ donors [18]. In 54 blood donors, WNV RNA no longer was detectable in plasma 3 weeks after the donation that tested positive for WNV RNA. However, in 42% of the donors, WNV RNA remained detectable in whole blood up to 3 months after the index donation. In this phase, WNV is bound to erythrocytes, but – except for one case – blood components of the donors involved are not infectious for the recipients, probably due to the presence of neutralizing antibodies [18]. In contrast, organs from two donors in the later phase of infection (both testing positive for WNV IgG antibodies; one testing positive for WNV RNA in serum, one negative) caused WNV infection in their recipients [19].

Blood donors may silently harbor acute parvovirus B19 (B19V) infection. After acute infection, decreasing levels of parvovirus DNA are detectable during months to years. Once the parvovirus DNA level drops below 100,000 IU/mL (ref. 20) or 10,000 IU/mL [21], donors do not transmit B19V to their recipients, which is attributed to concurrent neutralizing antibodies or to a noninfectious amount of transfused virions. However, recently, an alternative explanation was reported [22]. Studying ten donors up to 22 months after acute asymptomatic B19V infection, viral DNA remained detectable for more than 1 year. After 150 days post-infection, the B19V DNA of the donors became degradable by endonucleases, indicating that this concerned naked DNA, not the protected, encapsidated DNA as present in intact B19V virions. Hence, potentially infectious B19V viremia is only present during the first months of a much longer episode of B19V "DNA-emia" as detected by PCR.

Lasting Impact of vCJD

Considering the assessment of blood-borne threats to public health, possibly the most difficult task is to estimate the remaining threat of variant Creutzfeldt-Jakob disease (vCJD), as posed by blood donors with possible subclinical vCJD infection. As reviewed by Seed and colleagues, several studies indicate that the classic, sporadic form of CJD is no threat to the safety of transfusion, but three fatal cases of vCJD and one subclinical infection have been attributed to transmission via blood transfusion [23]. Since the outbreak of mad cow disease (BSE) in Great Britain, with subsequent cases of vCJD in humans, many blood banks maintain safety measures to prevent transmission of vCJD via blood transfusion and blood products. Examples of safety measures are the exclusion of blood donors who stayed at least 6 months in the UK during 1980–1996 and the exclusion of donors who themselves were transfused. Is it time to lift these restrictions? Until recently it seemed that the outbreak of vCJD had ended. Unfortunately in 2016 a new vCJD patient was reported. This patient was found to be heterozygous (methionine/valine) for codon 129 of the human prion gene. This is alarming, because so far all vCJD patients were methionine homozygous (Fig. 2.2, lower panel). Possibly this first heterozygous patient reflects the start of a second wave of vCJD cases, with longer incubation times than the former homozygous cases. Apparently, people may harbor the infection during many years and, regarding blood banking, could be seen as asymptomatic but possibly infectious carriers. Studies of archived appendices suggest that indeed roughly 1 in 2500 British appendices tests positive for the vCJD agent. The first and second appendix studies involved 12,674 resp. 32,441 appendices, from persons born between 1961 and 1985 resp. 1941–1985

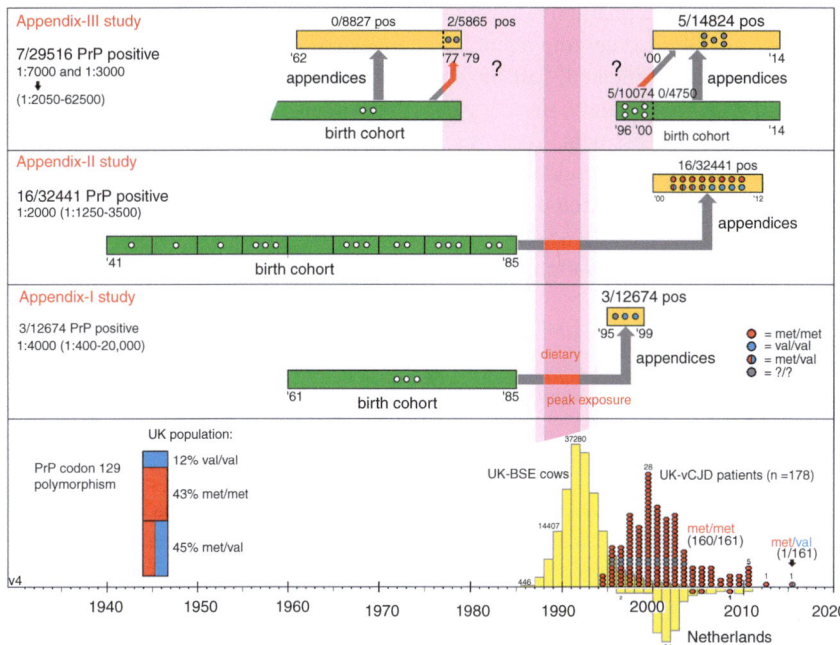

Fig. 2.2 Course of the BSE and vCJD outbreaks in the UK and in the Netherlands and findings of the Appendix I-III studies. (Reproduced with permission by the Sanquin Blood Supply Foundation)

[24, 25]; see the two middle panels in Fig. 2.2. These persons experienced dietary exposure to the vCJD agent around 1990; and their appendices were removed in 1995–1999 resp. 2000–2012; in which 3 resp. 16 vCJD-prion-positive appendices were found. Is this finding really linked to dietary exposure to the vCJD agent in the 1980s and 1990s, or is there an unrelated, harmless, and natural background presence of the protein in appendices? The Appendix-III study included appendices and persons who did not live in the late 1980s and early 1990s [26]. The upper panel in Fig. 2.2 shows the confusing findings of the Appendix-III study: is the period of dietary exposure larger than assumed? Or is there no connection to the BSE/vCJD outbreak? Currently it seems wise not to abandon vCJD blood safety measures yet.

Summary and Conclusion

When a threat to the safety of blood occurs, one must find a balance between the time it takes to collect and report relevant information and the urgency to start mitigating interventions. This chapter described three methods for assessing the impact of transfusion-transmitted infections for public health, in order of increasing precision and increasing labor intensity:

1. A blueprint for a qualitative inventory and a report, describing the relevant characteristics of the emerging agent, is offered in tables 2.1 and 2.2.
2. Two more sophisticated, "off the shelf" methods for the quantitative analysis of a threat to blood safety, the Biggerstaff-Petersen model and the European Up-Front Risk Assessment Tool (EUFRAT), are described. The output of the Biggerstaff-Petersen model is the number of potentially infectious donations, while EUFRAT additionally takes into account the components prepared from donations and the efficacy of mitigating interventions such as donor screening and pathogen inactivation, enabling an estimation of the consequences for recipients.
3. Examples of sophisticated quantitative studies of specific agents are mentioned: a donor-recipient transmission study [16] and a cost-benefit modeling study [15]. For this kind of analysis, no standardized recipe is available; the studies involved are defined by specific properties of the emerging agent and the local situation.

In an urgent situation, steps 1 and 2 will be started more or less simultaneously, and results may become available soon after. Sometimes an additional detailed cost-benefit analysis is needed. Only the implementation of partial or universal donor screening may generate sufficient data to precisely calculate the impact of the agent, facilitating the decision whether donor screening indeed is useful (in hindsight). In real-life blood banking, once safety measures have been implemented, it often is hard to stop them, even when the cost-benefit ratio is found to be very poor. Therefore, when a new threat arises, it must be considered to start donor screening only for a limited period [27]. This serves two purposes: it helps to prevent transmissions in an uncertain situation and maintains the public trust in blood transfusion, and it generates valuable data. When the period of temporary donor screening has ended, it can only be extended by an active decision to do so, based on the analysis of data that have become available in the meantime. This approach prevents the accumulation of inefficient preventive blood safety measures over time.

The impact of an emerging transfusion-transmitted infection on public health is only one of several factors that shape the policy regarding blood safety. In case of zoonoses (vCJD, Q-fever, and HEV genotype 3), agro-economic interests sometimes hindered effective safety measures. For other emerging agents, the emotional impact of the infection (e.g., of Zika-induced microcephaly), the societal trust in blood banking, and political liability (e.g., after local HIV or HCV "scandals") may be more important for the introduction of blood safety measures than exact figures for transfusion-induced morbidity and mortality.

References

1. Kiely P, Gambhir M, Cheng AC, McQuilten ZK, Seed CR, Wood EM. Emerging infectious diseases and blood safety: modelling the transfusion-transmission risk. Transfus Med Rev. 2017;31(3):154–64.

2. Biggerstaff BJ, Petersen LR. Estimated risk of West Nile virus transmission through blood transfusion during an epidemic in Queens, New York City. Transfusion. 2002;42(8):1019–26.
3. Biggerstaff BJ, Petersen LR. Estimated risk of transmission of the West Nile virus through blood transfusion in the US, 2002. Transfusion. 2003;43(8):1007–17.
4. Brouard C, Bernillon P, Quatresous I, Pillonel J, Assal A, De Valk H, et al. Estimated risk of chikungunya viremic blood donation during an epidemic on Reunion Island in the Indian Ocean, 2005 to 2007. Transfusion. 2008;48:1333–41.
5. Appassakij H, Promwong C, Rujirojindakul P, Wutthanarungsan R, Silpapojakul K. The risk of blood transfusion-associated chikungunya fever during the 2009 epidemic in Songkhla Province. Thailand Transfusion. 2014;54:1945–52.
6. Liumbruno GM, Calteri D, Petropulacos K, Mattivi A, Po C, Macini P, et al. The chikungunya epidemic in Italy and its repercussion on the blood system. Blood Transfus. 2008;6:199–210.
7. Faddy HM, Seed CR, Fryk JJ, Hyland CA, Ritchie SA, Taylor CT, et al. Implications of dengue outbreaks for blood supply, Australia. Emerg Infect Dis. 2013;19:787–9.
8. Seed CR, Hoad VC, Faddy HM, Kiely P, Keller AJ, Pink J. Re-evaluating the residual risk of transfusion-transmitted Ross River virus infection. Vox Sang. 2016;110(4):317–23.
9. Perevoscikovs J, Lenglet A, Lucenko I, Steinerte A, Payne Hallstrom L, Coulombier D. Assessing the risk of a community outbreak of hepatitis A on blood safety in Latvia, 2008. Euro Surveill. 2010;15:19640.
10. Oei W, Janssen MP, van der Poel CL, van Steenbergen JE, Rehmet S, Kretzschmar ME. Modeling the transmission risk of emerging infectious diseases through blood transfusion. Transfusion. 2013;53(7):1421–8.
11. Mapako T, Oei W, van Hulst M, Kretzschmar ME, Janssen MP. Modelling the risk of transfusion transmission from travelling donors. BMC Infect Dis. 2016;16:143.
12. Oei W, Kretzschmar ME, Zaaijer HL, Coutinho R, van der Poel CL, Janssen MP. Estimating the transfusion transmission risk of Q fever. Transfusion. 2014;54:1705–11.
13. Oei W, Lieshout-Krikke RW, Kretzschmar ME, Zaaijer HL, Coutinho RA, Eersel M, Jubithana B, Halabi Y, Gerstenbluth I, Maduro E, Tromp M, Janssen MP. Estimating the risk of dengue transmission from Dutch blood donors travelling to Suriname and the Dutch Caribbean. Vox Sang. 2016;110(4):301–9.
14. Borkent-Raven BA, Janssen MP, van der Poel CL, Bonsel GJ, van Hout BA. Cost-effectiveness of additional blood screening tests in the Netherlands. Transfusion. 2012;52(3):478–88.
15. de Vos AS, Janssen MP, Zaaijer HL, Hogema BM. Cost-effectiveness of the screening of blood donations for hepatitis E virus in the Netherlands. Transfusion. 2017;57(2):258–66.
16. Hewitt PE, Ijaz S, Brailsford SR, Brett R, Dicks S, Haywood B, et al. Hepatitis E virus in blood components: a prevalence and transmission study in Southeast England. Lancet. 2014;15;384(9956):1766–73.
17. Borkent-Raven BA, Janssen MP, van der Poel CL, Schaasberg WP, Bonsel GJ, van Hout BA. The PROTON study: profiles of blood product transfusion recipients in the Netherlands. Vox Sang. 2010;99(1):54–64.
18. Lanteri MC, Lee TH, Wen L, Kaidarova Z, Bravo MD, Kiely NE, et al. West Nile virus nucleic acid persistence in whole blood months after clearance in plasma: implication for transfusion and transplantation safety. Transfusion. 2014;54(12):3232–41.
19. Nett RJ, Kuehnert MJ, Ison MG, Orlowski JP, Fischer M, Staples JE. Current practices and evaluation of screening solid organ donors for West Nile virus. Transpl Infect Dis. 2012;14:268–77.
20. Hourfar MK, Mayr-Wohlfart U, Themann A, Sireis W, Seifried E, Schrezenmeier H, Schmidt M. Recipients potentially infected with parvovirus B19 by red blood cell products. Transfusion. 2011;51(1):129–36.
21. Juhl D, Özdemir M, Dreier J, Görg S, Hennig H. Look-back study on recipients of parvovirus B19 (B19V) DNA-positive blood components. Vox Sang. 2015;109(4):305–11.
22. Molenaar-de Backer MW, Russcher A, Kroes AC, Koppelman MH, Lanfermeijer M, Zaaijer HL. Detection of parvovirus B19 DNA in blood: viruses or DNA remnants? J Clin Virol. 2016;84:19–23.

23. Seed CR, Hewitt PE, Dodd RY, Houston F, Cervenakova L. Creutzfeldt-Jakob disease and blood transfusion safety. Vox Sang. 2018;113:220. https://doi.org/10.1111/vox.12631. (Epub ahead of print).
24. Hilton DA, Ghani AC, Conyers L, Edwards P, McCardle L, Ritchie D, Penney M, Hegazy D, Ironside JW. Prevalence of lymphoreticular prion protein accumulation in UK tissue samples. J Pathol. 2004;203(3):733–9.
25. Gill ON, Spencer Y, Richard-Loendt A, Kelly C, Dabaghian R, Boyes L, Linehan J, Simmons M, Webb P, Bellerby P, Andrews N, Hilton DA, Ironside JW, Beck J, Poulter M, Mead S, Brandner S. Prevalent abnormal prion protein in human appendixes after bovine spongiform encephalopathy epizootic: large scale survey. BMJ. 2013;347:f5675.
26. Summary results of the third national survey of abnormal prion prevalence in archived appendix specimens. Public Health England Infection report (weekly). 2016;10(26).
27. Kramer K, Verweij MF, Zaaijer HL. Are there ethical differences between stopping and not starting blood safety measures? Vox Sang. 2017;112(5):417–24.

Chapter 3
Assessing the Threat: Public Concern

Anne Wiles, Judie Leach Bennett, and Dana Devine

Introduction

When assessing blood safety threats and addressing public concern, several aspects of the risk management context are important. The first is that the blood system is inherently complex, characterized by a range of functions and responsibilities and by competing needs, constraints, and priorities from clinical, regulatory, industry, stakeholder, and public perspectives. Considerations also include patient and donor risks and benefits, blood operator performance and resource accountabilities and risks, and, more generally, societal ethics and values. However, an overriding consideration within blood systems over the last three decades has been the need to build trust in the blood system and confidence in the blood supply. As a result of a series of blood system risk management failures in the 1980s and 1990s, the blood sector adopted a risk management approach of significant precaution, with little regard to opportunity cost. This response created a secondary set of challenges, namely, an inclination towards a zero-risk management approach, which proved unsustainable and challenged the viability of operations within available resources.

Questions emerged as to what constitutes a tolerable level of risk and who decides. Such debates and analyses can find a home in the discipline of risk-based decision-making (RBDM), where optimizing safety can be considered together with healthcare resource opportunity cost and a full range of societal values. The

A. Wiles
Risk Sciences International, Ottawa, ON, Canada

J. L. Bennett (✉)
Canadian Blood Services, Ottawa, ON, Canada
e-mail: judie.leach.bennett@blood.ca

D. Devine
University of British Columbia Centre for Blood Research and Canadian Blood Services, Vancouver, BC, Canada

risk-based decision-making framework for blood safety [1] articulates the issue as follows:

> The first purpose of the Framework is to optimize the safety of the blood supply by enabling the proportional allocation of finite resources to mitigate the most serious risks, recognizing that the elimination of all risk is not possible. ... The second purpose of the Framework is to analyze and account for a series of contextual, often qualitative, factors that affect decision making in the management of blood risks. The Framework takes a societal perspective, supporting consideration of social, economic, and ethical perspectives, which go beyond quantitative calculations of risk and which can alter risk tolerability.

Inherent in this approach are four interrelated sets of principles and practices, in the domains of risk perception, risk communication, stakeholder engagement, and risk tolerability. When assessing blood safety threats with a particular focus on public concern, the techniques of risk-based decision-making become especially relevant. This chapter will explore these four areas, including the way in which they are made manifest in the Alliance of Blood Operators (ABO) RBDM Framework (Fig. 3.1), which is premised on seven risk management principles. The following three principles are particularly pertinent to the subject matter of this chapter:

> *Fairness:* Safety decisions must be timely, fair, independent, and sensitive to cultural values. Risks that are unacceptable to society are not imposed, and the risk is distributed as equitably as possible.
> *Transparency:* The decision-making process must be transparent and accessible to stakeholders and members of the public. People involved in making decisions must declare all relevant conflicts of interest.
> *Consultation:* Stakeholders must be consulted on relevant issues that affect them or present a significant social concern. The consultation process must give stakeholders an opportunity to provide input [1].

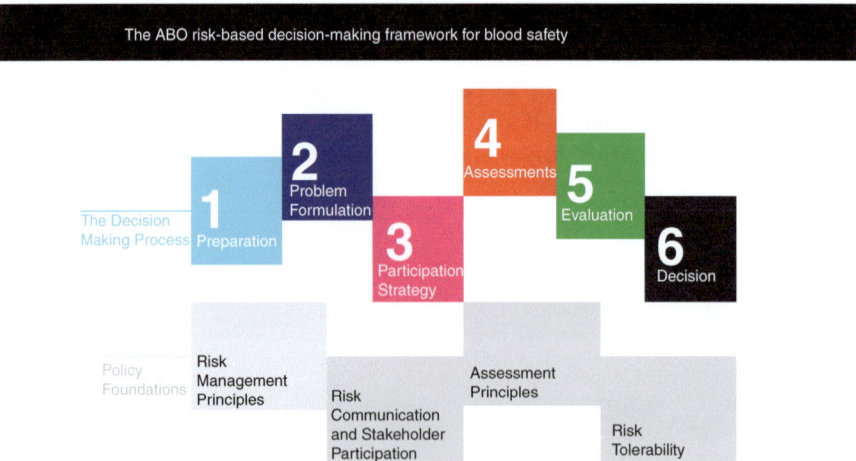

Fig. 3.1 The ABO risk-based decision-making framework for blood safety [1]

Risk Perception: General Principles

An increasingly diverse body of research from several disciplines, including cognitive and social psychology, sociology, anthropology, and even political science and geography, is investigating the way in which people make judgements about different risks and the factors that they consider in these judgements. The task has been to understand the perceptual processes by which non-experts understand and misunderstand risk probabilities and severities, in the presence and absence of expert estimates. Risk perception research has demonstrated that people's risk judgements reflect not only a sense of the significance of harm and potential benefits but also social values and priorities that are relevant to risk management policy. These judgements are affected by several factors, including qualitative assessments such as "dread" and "unknown" risk, some fundamental perceptual dynamics, collective risk judgement processes, and trust in risk management.

Qualitative Risk Factors

For some aspects of risk judgements, people rely on intuitive perceptual processes to construct (sometimes inaccurate) beliefs about the nature and significance of a potential event or outcome and the likelihood that it will occur. The consequences of a risk are more influential in perceptions than are the probabilities of its occurrence—even when these probabilities are extremely small. People typically have trouble understanding probabilities and uncertainties, which is a concern in contexts such as the risks and benefits of treatment options, or similarly in doses or exposures.

Many of the qualitative factors that people associate with risks relate to associations that are elicited by particular risk sources or outcomes that they might produce, while others are widely held or intuitive assumptions about biological or physical processes [2]. Many common qualitative associations that contribute to risk perceptions have been consolidated into two factors that lead to increased levels of concern [3]. Dread risk encompasses characteristics such as the quality of being imposed or uncontrollable, globally catastrophic, fatal, not equitable, and/or posing a risk to future generations. Unknown risk captures risks that are unfamiliar, emerging or are new to science, and are seen as higher risk than those that are familiar [3].

Risk Perception Dynamics

There are a number of psychological processes that contribute to the construction of a risk and the way that individuals integrate risk information and judgements into their larger stores of knowledge, value systems, and identities. These include a reliance on heuristics, framing processes and effects, and the selection of information that is brought to bear on a risk judgement to align with the individual's existing values and beliefs.

Heuristics are "rules of thumb" that people use as a shortcut to replace systematic and more effortful thinking and that rely on past experience with similar risks, risk contexts, managers, or information sources. Several types of heuristics have been identified that commonly lead risk judgements to diverge from assessed levels. The availability heuristic refers to the ease with which people can recall a risk type or event, often reflecting recent media coverage of an event, for example; it often leads to an assumption that the risk is more likely or frequent than is accurate [4]. Another is the affect heuristic, in which an emotional association that people have with a risk source or outcome dominates judgements on similar risks [5].

People tolerate higher risks from activities with which they perceive a benefit. However as it can be uncomfortable to engage in an activity that involves both benefit and risk, people often downplay the risks of an activity that they value, for example, to arrive at an overall "benefit-dominated" perspective on an activity or other risk agent [6]. The converse occurs when people focus on the risks of an activity from which they do not perceive a benefit, or that they dislike for other reasons. This effect is stronger when a strongly held risk attitude becomes associated with an emotion: the risk-benefit perspective becomes more polarized, with any potential benefits denied in a risk-based frame, and potential risks not acknowledged in a benefit-framed situation [7].

Finally, people's knowledge about a risk shapes their perceptions; however, the assumption that a lack of scientific understanding accounts for risk judgements that are inconsistent with technical assessments has been discounted [8]. People bring to bear their own knowledge on their risk judgements, which will be consistent with their existing belief structures and values and may not accord with scientific evidence. Several processes have been described as part of this process, including confirmation bias, in which we agree with information that is consistent with our prior beliefs, and scepticism bias, in which we discount information that challenges our prior beliefs [9].

These processes apply to experts and non-experts alike, as people select the information to which they pay attention, and find credible, in order to maintain coherence among their specific beliefs, larger knowledge, and attitudes and values. The concept of risk perception is much broader than probabilities of occurrence and legitimately incorporates many value-based and sociopolitical factors.

Collective Risk Judgement Processes

Many risk judgements are formed in social contexts that build on or alter individual perceptions and processes: the social context in which a risk occurs and the collective knowledge which circulates about it, constitute a frame that shapes the way the risk is considered in society and public responses are decided. A process called social amplification can raise public awareness of, and concern about a risk, and in some cases can result in persistent and generalized social assumptions about an issue. Social amplification of a risk occurs when information and information sources and channels of dissemination, institutional structures, social group behaviour, and individual responses combine to influence individual and collective awareness of, and response to, a risk [10].

Research on the social amplification of risk framework [10] has considered many factors that influence public perceptions of risks and risk issues. A key factor is media coverage, which both serves as an important source of information and also frames issues in a way that may shape social knowledge and attitudes about a risk [11–13]. Certain aspects of media coverage have been found to affect social awareness and perceptions of risks, including the amount or volume of coverage, pre-existing social debate on the issue, and the degree to which negative consequences of a risk are dramatized [13]. Several other factors and processes have also been identified as influential in the shaping of social awareness and beliefs, including discussions among individuals of media coverage and other information on risk issues [14] and, more recently, the effects of online information and social media [15–17].

Trust in Risk Management

Studies have found that perceptions of a risk are related to trust in the authorities who manage it, and the degree of trust in institutions responsible for risk management strongly influences the perception of an activity or technology or the source of risk itself [18, 19]. Judgements that a risk manager is not competent, or is otherwise not trustworthy, will be associated with an elevated perceived risk of an activity or technology [19].

While individuals delegate functions to expert systems, they also monitor the performance of those functions. This concept has been called active or critical social trust and incorporates monitoring of activities and institutions as an essential complement to the delegation of risk management responsibility [20]. This kind of trust functions both to monitor the competence of those entrusted to manage the risk and to ensure that they remain aligned with social values and expectations.

Risk Perception: Blood Safety Context

The perceptual patterns and influences described by risk perception researchers apply to judgements of the risks of blood products and blood donation. As with all risks, however, many of these processes and patterns are activated more or less strongly by characteristics and contextual factors that are specific to the way in which the blood products appear in society and in an individual's life, and this context changes over time.

Blood Products

In terms of underlying perceptions of risk, laypersons have tended to overestimate disease transmission rates (e.g. human immunodeficiency virus (HIV)) [21]. Not surprisingly, surveys conducted in the US in 1997 and 1998 found that a "substantial proportion" of respondents did not think the US blood supply was safe and would not accept a transfusion [5]; Lee found, in 2006, that transfusion registered as an intermediate dread risk and unknown risk [21]. A desire for retaining an element of personal control was reported, leading some to pursue autologous donation [22, 23]. Countering the perceived risks of blood transfusions, however, is the awareness that transfusions have a high benefit, and higher risk perceptions were reported among those who had not received a transfusion themselves [5]. Improved public trust and confidence in blood systems is associated with a decline in perceived risks [21]. Blood transfusion scored the lowest of ten risks rated for dread and unknown risk characteristics in 2013 [23], and in 2016 three quarters of Canadians rated the safety of the blood supply as a 7 or higher (with 10 being "very safe") [24].

Levels of knowledge tend to be low among members of the public on several aspects of blood, including the risk profile associated with transfusion and with donation, infection risks, and newer blood technologies such as pathogen inactivation. Due to media coverage and social amplification of issues related to the tragedies of HIV and hepatitis C transmission through blood products, however, most members of the public became well acquainted with and formed judgements on those risks. Heuristics and collective judgement influence social awareness and concern and subsequently policy; media is an important component in an amplification process, and the attitudes and biases of messages reflected in the coverage will become part of the social conversation and potentially of policy considerations [25].

There is evidence of some fundamental intuitive perceptions and framing effects on risk perceptions of pathogen inactivation technology; however, perhaps due to the clear benefits of transfusions, most agree that they would accept pathogen-inactivated blood products [24]. A strong framing effect has been observed, as those presented with a "gain-framed" scenario (in which 1,999,999 people will not contract HIV from two million transfused units) reported a higher level of confidence than those presented with a loss-framed scenario (1 case of HIV among two million units).

Blood Donors and Donation

Risk perceptions of blood donors are also relevant to a viable and safe blood system. Perceived risks have been associated with hesitancy in donating blood, primarily the fear of infection, of needles and of pain, as well as concerns about inconvenience and loss of time [26–28]. Risk perceptions on this issue can also be affected by framing effects: study participants who had been "cued" by a question on a questionnaire were significantly more likely to believe they could acquire HIV through donating blood than were those who had not been so cued [26].

Value-based and ethical issues have arisen in the area of donor relations, with the issue of the blood donor deferral of men who have sex with men (MSM) being one of the most contentious. In the late 1980s, most countries implemented an indefinite deferral of MSM donors as high-risk for HIV transmission; this was the subject of controversy and became an ethical risk with the potential stigmatizing of gay men [29, 30]. With improved testing technologies and process controls, and updated risk modelling, many countries have implemented less restrictive policies, with ongoing monitoring. Central to these change efforts has been the engagement and input of stakeholders on all aspects of the issue [31], perceived as relevant and instructive for policy development and regulatory decision-making [32, 33].

The principles of risk perception not only affect the assessment of blood safety threats and public concern but also inform effective risk communication and stakeholder engagement regarding those threats. In this regard, the goal is to ensure that concerned, interested, and affected individuals and groups are informed on key issues, enabling them to make informed decisions and to contribute to larger institutional decisions on matters that affect them.

Risk Communication

Risk communication is an exchange of risk information between interested parties, primarily including experts, stakeholders, and the general public. It usually involves conveying technical matters to non-technical audiences, focussing on message content and style appropriate to listeners' interests in the matter, their existing knowledge and level of comprehension, and the use to which they will put the information. Risk communication principles can be integrated into communications that take place between individuals, for example, by a physician wanting to ensure that patients have a clear understanding of treatment options, or the approach can be a more concerted organizational program to address specific risks or safety concerns or provide information on the rationale for a risk management or policy decision. The purpose of risk communication is generally to enhance audience understanding of a risk to their health or safety often in relation to benefits or protective measures, so they can make informed decisions. The goals of risk communication include sharing information, changing beliefs, and changing behaviour [2], but not all goals will apply equally to each application. There are many possible applications of risk communication, such as ongoing risk communications programs, or incident-based communications, such as those stemming from the identification of a defect or error [34].

Risk communication is generally concerned with an accessible and relevant presentation of scientific evidence or an explanation to an interested audience that does not have this knowledge or associated analytical skills. It is an exchange, even when used in relatively one-way settings, in that messages respond to information needs and interests of the intended audience. Attention to this interactive aspect is growing as its importance is recognized. The Council of Canadian Academies [34] describes risk communication as "fundamentally a socially and politically interactive process" that is increasingly seen as a relationship that builds and fosters trust over time. As such, a critical function in the development, updating, and revising of risk communication messages and materials is learning about audience information needs, evaluating the effectiveness of the messages for that audience, and receiving feedback and approaches from audiences so that corrections and improvements can be made [2, 34–36].

As noted above, effective risk communication is guided by the principles of risk perception; the preparation of risk communication messages draws on general risk perception patterns and specific perceptions of the risk at issue. It also requires an understanding of the audience and the context in which the audience will use the information, so that the specific messages and level of evidence can be tailored to their needs for the information. Risk communication may be conducted by professionals working in many different aspects of the blood system and may involve a spectrum of communications ranging from core risk and benefit considerations to ethical implications and system-wide policy issues.

Risk Communication Process

In many cases risk communication will be developed by an organization as part of a program and designed and conducted through a systematic process. The process broadly consists of goal definition and program design; audience identification and needs assessment; message preparation and delivery; and program implementation, including testing, monitoring, and revising the effectiveness of the messages for the audience.

The first step is the identification of the purpose of the risk communication program and the objectives of any particular message development. A determination must be made as to whether the messages are meant to be informative, that is, to enhance audience understanding so they are better equipped to make their own decisions, or whether the messages are meant to be persuasive, that is, to encourage a change in beliefs about a subject or, a more challenging objective, to change behaviours. Objectives could include responding to requests for certain risk information to enable a decision, providing comprehensive risk information about a procedure to ensure a patient or a blood donor is sufficiently informed, correcting misconceptions, encouraging healthy behaviours for blood donors, or providing basic education about blood risk management for the general public in an effort to be transparent and improve knowledge and confidence in the blood supply.

Based on the objectives of the risk communication, audiences are identified that may need the risk information, such as those who may be vulnerable to the risk or those who have an interest in the issue. An understanding is also developed regarding an audience's baseline knowledge, level of comprehension, existing concerns, and any contextual or value issues that could affect their interest in or response to the information, as may be catalogued in a systematic process such as a social concern assessment [1]. At the societal scale, a number of factors can shape attitudes to a risk and those responsible for its management. It is important to consider any existing societal concern or other contextual factors in the development of risk communication.

Messages are prepared for the audience and their needs, with attention to framing effects in the way that options are presented. People are particularly vulnerable to these effects when they are not familiar with the subject matter and may be facing difficult choices [2]. The use of gain- or loss-framed information can exert an influence on risk or safety perception that may or may not be appropriate, depending on the context. For example, both donors and non-donors who received information presented in a gain frame reported higher levels of confidence in blood safety for transfusion [37]; this effect may be approached differently, however, by a clinician providing information for a patient's own treatment decision [38]. Researchers and practitioners have given considerable attention to the most effective way of expressing technical information so that it is best understood by non-technical audiences. Probabilities and uncertainties may be important in a health risk context but are often not well understood, particularly with respect to level of risk and the risk-benefit balance of an option. The use of numbers can be important but is more effective with other aids such as graphics to assist comprehension [2, 34].

Finally, whenever possible, risk messages should be tested on a representative audience to evaluate their effectiveness and modified if the messages are not understood or credible. Their effectiveness once they are disseminated should also be monitored, with revisions and updates made as necessary to correct misunderstandings or update responses to issues of concern.

Applications

Discussions between physicians and patients, or their families, are likely to centre on core risk and benefit considerations of the use of blood products. These applications are more likely to be interpersonal interactions in which a clinician has personal knowledge of the recipient of the information, and in which there is likely a degree of trust present as a result of this personal attention and interaction. Even with an established professional relationship, the physician might inquire about the patient's primary risk concerns and any particularly hoped-for outcomes, clarifying these with evidence and experience of likely outcomes.

In contrast, risk communication messages for the broader public may be of two main types: notifications of health or safety risks that are broad enough to warrant dissemination to the general public and risk management education that includes elements of risk communication. Risk notifications should be prompt and complete, to ensure that vulnerable groups are protected and to ensure transparency [39].

These messages identify the product at issue, those who might be at risk and what people who might have been exposed should do. More generally public risk communication messages may be prepared to inform members of the public of the safety of the blood supply and the measures being taken to ensure that risks are minimized, the products are safe, and the supply is adequate. The overall goal is to educate the public about safety and risk management measures and to build confidence in the safety of blood products and the blood system.

Risk communication approaches are equally important to developing blood donor messages. For donors, risk-focussed public messages include notifications and explanations of new or revised donor deferral policies, implemented for reasons of patient safety (e.g. travel deferral for Zika virus) or donor safety (e.g. donor iron). These communications range in focus from basic risk information to policy decisions that have ethical implications. Research on donor knowledge and risk perceptions can direct communicators to provide information particularly tailored for donors and to be oriented with a recognition of the altruistic motivation and social value of these donations.

Whether the focus is patient or donor safety, risk communication is highly related to effective stakeholder engagement. In the ABO RBDM Framework, both concepts form one of the key policy foundations underlying the risk-based decision-making process and are also specifically addressed in stage three of the decision process, which focuses on the development and implementation of a participation strategy for the risk decision (Table 3.1).

Stakeholder Engagement

Stakeholder engagement is a systematic discipline with defined principles and responsibilities, aimed at building and maintaining relationships with stakeholders, including stakeholders in decisions that affect them, building trust, and developing risk management measures and decisions that reflect stakeholders' priorities. Such engagement may range from information gathering or exchange, to participation on working groups and collaboration on the development of risk management options. These approaches can build trust among stakeholders, through enabling participation and generating a sense of ownership of processes and decisions and through the development of relationships via direct interactions and engagement. Unlike risk communication, stakeholder engagement is oriented towards partnership with individuals and groups with interest and influence in specific policy directions. The input required in a stakeholder engagement exercise will be determined by the parameters of the decision under consideration, the priorities which must be addressed, and the risk management options which are being considered. Engaging stakeholders does not mean that an institution bearing the responsibility for the decision abdicates its decision-making obligation and authority. Care must be taken to ensure that participants in an engagement process understand the roles and

Table 3.1 Risk-based decision-making framework for blood safety [1]

Framework structure	
Stage 1: Preparation	Task 1: Review the purpose of the framework
	Task 2: Review risk management foundations
	Task 3: Understand how the framework is organized
Stage 2: Problem formulation	Task 1: Characterize the issue
	Task 2: Identify the decision driver
	Task 3: Formulate the assessment question
	Task 4: Identify preliminary risk management options
	Task 5: Determine the required assessments for Stage 4
Stage 3: Participation strategy	Task 1: Review best practice considerations for risk communication and stakeholder involvement
	Task 2: Define the need for stakeholder participation
	Task 3: Identify and assess stakeholder audiences
	Task 4: Develop a participation plan
	Task 5: Initiate the plan
Stage 4: Assessment [Note: It may not be necessary to carry out all assessments]	Task 1: Review assessment principles
	Task 2: Screening assessment
	Task 3: Blood safety risk assessment
	Task 5: Operational risk assessment
	Task 6: Contextual assessment
	Task 7: Summary of assessments
Stage 5: Evaluation	Task 1: Use assessment results to evaluate risk management options
	Task 2: Involve stakeholders and incorporate their feedback
	Task 3: Evaluate the risk tolerability of each option
	Task 4: Rank the risk management options
Stage 6: Decision	Task 1: Prepare a report of risk management options
	Task 2: Develop and present a recommendation
	Task 3: Share the decision
	Task 4: Create a decision implementation plan

obligations of the parties in the engagement, the opportunities for input, and the limits inherent in the process.

There are many rationales cited for stakeholder engagement in the context of assessing blood safety threats and addressing public concern. Stakeholders have a right to have a say in decisions that affect them and to expect that their legitimate needs will be addressed in decisions. In addition, better decisions result when gaps, opportunities, and possible solutions are identified as part of a full spectrum of perspectives. Stakeholders may also contribute influence, networks, and other resources to risk communication and to risk management and decision-making, in the context of a genuine partnership. Conversely, stakeholders who are not engaged, or feel that engagement was not genuine or adequate, can undermine efforts to manage and communicate risk. Optimal stakeholder involvement includes two components: stakeholder discovery and stakeholder engagement.

Stakeholder Discovery

Stakeholder discovery involves identifying and characterizing key categories of stakeholders who should be engaged, based on relevance, interest, and influence. It is important to clarify why stakeholders need to be involved, whether they expect to be involved and how, the roles they will play, how their involvement might impact the decision, how their input could fill information gaps, their ability to influence others, and whether there are any regulatory expectations for stakeholder involvement. In order to identify and prioritize the stakeholders to be included in the decision process, it is optimal to consider a wide variety of categories of stakeholders, such as patient groups, affected individual patients, blood donors, health professionals, researchers, health institutions, professional associations, funders, regulators, industry partners, suppliers, and the general public. There may be groups interested in participating in decisions on certain issues, or whose participation could be particularly valuable in implementing a decision. Another category of potential stakeholders or participants to be considered is that of "thought leaders", who are individuals involved in health policy or academic research and can elucidate key concepts or principles that would be implicit or at stake in an issue.

Each stakeholder would then be assessed according to level of interest and influence. The guidance offered by the ABO RBDM Framework is to locate the stakeholder, in accordance with levels of interest and influence, in a quadrant of a matrix, thus triggering varied types of engagement. For example, stakeholders who are assessed as low in interest and influence will be kept informed, whereas those who have high interest but lower levels of influence may be consulted, while collaboration would be sought with those who display high levels of interest and influence (Fig. 3.2) [1].

Stakeholder Engagement

The second component is engagement, the practice of facilitating opportunities to participate in a decision for potentially interested parties. Stakeholder engagement may be conducted in a number of ways, according to the type of issue on which input is sought. The type of engagement will be appropriate to the objectives and subject area of the decision, such as decisions on blood safety and supply, ethical challenges in donor management, or policy decisions with regulators and funders.

Some engagement processes may be relatively routine processes in which certain stakeholders are involved on an ongoing basis, participating, for example, in standing committees which meet periodically to review or work on issues as they emerge. Others may be planned to gather input on specific decisions or on the development of specific initiatives; methods include online consultations, workshops, or meetings, structured to capture and assess participants' feedback. For engagement on

3 Assessing the Threat: Public Concern

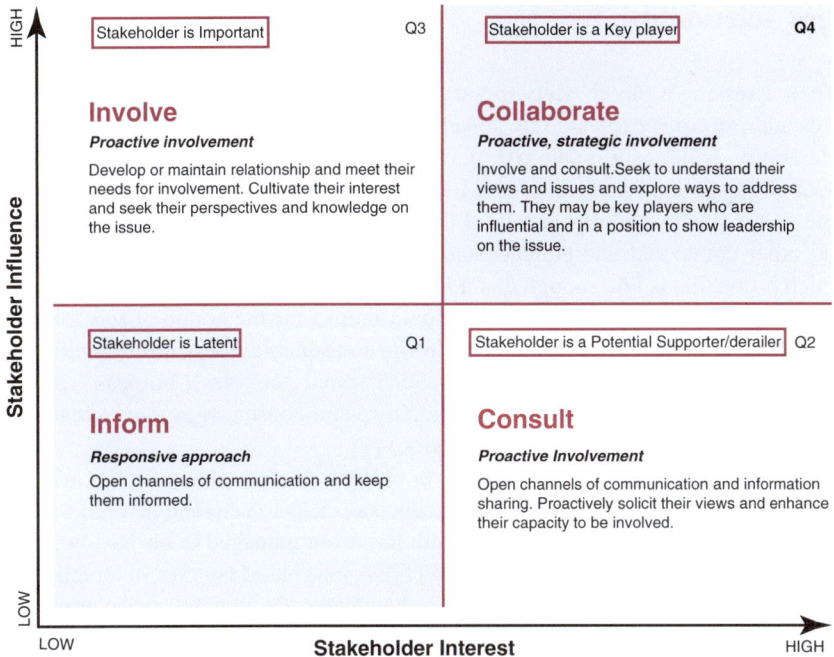

Fig. 3.2 Stakeholder identification tool [1]

risk decisions, there are certain points in the decision process at which engagement is most appropriate, such as in assessing the risk and the contextual factors surrounding the risk, in the generation of risk management options, and in conducting the evaluation aimed at selecting from among the options. For example, blood operators in various jurisdictions have reported assessing and/or facilitating stakeholder participation on a variety of risk issues, including emerging infectious disease risks (e.g. *Babesia microti,* hepatitis E); donor testing strategies (e.g. cytomegalovirus, human T-lymphotropic virus); donor deferral criteria (e.g. donor iron, MSM) [31]; security of supply risks (e.g. plasma for immunoglobulin products to meet patient need); and adoption of new technologies (e.g. pathogen inactivation technology for platelets).

In all cases, the purpose and objectives of the engagement are stated—the opportunities but also the limits—along with a clear articulation of the issues on which input is requested. Any documents prepared for stakeholders should follow the principles of risk communication, tailoring the content and style to stakeholders' interests, clarifying the issues on which their input is requested, and building trust by demonstrating shared values and objectives for the decision. Ideally, the proceedings of the consultation are documented and summarized in a report, which is shared with stakeholders to enable them to verify its accuracy. After the decision is made, the institution reports back to all stakeholders on the decision and its rationale, and the use that was made of their input.

Risk Tolerability

When assessing a blood safety threat and associated public concern, the perspectives and priorities expressed by stakeholders are relevant to the evaluation of risk tolerability, which is a public risk management principle concerned with a judgement of the appropriate level of risk to the public from a managed activity. A tolerable risk is a managed risk at a level that is appropriate in view of benefits gained and other contextual and ethical factors; this is distinct from an acceptable risk, which is one that is low enough that no management is needed [40]. At a theoretical level, there are several philosophical underpinnings for the notion of risk tolerability, including human rights (protection from unreasonable risks), utility (individuals are expected to accept risks from beneficial social activities), fairness (risks are justified by benefits and distributed equitably), and consent (generally satisfied by transparency and access to risk information) [1].

Risk tolerability is thus a system-level evaluation that is based in the acknowledgement that society cannot afford to reduce all risks to zero and that risks vary in the ease with which they may be reduced. Risks are managed to be "as low as reasonably achievable" (ALARA) (Fig. 3.3 [1]). A risk-based concept, tolerability is a problem of trade-offs [41] which is why risk perception principles, risk communication, and stakeholder engagement are highly relevant to the assessment of public risks, alongside quantitative risk assessment and economic factors in the cost-effective management and reduction of risk.

Blood safety risks, borne by the public and managed on the public's behalf by blood operators and others in the system from "vein to vein", are more fully understood in the light of an assessment of risk tolerability. As such, the evaluation stage of the ABO RBDM Framework (Stage 5, Fig. 3.1; Table 3.1) incorporates an approach for making a qualitative judgement of relevant societal and contextual factors, integrated with assessed risk levels, health benefits, and economic costs of each proposed risk management option or scenario. The risk tolerability evaluation process is a comparison of risk management options through a systematic approach which synthesizes the outputs of assessments of blood risk, operational impact, health economics and outcomes, as well as other assessments such as a social concern assessment and the outcomes of stakeholder consultation processes, as necessary. A tolerability assessment may be concerned not only with the various degrees to which the different options may reduce risk and incur system costs but also with management options that pose concerns to some stakeholders, surface political or social value questions, or raise ethical considerations in the distribution of risks and benefits. The risk tolerability evaluation is a comprehensive, qualitative evaluation of the various risk management options. It is tailored for the factors that are relevant for each decision, taking into account several perspectives; given the balance of factors, the outcome may differ somewhat from the conclusions of technical assessments alone but also from the expressed preferences of stakeholders or the public.

For example, with respect to the revision by many countries of the indefinite deferral of MSM donors, this revised approach was a carefully considered balance

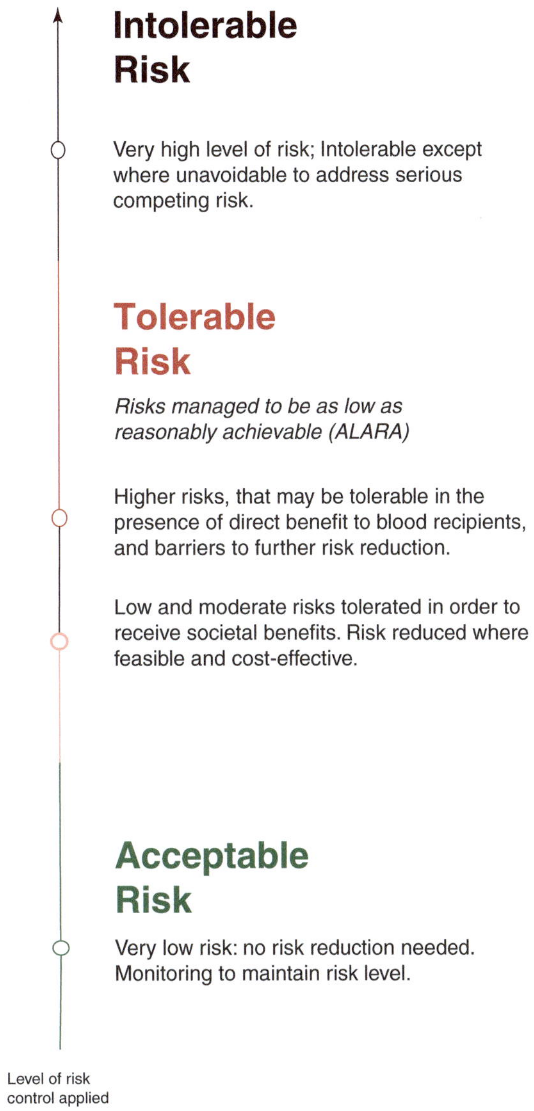

Fig. 3.3 Risk tolerability evaluation [1]

Intolerable Risk

Very high level of risk; Intolerable except where unavoidable to address serious competing risk.

Tolerable Risk

Risks managed to be as low as reasonably achievable (ALARA)

Higher risks, that may be tolerable in the presence of direct benefit to blood recipients, and barriers to further risk reduction.

Low and moderate risks tolerated in order to receive societal benefits. Risk reduced where feasible and cost-effective.

Acceptable Risk

Very low risk: no risk reduction needed. Monitoring to maintain risk level.

Level of risk control applied

of both risk and ethical issues that goes to the core rationale of risk tolerability evaluation:

> The overriding consideration should be that a change in policy should not increase risk to transfusion recipients. However, de minimus changes in risk may be acceptable in the context of larger societal benefits. Social factors affecting the overall safety and adequacy of the blood supply such as compliance with deferral criteria and public willingness to donate blood may be part of the assessment of risks and benefits of a policy change. The discussion should include whether the public is prepared to accept some added risk of transfusion for a possible benefit of reducing a perceived discrimination against MSM [32].

In a single-risk situation, the risk tolerability of various risk management options can be compared to a "baseline" risk situation or a status quo option as well as to other potential mitigation options. More complex evaluations involve multidimensional risk issues in which mitigation options may have different types of risks and benefits and also invoke a range of different policy implications, public concerns, or stakeholder conditions. In either case, the evaluation may result in the selection or elimination of a particular management option. Alternatively, it may lead to an adjustment in the way an option is implemented, by identifying societal concerns associated with the option as initially presented. The risk tolerability evaluation provides a comprehensive perspective on each option and alerts decision-makers to any contextual issues that could cause a blood safety risk management approach to enhance or undermine public trust.

Conclusion

Formal processes to assess quantitative blood safety risk are well established. However, the evolving use of risk-based decision-making has facilitated a broader evaluation of both quantitative and qualitative factors pertinent to blood safety questions. This approach enables risk decision-makers to incorporate public concern into risk assessment and into the evaluation of risk management options. Informed by risk perception principles, the practices of risk communication and stakeholder engagement provide valuable input on ethical issues and social concerns and ultimately in the evaluation of risk tolerability. Blood safety risks are borne by the public; hence engagement of the public is an essential step.

References

1. Alliance of Blood Operators. Risk-based decision-making framework for blood safety. 2015. https://www.allianceofbloodoperators.org/abo-resources/risk-based-decision-making.aspx. Accessed 13 April 2018.
2. Fischhoff B. Communicating risk and benefits: an evidence-based User's guide. Food and Drug Administration. 2011, Chapter 8, Pages 71–81.
3. Munier B. The Perception of Risk: Paul Slovic. London: Earthscan; 2004. 2000, 473 + xxxvii pp., Bibliography, Index, Foreword by G. White, [UK pound]19.95 paperback, ISBN 1-85383-528-5," Journal of Behavioral and Experimental Economics (formerly The Journal of Socio-Economics), Elsevier, vol. 33(1), pages 128–131, March.
4. Tversky A, Kahneman D. Judgment under uncertainty: heuristics and biases. Science. 1974;185(4157):1124–31.
5. Finucane ML, Slovic P, Mertz CK. Public perception of the risk of blood transfusion. Transfusion. 2000;40(8):1017–22.
6. Alhakami AS, Slovic P. A psychological study of the inverse relationship between perceived risk and perceived benefit. Risk Anal. 1994;14(6):1085–96.

7. Peters E. Affect and Emotion. In: Fischhoff B, Brewer NT, Downs JS, editors. Communicating risks and benefits: an evidence-based user's guide: US Department of Health and Human Services: Food and Drug Administration; 2011. https://www.fda.gov/downloads/AboutFDA/ReportsManualsForms/Reports/UCM268069.pdf. Accessed 30 April 2018.
8. Bauer MW, Allum N, Miller S. What can we learn from 25 years of PUS survey research? Liberating and expanding the agenda. Public Underst Sci. 2007;16(1):79–95.
9. Gluckman P. Making decisions in the face of uncertainty: understanding risk O.o.t.P.M.s.C.S. Advisor, Editor. Office of the Prime Minister's Chief Science Advisor. 2016.
10. Kasperson RE, et al. The social amplification of risk: a conceptual framework. Risk Anal. 1988;8(2):177–87.
11. Ji BC, Gi WY. Media and social amplification of risk: BSE and H1N1 cases in South Korea. Disaster Prevention Manag: An Inter J. 2013;22(2):148–59.
12. Frewer LJ, Miles A, Marsh R. The media and genetically modified foods: evidence in support of social amplification of risk. Risk Anal. 2002;22(4):701–11.
13. Rossmann C, Meyer L, Schulz PJ. The mediated amplification of a crisis: communicating the a/H1N1 pandemic in press releases and press coverage in Europe. Risk Anal. 2018;38(2):357–75.
14. Binder AR, et al. Interpersonal amplification of risk? Citizen discussions and their impact on perceptions of risks and benefits of a biological research facility. Risk Anal. 2011;31(2):324–34.
15. Bucher HJ. Crisis communication and the internet: risk and trust in a global media. First Monday. 2002;7(4). Retrieved 10 Aug, 2018, from http://firstmonday.org/ojs/index.php/fm/article/view/943.
16. Vijaykumar S, Jin Y, Nowak G. Social media and the virality of risk: the risk amplification through media spread (RAMS) model. J Homeland Sec Emerg Manag. 2015;12(3):653–77.
17. Ng YJ. Noisy haze, quiet dengue: the effects of mass media, interpersonal interactions and social media on risk amplification. Buffalo: Department of Communications. State University of New York; 2014.
18. Slovic P. Trust, emotion, sex, politics, and science: surveying the risk-assessment battlefield. Risk Anal. 1999;19(4):689–701.
19. Siegrist M, Cvetkovich G. Perception of hazards: the role of social trust and knowledge. Risk Anal. 2000;20(5):713–20.
20. Taylor-Gooby P. Social divisions of trust: Scepticism and democracy in the GM nation? Debate. J Risk Res. 2006;9(1):75–95.
21. Lee D. Perception of blood transfusion risk. Transfus Med Rev. 2006;20(2):141–8.
22. Lee DH, Mehta MD, James PD. Differences in the perception of blood transfusion risk between laypeople and physicians. Transfusion. 2003;43(6):772–8.
23. Ngo LT, Bruhn R, Custer B. Risk perception and its role in attitudes toward blood transfusion: a qualitative systematic review. Transfus Med Rev. 2013;27(2):119–28.
24. Gray N, et al. Public perceptions of pathogen reduction Technology in the Canadian Donor Blood Supply. ISBT Science Series. 2016;11(1):14–23.
25. Wilson K, et al. The reporting of theoretical health risks by the media: Canadian newspaper reporting of potential blood transmission of Creutzfeldt-Jakob disease. BMC Public Health. 2004;4(1):1.
26. Farrell K, et al. Public perception of the risk of HIV infection associated with blood donation: the role of contextual cues. Transfusion. 2002;42(6):679–83.
27. Ferguson E, et al. Trustworthiness of information about blood donation and transfusion in relation to knowledge and perceptions of risk: an analysis of UK stakeholder groups. Transfus Med. 2004;14(3):205–16.
28. Barkworth L, et al. Giving at risk? Examining perceived risk and blood donation behaviour. J Mark Manag. 2002;18(9–10):905–22.
29. Duquesnoy A, et al. Context and social perceptions of blood donation in donors found positive for human immunodeficiency virus in France. Transfusion. 2017;57(9):2240–7.
30. Go SL, et al. The attitude of Canadian university students toward a behavior-based blood donor health assessment questionnaire. Transfusion. 2011;51(4):742–52.

31. Goldman M, et al. Donor criteria for men who have sex with men: a Canadian perspective. Transfusion. 2014;54(7):1887–92.
32. Epstein J, Ganz PR, Seitz R. A shared regulatory perspective on deferral from blood donation of men who have sex with men (MSM). Vox Sang. 2014;107(4):416–9.
33. Advisory committee on the safety of blood tissues and organs. Donor selection criteria report. 2017. https://www.gov.uk/government/uploads/system/uploads/attachment_data/file/631626/SaBTO_donor_selection_criteria_report.pdf. Accessed 13 April 2018.
34. Council of Canadian Academies. Health product risk communication: is the message getting through? The expert panel on the effectiveness of health product risk communication. Ottawa: Council of Canadian Academies; 2015.
35. Renn O. Risk communication: towards a rational discourse with the public. J Hazard Mater. 1992;29(3):465–519.
36. Leiss W. Effective risk communication practice. Toxicol Lett. 2004;149(1):399–404.
37. Farrell K, et al. Confidence in the safety of blood for transfusion: the effect of message framing. Transfusion. 2001;41(11):1335–40.
38. Hossenlopp C. The risk debate in blood transfusion: how perceptions, beliefs and behaviours can be shaped by an efficient communication. Transfus Med. 2001;11(2):124–9.
39. Barlow S, et al. Transparency in risk assessment - scientific aspects guidance of the scientific committee on transparency in the scientific aspects of risk assessments carried out by EFSA. Part 2: general. 2018.
40. Bouder F, Löfstedt R. Tolerability of risk approach and the management of pharmaceutical risks. Expert Rev Clin Pharmacol. 2008;1(2):187–90.
41. Kletz T. Reducing risks, protecting people—HSE's decision making process. HSE Books. 2001;81(2003):53–4.

Chapter 4
Health Economics in Blood Safety

Brian Custer

Part I: Health Economics

The health economics of blood safety interventions is differentiated from other healthcare disciplines by the context of transfusion medicine, including the role of blood donors and the characteristics of the blood recipient population, as well as the history of transfusion-transmitted infections (TTI) with a resulting high level of risk aversion present today [1, 2]. The blood supply can be classified as a public good, and therefore consideration of economics in terms of welfare economics is endorsed [3]. Economics studies efficiency. In healthcare, efficiency is directly related to social welfare and utilitarianism – seeking to maximize health benefits to the largest proportion of society as achievable [4, 5]. However, it is not possible to maximize health benefits for all because of limited resources. The process of decision-making when competing priorities are present leads to accrual of benefits for some and lost opportunity of benefits for others. For medical, ethical, and legal reasons, healthcare resources in any society are not distributed solely according to efficiency [6]. These factors drive decision-making for microbial safety in transfusion in ways which are unique to this sector of healthcare.

Health economics is distinct from general economics because of the specific quantitative methods which are used to assess interventions in health and medicine. The presence of economics in healthcare and public health policy decision-making is controversial but unavoidable because no healthcare system has enough human and financial resources to do everything it might wish to do. The principles that underpin health economic assessments are the same as general economics, beginning

---

B. Custer
Epidemiology and Health Policy Science, VP Research and Scientific Programs,
Blood Systems Research Institute, San Francisco, CA, USA

Department of Laboratory Medicine, University of California San Francisco,
San Francisco, CA, USA
e-mail: bcuster@bloodsystems.org

with the concepts of scarcity, choice, and opportunity cost [3]. Scarcity is the recognition that resources are limited. No country, healthcare service provider, or blood system has an unlimited budget for blood safety. Choice is the direct consequence of limited budgets where decisions have to be made as to where to invest resources and in selecting between competing alternatives. Even relatively well-resourced healthcare systems have to choose between interventions which might substantially achieve the same outcomes. Opportunity cost is a consequence of choice. Opportunity cost is a somewhat elusive concept. It represents benefits not realized from choosing to spend healthcare resources in specific ways and thereby knowingly foregoing the benefits which cannot accrue because the available resources have been expended on other interventions. In practical terms for microbial safety in transfusion, the resources used to screen for or prevent specific transfusion-transmissible viral, bacterial, and parasitic agents are not available to screen for or prevent other recognized infectious agents.

Healthcare policy decision-makers must consider two broad objectives related to economics, a simpler one of remaining within available finances or budgets and a more complex one of seeking to maximize efficiency [7]. These two objectives are not always consistent. Decision-making that stays within the available budget won't necessarily maximize health benefits to the transfused population. Maximizing health benefits under a fixed budget requires careful consideration of and selection between interventions. In the context of blood safety, the Risk-Based Decision-Making (RBDM) framework for blood operators was developed and is discussed elsewhere in this book [8, 9]. The RBDM framework includes explicit consideration of costs and potential cost-effectiveness as inputs to the decision-making process in blood safety [3].

Health Economic Analysis Study Designs and Methods

Health economics, like all disciplines, has specific terminology defining methodologies and concepts. Persons unfamiliar with the discipline may misuse terms or simplify intended meaning to the point of introducing inaccuracy or mistaken meaning. Guidelines for conducting health economic analyses exist for a number of countries, and this chapter does not seek to define and describe all of methods used in health economics research or the specific requirements for health economics or health technology assessments in different countries. The International Society for Pharmaceutical Outcomes Research (ISPOR) maintains a web-based compendium of methods guidance recommendations, glossary of terms, as well as country-specific requirements available in different languages [10]. This resource will help to defined country-specific analysis designs and methodological requirements.

The methods available for health economic assessments start with simple cost accounting studies which seek to measure the economic consequences (ranging from increased expenditures to cost savings that accumulate) and health outcomes (reduced morbidity and mortality or identification of unexpected adverse events) that result from different interventions. The first economic evaluation method used in healthcare was cost of illness (COI) which sought to measure the economic burden of illness [11]. These studies remain important for defining the expenditures which result from treating illness but also have substantial limitations [12, 13]. These studies alone are inadequate for decision-makers because treating disease is not the same as paying to prevent or reduce the impact of disease. Decision-making in health policy is often focused on what interventions should be considered to prevent disease and mitigate disease outcomes [14, 15]. Prevention of microbial threats in transfusion medicine is paramount, especially the prevention of TTI.

Consistent with broader developments in health economics, comprehensive economic assessment of a new healthcare intervention is necessary when considered for adoption [16]. In transfusion safety similar recommendations were included as part of RBDM for blood safety. Assessment of microbial threats in blood safety should involve at least two different economic analyses: a budget impact analysis (BIA) and a cost-effectiveness analysis (CEA or CUA). Budget impact analysis examines the issue of affordability or the cost of adopting a new intervention. Budget impact analysis is an expansion of cost of illness to consider more than treatment. Affordability is not the same as cost of illness because the cost offsets of prevented adverse events are included in BIA. All costs are measured in currency units, meaning dollars, Euros, Yen, etc. A BIA takes the estimated unit cost of an intervention and multiplies it by the number of people affected by the intervention along with the estimated unit cost of prevented adverse events by the number of people expected to experience those events, to calculate the total budget required to fund the intervention [17]. BIA is a cost accounting study focused on the cost to implement or maintain a healthcare intervention over a relatively short time horizon, typically 1 to 5 years. The short time horizon coupled with a focus on currency units means BIA includes direct costs (see below).

Methods for conducting cost-effectiveness analyses in the blood safety context have been described in previous publications [3, 18–22]. Review papers published in the last 20 years have also sought to consider the available evidence and role of cost-effectiveness in transfusion medicine [23–25]. One point of potential confusion is that cost-effectiveness analysis is both a specific term and used as general term used to cover an array of studies from cost-minimization analysis (CMA) to cost-effectiveness analysis (CEA), to cost-utility analysis (CUA), and to cost-benefit analysis (CBA). All costs are measured in currency units. Each of these study designs seeks to compare the ratio of costs to benefits, including at least two different interventions, but does so under different assumptions about either costs or benefits under a longer-term time horizon. Interventions included in the analyses can include a comparison to no intervention (the so-called "do nothing" strategy), the currently adopted intervention ("status quo"), and various alternate similar or dissimilar interventions. For example, in responses to microbial safety in transfusion medicine, evaluations could include no intervention to various approaches for directly or indirectly screening for specific pathogens to remove infected units from the supply to the use of pathogen reduction technologies which seek to nonspecifically "sterilize" components by inactivating pathogens. In CMA, health effects (benefits and adverse events) are assumed or expected to be identical between competing interventions, and so only costs are compared with the objective to identify the intervention with the lowest overall cost. There are no published studies of microbial safety in transfusion using a CMA design. This is understandable because rarely do interventions in blood safety generate the same level of effectiveness (health benefit). In fact it is the careful evaluation of trade-offs in effectiveness that are often the key considerations of the interventions which are adopted to address microbial threats in transfusion. Likewise CBA is also uncommon in health economic analyses because both cost and effects are expressed as currency units. Results are reported as a ratio of cost incurred to costs saved by use of the intervention. This type of analysis specifically requires placing a monetary value on each human life which remains controversial [26]. In microbial safety of transfusion, health economic assessments of use of alanine aminotransferase (ALT) as a surrogate marker of TTIs, anti-HIV screening, and HBV vaccination have used CBA [27–30]. Most of these studies were conducted in the 1980s and 1990s with one reported in 2010.

The main study types used in most economic evaluation of healthcare are cost-effectiveness (CEA) and cost-utility analysis (CUA) in which the difference in costs of an intervention is divided by the difference in health benefits to generate a cost-effectiveness ratio (CER). For CEA, the results are in terms of cost per natural units such as infections avoided or life years gained, and for CUA, results are in terms of cost per quality-adjusted life years gained (QALYs) or disability-adjusted life years averted (DALYs). QALYs are estimated using health-state preference weights bound by values between 0 (equivalent to death) and 1 (perfect health) to adjust an entire year of life of the so-called perfect health downward according to the severity or loss of function from disease [31, 32]. DALYs are estimated by adding the years of life lost from disease with the adjusted years lived with disease. The sum of DALYs over the population is a measure of the burden of disease measures in terms of the gap between current health status and the counterfactual scenario of the entire population living to advanced age, free of disease, and disability [33]. Disability weights reflect the severity of the disease on a scale from 0 (perfect health) to 1 (equivalent to death). As implied by the QALY and DALY acronyms, these analyses use a long-term time horizon, typically lifetime. While QALYs and DALYs represent different conceptualizations of effects and effectiveness, for CUA the same analysis approach is used because both are aggregate measures of health benefits accrued or lost. Cost-effectiveness or cost-utility ratios are expressed as net costs per unit of effectiveness by comparing a new intervention with current practice or another potential intervention. The primary result of a CEA or CUA is the incremental cost-effectiveness ratio (ICER).

In blood safety results of analyses have been reported as CERs and ICERs. The cost-effectiveness ratio of each competing intervention relative to a common baseline such as no screening or the status quo is the best way to determine the cost-effectiveness of adopting an intervention for which no intervention is currently in place. Formally, the ICER is the true measure of the benefit achieved for the additional resources expended as increasingly resource-intensive or health benefit-producing interventions are compared. Unlike the comparison to a common baseline, ICERs are calculated in a stepwise manner where each more effective and/or more expensive intervention is compared to its closest (less costly and/or less effective) neighboring intervention to determine the increment of cost-effectiveness achieved. A summary of differences between BIA and CEA/CUA is provided in Table 4.1.

Perspective

The perspective defines which costs and effects are explicitly included or excluded from the evaluation. The major categories of perspective are the societal, third-party payer (insurer), employer, and patient/client perspectives. Depending on the analysis perspective, analyses include *direct* costs for healthcare paid by the health system, insurance, communities, and so-called "out of pocket" expense incurred by patients and their families. Direct costs are the clinical services, medications, hospitalizations, and other direct expenditures for care. Direct costs include the cost of labor. Direct costs can also include nonmedical costs such as transportation to attend an appointment at a healthcare clinic and child care or costs incurred to allow for a clinic visit to occur. *Indirect* costs are costs such as time away from work or lost productivity. Indirect costs are controversial and hard to measure [35]. There are many considerations that must be addressed in selecting the analysis perspective and then within that perspective defining which direct and indirect costs are included [36, 37]. The consensus in health economics, including blood safety economics, is that a more complete assessment of cost-effectiveness is achieved with the use of a societal perspective because relevant costs and consequences for different parts of society can be considered [3]. The costs and outcomes to blood centers, hospitals, donors, and mostly importantly blood recipients are reflected in the societal perspective. An analysis conducted using a societal perspective can also be modified to reflect a more limited perspective, so that the costs and consequences for different groups, such as for only payers/insurers or patients, can be identified and

Table 4.1 Summary of key methodological differences for budget impact compared to cost-effectiveness/utility analysis, adapted from [34]

Methodologic topic	Budget impact analysis	Cost-effectiveness/utility analysis
Typical perspective	Payer	Societal
Time horizon	Short-term (1–5 years)	Long-term/lifetime
Size of population	Includes	Ignores
Model inputs	Payer-specific	Population-average
Model output	Cost	Cost and health outcomes
Discounting	No	Yes
Include overhead costs	No	Yes

understood distinctly from other cost and outcome streams. Note that costs rather than charges are used in health economic analyses [38]. For example, hospital charges for specific procedures may not always be the same multiplier of cost and are widely variable by geographic location and hospital [39]. Cost-to-charge ratios are most relevant in market-driven healthcare systems, like in the USA, and may not be applicable in all jurisdictions.

Discounting

Discounting is a method to adjust future costs and benefits to their presumed present value. This is a reflection of time preference for both money and health. Economists have empirically measured preference for money and health today rather than in the future; therefore costs and benefits are weighted (adjusted to be less) the farther in the future they occur. Country-specific discount rates are typically specified in guidelines for health economic research. For example, some recommendations include discounting cost and effects as the same rate. In the USA and Germany, the recommend rate is 3.0% for both costs and effects, in the United Kingdom 3.5%, and in Australia and Canada 5% [40–42]. Other jurisdictions recommend different rates. In the Netherlands, discount rates of 4.0% costs and 1.5% for effects have been used [42]. Discount rates may change over time or be redefined by healthcare authorities.

CE Plane

Results of CEA/CUA are in terms of the cost and effectiveness of each intervention. Because each intervention will have separate cost and effectiveness point estimates, the overall results of CEA/CUA analyses can be plotted as Cartesian coordinates, creating the cost-effectiveness (CE) plane (Fig. 4.1). This approach to graphically displaying the results provides several insights into the relative efficiency of each of the interventions included in the analysis. The diagram shows how the ICER comparing "Intervention B" to "Intervention A" can be represented graphically as a ray from the origin and also shows a ray from the origin representing a defined cost-effectiveness threshold (see below). Depending on which quadrant the results for each intervention are in, certain conclusions can be made about the value of the intervention relative to its comparators. Interventions which are more costly and more effective will appear in the upper right quadrant (NE). Interventions which are less costly and more effective will appear in the lower right quadrant (SE). Interventions which are less costly and less effective will appear in the lower left quadrant (SW). Finally, interventions which are more costly and less effective will appear in the upper left quadrant (NW). Depending on budget impact or ability to fund, any intervention which is less costly and more effective would be appropriate

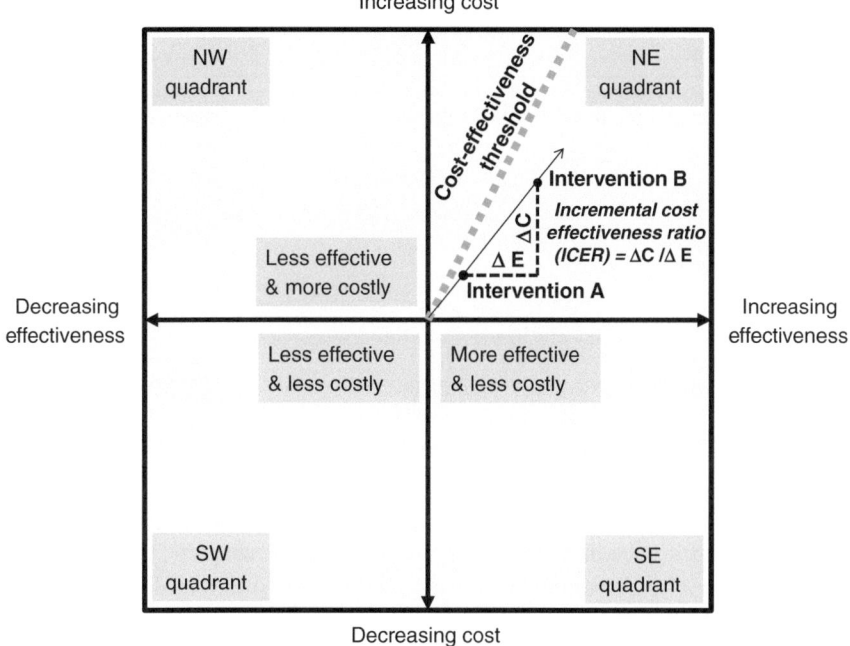

Fig. 4.1 Cost-effectiveness plane with rule of thumb decision guides

to adopt because the net impact to the healthcare system is greater health at overall lower cost. Interventions which fall in the SW and NW quadrants raise challenging questions, but although less effective may still be candidates for adoption [43]. Even when all results fall within the same quadrant (typically NE), graphing them provides a visual method for comparison, including the concepts of dominant or dominated strategies. Interventions with lower net costs and at least zero or net health benefits are considered dominant interventions and should be candidates for adoption.

Cost-Effectiveness Thresholds

To determine whether implementation is justified, the cost-effectiveness ratio should be compared to acceptability thresholds, if available. Typical thresholds for what is considered "cost-effective" in health and medicine are in the range of US$50,000 to 100,000/QALY [18, 23] or similar values in currencies as shown for some other developed countries (Table 4.2). Efforts to align acceptable CUA thresholds with reported ratios from healthcare authorities do overlap with empirically measured willingness to pay values. No such research has been conducted specific to blood transfusion interventions, and so it is unknown if the willingness to pay per QALY

Table 4.2 Threshold cost-effectiveness ratios defined as cost-effective in different scenarios compared to willingness to pay per QALY from studies conducted in each country and the WHO suggested guideline

Country	Specified range of cost/QALY ratio in local currency [46]	Empirically measured willingness to pay (cost/QALY ratio) [47]	Threshold cost/DALY based on 3 × Current GNI
Australia	AUS$42,000–76,000/life year	AUS$64,000/QALY	AUS$168,000/DALY
Canada	CAN$20,000–100,000/QALY	–	CAN$151,000/DALY
Japan	–	JPY 5 million/QALY	JPY 12,950,000/DALY
Netherlands	20,000–80,000 €/QALY	–	113,000 €/DALY
New Zealand	NZ$3000–15,000/QALY	–	NZ$166,000/DALY
United Kingdom	£20,000–30,000/QALY	£23,000/QALY	£93,000/DALY
United States	US$50,000/QALY	US$ 62,000/QALY	US$ 170,000/DALY

in any society is different for transfusion medicine, but the willingness to pay per QALY is assumed to be different as discussed later in the chapter.

Another approach to defining a cost-effective threshold is according to the gross domestic product (GDP) or gross national income (GNI) per person in each country. The WHO has recommended this approach where interventions with cost-utility ratios results above three times the GNI are classified as not cost-effective [44]. This approach directly adjusts thresholds to the size of the economy and average economic productivity of the population, making the threshold specific to the economic development level of the country. Recently, the WHO has further refined some of the ideas around appropriate thresholds to account for intangible aspects of the true GNI for a country as well as formally including consideration of budget impact, feasibility, and acceptability in addition to cost-utility results [45]. Table 4.2 provides various thresholds from healthcare authorities or assessment bodies, as measured according to willingness to pay and in terms of the approach recommended by WHO. Admittedly the WHO guideline is considered most applicable to low- and middle-income countries. For the high-income countries listed in the table, this threshold may be high relative to accepted thresholds.

Uncertainty and Sensitivity Analysis

Uncertainty and sensitivity are not the same. There are several levels of uncertainty in health economics. The first is stochastic uncertainty (first order) in the input parameter values for models. This type of uncertainty is from traditional statistical measures such as confidence intervals or standard deviations. Less familiar to many medical and scientific professionals is second-order uncertainty also known as parameter uncertainty which comes into consideration as part of modeling of complex systems. Feasible ranges of possible values coupled with known stochastic uncertainty are defined and then assessed for how the parameter uncertainty influences the BIA or CEA/CUA results. At the level of decision-making, it is the consideration of uncertainty in health economics and other evaluations that contribute to the overall confidence in BIA and CEA/CUA results. This level of uncertainty is assessed through sensitivity analysis.

Sensitivity analysis is an important tool to investigate how assumptions and numerical values used in the analysis influence the results. Health economic analyses are performed using models. These models require numerical inputs. The model parameters may be derived from clinical trials, observational studies, expert opinion, or assumptions. Few of these parameters are known with a high-degree precision and accuracy. There are two categories of sensitivity analysis: deterministic and probabilistic. Deterministic sensitivity analysis serves to highlight which numerical inputs are most influential and which specific model parameters are critical to driving a decision, whereas probabilistic sensitivity analysis provides an indication of the overall parameter uncertainty. Both are necessary to understand and report as part of an evaluation. Tornado diagrams, threshold plots, and two-way and three-way analyses are all appropriate ways of reporting results from deterministic sensitivity analyses [48]. Probabilistic sensitivity analysis is conducted using Monte Carlo simulation. Analyses are run 1000s of times with values drawn randomly from the uncertainty distributions of the model parameters. The paired distribution of costs and effectiveness from each iteration can be represented as a series of coordinate points on the CE plane. These data are also used to estimate 95% credible intervals, which are 95% confidence interval approximations. Ninety-five percent credible intervals are the simulation results of the analysis representing the 2.5th and 97.5th percentile of the distribution of all results from the Monte Carlo simulation. The results of each iteration of a simulation when plotted on the CE plane visually display the full potential range of the joint uncertainty of cost and effects. These figures are often referred to as cloud diagrams.

The inherent correlation structure of the model parameters can also be accounted for in probabilistic sensitivity, and the lack of such consideration has been identified as a limitation of many previous publications [49]. Not accounting for correlated parameters could lead to conflation and over estimation of uncertainty. Probabilistic sensitivity analysis provides a measure of the overall uncertainty of the costs, effectiveness, and cost-effectiveness results depending on whether BIA or CEA/CUA is being conducted.

Cost-Effectiveness Acceptability Curves

One of the most relevant current methods to more accurately incorporate uncertainty into the results reporting is to generate a cost-effectiveness acceptability curve (CEACs). The CEAC is a graph summarizing the impact of uncertainty from probabilistic sensitivity analysis on the result of an economic evaluation, frequently expressed as an ICER in relation to possible values of the cost-effectiveness threshold [50]. There are "textbook" versions of CEACs where the results are shown as sigmoid curves. This type of results display occurs only when all of individual iteration results fall into the NE quadrant of CE plane, i.e., when the intervention is always both more costly and more effective. A CEAC can take many shapes and forms because it is a graphic display of the probabilistic sensitivity analysis results transformed from the CE plane, where incremental costs and effects may cross quadrants resulting in discontinuous curves and asymptotes [51]. The CEAC is a useful tool in describing and quantifying uncertainty around the ICER, especially in combination with other tools such as plots on the CE plane and other related approaches to presenting health economic modeling results [52].

Considerations for Conducting and Reporting Analyses

The development of checklist approaches to review health economic and outcomes studies is useful for both subject matter experts and non-experts. The recently developed Consolidated Health Economic Evaluation Reporting Standards (CHEERS) are not intended to serve as a critiquing tool but can be used to assess if key aspects of the analysis are defined and reported in sufficient detail to help build confidence in the analysis and findings [53, 54]. If evaluating a published study is applicable to your setting, it is highly recommended to use CHEERS or formal critiquing approaches found in cost-effectiveness analysis textbooks to assess the strengths and limitations of an analysis.

Methodological Aspects of Health Economics Unique to Transfusion

Posttransfusion Survival

The mean age of the transfused population is variable across levels of development with more developed countries having a higher mean age of transfusion. Age at transfusion is linked to life expectancy which directly influences the cost-effectiveness of different interventions when calculated as cost per life years or QALYs. Even though posttransfusion survival is reduced when compared to the age-matched nontransfused population [55–59], there is a strong relationship between survival and the age of transfusion, as well as the number of components received [60]. Posttransfusion survival is also linked to the blood components received as these are directly related to the underlying indication for transfusion. Posttransfusion survival by component type has rarely been studied but is known to be an additional factor which will influence cost-effectiveness assessments [61, 62].

Such data are critical for the analyses of cost-utility because QALY calculations rely on accurate estimates of both short-term and long-term survival. Analyses which do not formally include posttransfusion survival are biased toward more favorable cost-effective ratios.

Residual Risk Calculations

Most microbial risks in transfusion medicine are rare. Directly measuring the risk is difficult, and in addition the factors which lead to transfusion-transmission are not simply the presence of the infectious agent. For these reasons, residual risk models are used to infer the risk of TTI [63–65]. Based on available hemovigilance data, the rates of actual transfusion-transmission appear to be even lower than residual risk estimates. The implications for health economics are that risk models and detection of infections in donors may overestimate clinically apparent TTI. Overestimated rates of TTI lead to more favorable cost-effectiveness ratios than would otherwise result.

Part II: Health Economics of Microbial Threats to Blood Safety

This section will review health economic evidence with respect to selected microbial threats to the blood supply. The examples are not exhaustive of all currently available health economic evidence in microbial threats in transfusion medicine. Rather the examples provide an overview of the range of health economic evidence for different safety threats. These findings are then used to discuss the scope and quality of health economic evidence in microbial threats to transfusion safety and to comment on implications for policy-makers.

Zika Virus

In 2015 Zika virus (ZIKV) became a re-emerging or recently emerged global pathogen [66]. Substantial effort to conduct research to understand the consequences of ZIKV infection to donors and blood recipients is ongoing [67]. Approaches to addressing TT ZIKV have been very different in different jurisdictions. The USA has taken the most aggressive response to the threat of TT ZIKV by adopting individual-donation (ID) nucleic acid testing (NAT) screening of every donation collected in the US states and some territories, such as Puerto Rico, since mid-2016.

The economic burden of ZIKV infection is of great concern with high potential consequence. Forecasts of the potential overall economic burden of ZIKV outbreaks across the six highest risk states in the USA (Alabama, Florida, Georgia, Louisiana, Mississippi, and Texas) showed that a population attack rate as low as 0.01% was estimated to cost $183.4 million to society ($117.1 million in direct medical costs and $66.3 million in productivity losses) [68]. Any higher attack rate would lead to even greater economic consequences. The potential impact was sufficient to spur adoption of a range of interventions to reduce the risk and prevent wider distribution of ZIKV infection. Cost-effectiveness of public health measures in vector (mosquito) control to reduce the risk of ZIKV appears to conform to accepted cost-effectiveness thresholds [69], whereas the implementation of blood screening interventions is unlikely to achieve such results. Cost-effectiveness of blood supply screening in the USA has not been reported. Cost projections (budget impact) for implementing screening have been reported and are sufficient to gain an understanding of the likely cost-effectiveness of blood screening. Screening all donations in the 50 states and the District of Columbia for ZIKV by ID-NAT was estimated to cost $137 million (95% confidence interval [CI], $109–$167) annually [70]. Given the observed yield of confirmed ZIKV infection in US donations of approximately 50 confirmed positive infections in blood donations from late 2016 to the end of 2017, the cost-effectiveness is roughly US$2.5 million per donor infection identified for the first year of ID-NAT screening of donations. For the cost-effectiveness to approach a threshold that could potentially be considered in line with accepted thresholds, the number of confirmed ZIKV infections in donors per year in the US states and the District of Columbia would have to be at least 2800 for a cost-effectiveness ratio of $50,000 per identified donor infection. No estimates are currently available for TTI prevention in terms of the cost per QALY, but such evaluations are certain to exceed the US$2.5 million per donor infection identified back-of-the-envelope calculation.

Human T-cell Lymphotropic Virus (HTLV)

Human T-cell lymphotropic virus is a TTI. The controversy in screening blood donors to prevent HTLV transmission lies in the relative cost-effectiveness of preventing transmission. A wide range of approaches to prevent TT HTLV have been adopted in different settings. These approaches are linked to the epidemiology observed in different jurisdictions. Where donor prevalence (and incidence) is low, the cost-effectiveness of screening all donations to prevent transfusion-transmission is far outside of accepted thresholds for cost-effectiveness. For high prevalence, endemic regions, no cost-effectiveness studies have been reported in the English language, peer-reviewed literature. In such locations, the cost-effectiveness of HTLV screening of all donors may be favorable and in line with accepted cost-effectiveness ratios.

Other safety measures in use in many jurisdictions contribute to a reduced risk of TT HTLV. Because HTLV is a cell-associated virus, leukoreduction plays an important role in reducing the risk of TTI [71]. Many high- and some middle-income countries have introduced universal leukoreduction of blood components [72]. Against this backdrop using the yield of infections identified in tested donations will overestimate the cost-effectiveness of donation screening because the actual risk of transmission will be low. Even before widespread leukoreduction, cost-effectiveness analyses of screening donated blood for HTLV were conducted; published results are summarized in Table 4.3. In none of the analyses except one from the late 1990s from France was screening all donors/donations less than a million donors (or equivalent in local currency) per QALY. The analyses conducted for France and Australia were CEA rather than CUA, providing results in terms of infections identified in donated blood. Regardless, health economic evidence suggests a limited justification for testing every donation because such testing is not cost-effective. Only one of the published studies addressed the issue of budget impact, reporting for the Netherlands a cost of screening of €25,700 for new donors screening and €589,000 for screening all donations [73]. The relative cost of screening is comparatively low and often included as an additional analyte on the high-throughput serology screening platform. This is one of the primary explanations for why HTLV screening of all donations is expected to continue in many jurisdictions, although the cost-effectiveness of screening for HTLV is not favorable.

Babesia

The primary species of concern with respect to transfusion-transmitted babesiosis is *Babesia microti* [76, 77]. While other spp. of *Babesia* are known to be transfusion-transmissible both in the USA and in other jurisdictions [78, 79], the focus is on interdiction of *B. microti* infection in endemic parts of the continental USA [80]. Currently, in the USA, there is no approved test for donor screening. Considerable

Table 4.3 Cost-effectiveness of serological screening of donors for HTLV from four different jurisdictions and varying time periods

Country or setting	Intervention (all are compared to no screening)	Cost-effectiveness ratio	Analysis year and reference
Australia	Anti-HTLV I/II screening of new donors	AUS$103,700/TT HTLV prevented	2014 [71]
	Anti-HTLV I/II screening of all donors/donations	AUS$1.4 million/TT HTLV prevented	
Netherlands	Anti-HTLV I/II screening of new donors	€2.23 million/QALY	2008 [73]
	Anti-HTLV I/II screening of all donors/donations	€45.2 million/QALY	
France	Anti-HTLV I/II screening of new donors	€237,000/ TT HTLV prevented	Before 1997 [74]
Norway	Anti-HTLV I/II screening of all donors	€930,000/QALY	Before 1996 [74, 75]

discussion of approaches to screening or other modes of prevention has been reviewed in the literature [76]. Three cost-effectiveness studies have been published focused on different approaches for donation screening for *Babesia microti* in terms of the mix of serological and/or polymerase chain reaction (PCR)-based assays and geographic locations of screening (Table 4.4).

Table 4.4 shows highly variable results for the cost-effectiveness of screening for *Babesia microti*. Result differences are attributed to different assumptions with

Table 4.4 Cost-effectiveness of screening US donors for *Babesia microti* according to the screening approach and geographic extent of testing

Geographic screening strategy	Intervention and comparator	Cost-effectiveness in US$/QALY	Cost-effectiveness in US$/QALY	Cost-effectiveness in US$/QALY
Analysis year and reference		2011 [81]	2013 [82]	Before 2015 [83]
4-state high endemic region[a]	Antibody screening compared to no testing	–	2,615,000	51,000
	PCR screening compared to no testing	–	5,006,000	Cost saving −63,600
	Antibody and PCR screening compared to no testing	–	5,210,000	251,000
	Recipient-targeted antibody and PCR screening compared to no testing	–	–	148,000
7-state endemic region[b]	Antibody screening compared to no testing	730,000	3,231,000	–
	PCR screening compared to no testing	–	6,394,000	–
	Antibody and PCR screening compared to no screening	1,222,000	6,582,000	–
	Recipient-targeted antibody and PCR screening compared to no testing	708,000	–	–
20-state potential risk region[c]	Antibody screening compared to no testing	–	6,685,000	–
	PCR screening compared to no testing	–	14,185,000	–
	Antibody and PCR screening compared to no testing	–	14,228,000	–

[a]4-state strategies are different in each analysis: Goodell et al. Connecticut, Massachusetts, New York, and Rhode Island; Bish et al. Connecticut, Massachusetts, Wisconsin, and Minnesota
[b]7-state: Connecticut, Massachusetts, Minnesota, New Jersey, New York, Rhode Island, and Wisconsin
[c]20-state includes states surrounding the 7-state endemic region

respect to localization of testing, i.e., how locally precise testing could be in high-risk regions, assumed rates of active and resolved babesiosis infection in donors, transmissibility to recipients, performance of the testing platforms, and the costs of testing. While there are identifiable methodologic differences between the analyses, it remains difficult to reconcile the different cost-effectiveness results from these analyses. Currently, development of new assays continues including NAT platforms [84] as well as clinical trials of these newer assays. Transfusion-transmitted *Babesia* remains a serious issue in the USA [85, 86]. The economic assessment of the newer assays designed for high-throughput blood donation screening laboratories may provide an important resolution of the disparate cost-effectiveness results published to date.

HIV, HBV, and HCV

These are the virus infections of broadest concern to the global blood supply because of the human-to-human spread of infection, relative ease of transmission, disease progression, and chronic nature of infection if untreated [87–89]. These pathogens are detectable by both serological and NAT testing methods. These infections are grouped together for discussion because these blood screening interventions are often performed in parallel on the same serology or NAT testing platforms. This multiplex approach achieves important efficiency in the testing laboratory. These three viruses remain highly important TTI threats, and with donor questioning for risk behaviors considered inadequate, prevention of TTI HIV, HBV, and HCV will continue to rely primarily on donation testing in virtually all settings [90–93]. Thus, there is worldwide interest in which combination of testing achieves acceptable prevention of HIV, HBV, and HIV in the context of a country or blood service's ability to pay for testing compared to TTI risk. The combination of the specific epidemiology (behavioral risk factors, prevalence, and incidence) of each viral infection in each country and the transfused patient population (age, health status, indication for transfusion) are drivers of decision-making with respect to screening approaches, and the cost-effectiveness of screening for these agents likewise is dependent on the local epidemiology, cost of screening, and specific characteristics of the transfused population.

The global concern for these agents coupled with relatively little expertise in health economic evaluation of blood safety threats was the key motivators for the development of a web-based tool to allow for local policy-makers to assess the budget impact (cost to screen) and cost-effectiveness of screening approaches for HIV, HBV, and HCV without having to have the expertise in health economics or access to specialized analysis software. The tool was developed by the Surveillance, Risk Assessment and Policy subgroup and funded by the Transfusion-Transmitted Infectious Diseases Working Party of the International Society for Blood Transfusion (ISBT). Publications describing the development and use of this tool can serve as guides for interested readers who wish to conduct similar analyses [94–96]. The web tool accounts for local blood collection factors such as the number of repeat versus first-time donors and performance of available assays and wherever accessible uses local donation testing and cost data. The tool has been used to conduct analyses for a range of countries with different levels of development, comparing the cost-effectiveness of different screening approaches to no screening and in incremental analyses. The tool also gives a total cost estimate of implementing a given strategy, providing a simplified budget impact analysis. Table 4.5 provides an example set of results comparing the cost-effectiveness of combination antigen and antibody serology assays, minipool (MP) NAT screening (in an arbitrary eight donation pooled format), and ID-NAT for six countries. Each intervention is compared to no screening, and ICERs are provided for MP-NAT relative to serology screening and ID-NAT relative to MP-NAT.

The results from this analysis show that in lower- and middle-income countries, serological screening compared to no screening is a dominant strategy, meaning it is cost saving and/or generates more health through the prevention of TTI disease. Likewise if MP-NAT or ID-NAT could be adopted without serology screening already in place, in many settings, each would also be a dominant strategy compared to no screening, and higher-income countries (the Netherlands and the USA) would be considered cost-effective, particularly relative to other adopted interventions in blood safety. While the incremental cost-effectiveness of adding NAT to serological screening for HIV, HBV and HCV has consistently been found to be cost-ineffective in developed countries, NAT is now inculcated into the safety paradigm for transfusion medicine.

The examples provided for Zika, HTLV, *Babesia microti*, HIV, HBV, and HCV represent results from analyses published in the peer-reviewed literature. Each of the studies was conducted at a specific point in time, and cost-effectiveness will change over time relative to changing dynamics of outbreaks and rates of infection in donors [97]. In addition, these results should not be considered definitive, and reporting the point estimate cost-effectiveness ratio results, as done here, without also including measures of uncertainty from deterministic and probabilistic sensitivity analysis, including the 95% credible intervals, can be potentially misleading. In this chapter this was done for expediency and with the specific intent to not overly complicate numerical results or to delve into too much detail with respect to each of these particular studies. When an actual decision or policy is to be made, the consideration of the sources of data and the uncertainty in the analyses, as displayed in a cloud diagram on the CE plane and also CEACs, are critical to making better-informed decisions.

Table 4.5 Cost of screening and cost-effectiveness reported using a common denominator per one million donations screened in US$ and US$/QALY for six countries with differing levels of development

Country	Screening strategy							
	Serology (antibody and antigen assays)		Minipool NAT (assumed pool size of 8)			Individual-donation NAT		
	Total cost	Cost-effective-ness compared to no screening (US$/QALY)	Total cost	Cost-effective-ness compared to no screening (US$/QALY)	ICER (US$/QALY)	Total cost	Cost-effective-ness compared to no screening (US$/QALY)	ICER (US$/QALY)
Brazil	9,796,000	Dominant	14,107,000	Dominant	171,500	19,570,000	Dominant	407,700
Ghana	7,135,000	Dominant	14,105,000	Dominant	6628	19,600,000	Dominant	10,669
Netherlands	8,056,000	12,200	17,650,000	36,300	8,480,000	28,600,000	64,000	96,900,000
South Africa	7,720,000	Dominant	14,464,000	Dominant	34,800	19,800,000	Dominant	44,300
Thailand	6,540,000	Dominant	13,600,000	Dominant	63,000	19,600,000	17	107,100
USA	14,708,000	97,800	16,333,000	110,000	1,532,000	25,500,000	177,000	31,950,000

Part III: Health Economics of Pathogen Reduction/Inactivation Technologies

Pathogen reduction/inactivation technologies protect blood recipients from the risk of known and unknown transfusion-transmissible agents, so long as the specific technology is capable of inactivating the microbial threat. These technologies are viewed as proactive because they prevent transfusion-transmission without directly identifying the presence of a microbial threat [98]. In this way, they are the technologies in blood safety that are closet in purpose to vaccines. There are several technologies, each with different mechanisms of action and inactivation capacity, which have been reviewed in detail in several previous publications [99–105]. Although red cell inactivation and whole blood inactivation technologies are in development [106–109] and some have been used to conduct studies demonstrating a safety benefit in clinical use [108, 110], health economic evidence has not been published for these methods.

For plasma, available technologies are solvent-detergent, methylene blue and visible light, amotosalen and UV light, and riboflavin and UV light treatment. A recent comprehensive review conducted for Italy compared plasma treated with each of the four technologies to fresh frozen plasma (FFP) on preparation methods, effectiveness, safety, and economic, ethical, social, and legal implications. The authors' summary of findings was that currently available evidence is not sufficient to state which of the techniques compared are superior in terms of efficacy, safety, and cost-effectiveness [111]. Several studies have been published examining the cost-effectiveness of pathogen reduction/inactivation methods for plasma (Table 4.6). A review of the published literature without detailed evaluation of all of the analysis assumptions and methodological approaches used in each study suggests that pathogen reduction/inactivation methods for plasma compared to current screening interventions, when focused on the life expectancy of the transfused population, have cost-effectiveness ratios expected to fall within the range of US$700,000–1,400,000/QALY regardless of the technology. Emerging agents will potentially shift the ratio to being more cost-effective than this range but may not approach accepted thresholds in health and medicine.

The situation for platelets is different. Estimated cost-effectiveness ratios of pathogen reduction/inactivation for platelets are highly dependent on the level of clinically apparent bacterial contamination and platelet preparation method in use in a given setting. Pathogen reduction/inactivation of apheresis platelet preparations with the attendant lower number of donor exposures is less cost-effective than reduction/inactivation of pooled products using either the buffy coat or random donor pooling methods. Without removal of bacterial culture and using hemovigilance data cost-effectiveness ratios are in the range of US$500,000–1,000,000/QALY. If all bacterial culture is discontinued, results may approach CERs of US$200,000/QALY or less. This level of cost-effectiveness would make pathogen reduction/inactivation of platelets a strong candidate for adoption, particularly assuming that sufficient cost offsets can be realized through discontinuation of

Table 4.6 Published cost-effectiveness results for different pathogen reduction/inactivation technologies in different settings. Results are reported in the local currency at the time the study was conducted

Country or setting	Intervention	Comparison intervention	Cost-effectiveness ratio (cost/QALY)	Analysis year and reference
Spain	Solvent-detergent-treated plasma	FFP in the pre-NAT era	US$ 2,200,000	1999 [114]
Canada	Solvent-detergent-treated plasma	FFP prepared after current screens	Dominant	2012 [115]
Canada	Solvent-detergent-treated plasma	FFP prepared after current screens	CAN$ 933,400	Before 2010 [116]
USA	Solvent-detergent-treated plasma	FFP prepared after current screens	US$ 16,159	2013 [117]
Poland	Riboflavin and UV light	FFP prepared after current screens	610,000€	2014 [118]
Spain	Methylene blue and visible light	Quarantine FFP	705,100€	2014 [119]
Canada	Riboflavin and UV light	Platelets and FFP	CAN$ 1,423,000	2007 [120]
Poland	Riboflavin and UV light	Platelets and FFP	348,000€	2014 [118]
USA	Amotosalen and UV light	Apheresis platelets with current screens without bacterial culture	US$ 2,675,000[a]	2001 [121]
	Amotosalen and UV light	Apheresis platelets with current screens including bacterial culture	US$ 12,975,000[a]	
	Amotosalen and UV light	Pooled platelets with current screens without bacterial culture	US$ 1,060,000[a]	
	Amotosalen and UV light	Pooled platelets with current screens including bacterial culture	US$ 3,250,000[a]	
Netherlands	Amotosalen and UV light	Pooled platelets with current screens including bacterial culture	554,000€ per life year gained	2003 [122]
Netherlands	Pathogen reduction	Pooled platelets with current screens without bacterial culture	382,000€	2002 [123]

[a]Simple average across four different patient populations

redundant safety measures. Analyses focused on this cost-offset approach are being published and are expected to increase in the near future [112, 113].

Use of pathogen reduction/inactivation for both platelets and plasma in addition to current screens was estimated to have a cost-effectiveness of US$1,400,000/

QALY in one study. Removal of interventions such as bacterial culture and gamma irradiation could shift the cost-effectiveness ratio with results approaching $500,000/QALY. As new threats emerge and are included in analyses, the CER for pathogen reduction/inactivation is expected to improve. Depending on the technology used, the cost per treated product varies from US$25 to US$100. The current cost per treated component may be too high for some jurisdictions, though this has not prevented the implemention in others. Therefore, it is the budget impact of the cost of treatment that may currently be the most important impediment to broader adoption in many jurisdictions.

Part IV: Implications for Health Economics in the Context of Blood Safety

The previous examples provide an opportunity for inferences about the acceptable health economic profile of interventions for microbial safety in transfusion. Each example is informative alone but, taken together, also reveals common themes regardless of the specific microbial threat or intervention. The health economics of adopted blood safety interventions in the majority of high-income countries speak for themselves: Blood safety interventions for microbial threats which are much less cost-effective (have high cost per effectiveness achieved) than many other areas of healthcare are tolerable. A large number of blood safety interventions have been adopted with cost-effectiveness ratio results above and sometimes exceedingly far above accepted or proposed thresholds for other sectors of health and medicine. From the perspective of the year 2018, ID-NAT testing for Zika virus in the USA is one of the most extreme examples of not including health economic analyses in the decision-making process. How studies on the cost-effectiveness of Zika screening in blood donors are included in future decision-making geared toward less intensive Zika screening will be telling with respect to improved policy-making processes in the USA for blood safety.

Health economics and technology assessment are challenging disciplines with many inherent controversies [124]. The reporting of the analyses and the transparency of modeling are recognized challenges in health economics. Cost-effectiveness analyses of two interventions covered in the previous section showed dissimilar results. Recent analyses of solvent-detergent-treated plasma and the analysis of *Babesia microti* screening are examples of inconsistent application of health economic analysis methods. These differences make it hard for policy-makers to have confidence in health economic evaluations. Guidelines for reporting have been developed. While use of such guidelines will not resolve result differences based on disease assumptions and performance of screening assays, the clear adherence to recommended reporting guidelines would improve the confidence in published studies [53, 54, 125–130].

Strong parallels exist between addressing microbial threats in blood safety and the use of vaccines. Vaccines reside in a complex multiscale implementation context that includes biological, clinical, behavioral, social, operational, environmental, and economical relationships [131]. Microbial safety in transfusion resides in this same complex realm. Both are focused on prevention and matters of broad public health. The vaccine development field has used new approaches for long-range planning. Other approaches to assessing economic impacts of emerging agents exist such as systems analysis for preparedness planning for infectious disease. Systems analysis is able to include important external factors beyond cost and therefore may be more useful as an overall guide to improve priority setting; use of this approach was seen as very important for understanding aspects of Ebola control efforts [132]. However, systems analysis requires cost-effectiveness results as part of the decision-making process. Many of the next-generation issues facing blood safety are similar to those of vaccines. Inclusion of broader sets of inputs to decision-making will improve the decision-making process [133] but will not circumvent the need for high-quality health economic analyses of current and future interventions for microbial safety. Any decision-making approach without explicit use of health economics results requires value judgments which have even less transparency. While all decision analyses have a subjective aspect, use of CUA at least establishes a common denominator for comparing the costs and health outcomes (in terms of QALYs or DALYs) of competing interventions to address the same microbial risk, as well as providing an approach for deciding between interventions which address different transfusion risks. The severity of the infection and the longer-term consequences of different types of agents and infections are very difficult to compare without use of a common denominator such as cost per QALY.

Acceptable thresholds must be placed in the context of societal expectations because prevention of some events, such as transfusion-transmission HIV, HCV, and other infections, is considered more important than prevention of other events, and even within the blood safety context-specific thresholds, distinguishing cost-effective from cost-ineffective interventions does not exist [3]. The lesson is that thresholds for acceptable costs per QALY gained that may be applicable in other healthcare settings do not apply in blood safety. Further, the revealed preferences of what is considered acceptable, regardless of the underlying reasons, suggest any intervention with a ratio of cost to health benefits of US$ one million/QALY is at least a candidate for adoption consideration [134]. While this threshold has never been formally set, cross-jurisdictional decisions support this as a working threshold for microbial threats in transfusion. The willingness to tolerate what can be classified as cost-*in*effective approaches to microbial threats continues to be evident.

Summary

Health economics measures the cost of illness and the cost of interventions to interdict or prevent disease as well as the health outcomes which result from choices made on which programs to implement. Both budget impact analyses, an assessment of cost to implement as well as any potential savings achieved in averted healthcare expenditures, and cost-effectiveness analyses which directly assess the health benefits achieved for the transfused population relative to costs are critical to evidenced-based policy. Microbial threats to transfusion will continue to exist and emerge. Improving blood transfusion safety with regard to interdicting pathogen transmission requires substantial monetary investment. This investment is coupled with evidence of small health gains when appropriate analyses of cost-effectiveness are conducted. The degree to which health economic evaluations may have a greater role in contributing to decision-making for microbial threats in transfusion medicine in the future remains an open question.

References

1. Allain JP, Stramer SL, Carneiro-Proietti AB, Martins ML, Lopes da Silva SN, Ribeiro M, et al. transfusion-transmitted infectious diseases. Biologicals. 2009;37(2):71–7. Epub 2009/02/24.
2. Alter HJ, Klein HG. The hazards of blood transfusion in historical perspective. Blood. 2008;112(7):2617–26.
3. Custer B, Janssen MP. Alliance of blood operators risk-based decision-making I. Health economics and outcomes methods in risk-based decision-making for blood safety. Transfusion. 2015;55(8):2039–47. Epub 2015/04/10.
4. Johannesson M. Theory and methods of economic evaluation of health care. Dev Health Econ Public Policy. 1996;4:1–245. Epub 1995/12/09.
5. Liljas B. On the welfare theoretic foundation of cost-effectiveness analysis-the case when survival is not affected. Eur J Health Econ. 2010;11(1):5–13. Epub 2009/03/04.
6. Cookson R, McCabe C, Tsuchiya A. Public healthcare resource allocation and the rule of rescue. J Med Ethics. 2008;34(7):540–4. Epub 2008/07/02.
7. Trueman P, Drummond M, Hutton J. Developing guidance for budget impact analysis. PharmacoEconomics. 2001;19(6):609–21. Epub 2001/07/18.
8. Leach Bennett J, Blajchman MA, Delage G, Fearon M, Devine D. Proceedings of a consensus conference: risk-based decision making for blood safety. Transfus Med Rev. 2011;25(4):267–92. Epub 2011/07/19.
9. Stein J, Besley J, Brook C, Hamill M, Klein E, Krewski D, et al. Risk-based decision-making for blood safety: preliminary report of a consensus conference. Vox Sang. 2011;101(4):277–81. Epub 2011/07/26.
10. International Society for Pharmaceutical Outcomes Research (ISPOR). ISPOR Good Practices for Outcomes Research Index. Lawrenceville, NJ: ISPOR; 2017 [cited 2017 12/31/2017]; Available from: https://www.ispor.org/.
11. Tarricone R. Cost-of-illness analysis. What room in health economics? Health Policy. 2006;77(1):51–63. Epub 2005/09/06.
12. Clabaugh G, Ward MM. Cost-of-illness studies in the United States: a systematic review of methodologies used for direct cost. Value in Health: The Journal of the International Society for Pharmacoeconomics and Outcomes Research. 2008;11(1):13–21. Epub 2008/02/02.
13. Heijink R, Noethen M, Renaud T, Koopmanschap M, Polder J. Cost of illness: an international comparison. Australia, Canada, France, Germany and the Netherlands. Health Policy. 2008;88(1):49–61. Epub 2008/04/15.
14. El Saadany S, Coyle D, Giulivi A, Afzal M. Economic burden of hepatitis C in Canada and the potential impact of prevention. Results from a disease model. Eur J Health Econ. 2005;6(2):159–65. Epub 2005/03/12.
15. Freedberg KA, Scharfstein JA, Seage GR 3rd, Losina E, Weinstein MC, Craven DE, et al. The cost-effectiveness of preventing AIDS-related opportunistic infections. JAMA. 1998;279(2):130–6. Epub 1998/01/24.

16. Mauskopf JA, Sullivan SD, Annemans L, Caro J, Mullins CD, Nuijten M, et al. Principles of good practice for budget impact analysis: report of the ISPOR task force on good research practices--budget impact analysis. Value in Health: The Journal of the International Society for Pharmacoeconomics and Outcomes Research. 2007;10(5):336–47. Epub 2007/09/25.
17. US Deparment of Veterans Affairs. Budget Impact Analysis. Washington, DC: U.S. Department of Health and Human Services; 2016 [updated 2/15/2016; cited 2017 12/27/2017]; Available from: https://www.herc.research.va.gov/include/page.asp?id=budget-impactanalysis.
18. Custer B, Hoch JS. Cost-effectiveness analysis: what it really means for transfusion medicine decision making. Transfus Med Rev. 2009;23(1):1–12. Epub 2008/12/06.
19. Kacker S, Frick KD, Tobian AA. The costs of transfusion: economic evaluations in transfusion medicine, part 1. Transfusion. 2013;53(7):1383–5. Epub 2013/04/09.
20. Kacker S, Frick KD, Tobian AA. Establishing a framework: economic evaluations in transfusion medicine, part 2. Transfusion. 2013;53(8):1634–6. Epub 2013/04/09.
21. Kacker S, Frick KD, Tobian AA. Constructing a model: economic evaluations in transfusion medicine, Part 3. Transfusion. 2013;53:1885–7. Epub 2013/04/09.
22. Kacker S, Frick KD, Tobian AA. Data and interpretation: economic evaluations in transfusion medicine, Part 4. Transfusion. 2013;53:2130–3. Epub 2013/04/09.
23. van Hulst M, de Wolf JT, Staginnus U, Ruitenberg EJ, Postma MJ. Pharmaco-economics of blood transfusion safety: review of the available evidence. Vox Sang. 2002;83(2):146–55. Epub 2002/08/31.
24. Custer B. Economic analyses of blood safety and transfusion medicine interventions: a systematic review. Transfus Med Rev. 2004;18(2):127–43. Epub 2004/04/07.
25. van Hulst M, Smit Sibinga CT, Postma MJ. Health economics of blood transfusion safety--focus on sub-Saharan Africa. Biologicals. 2010;38(1):53–8. Epub 2009/12/22.
26. Dolan P, Edlin R. Is it really possible to build a bridge between cost-benefit analysis and cost-effectiveness analysis? J Health Econ. 2002;21(5):827–43. Epub 2002/09/28.
27. Eisenstaedt RS, Getzen TE. Screening blood donors for human immunodeficiency virus antibody: cost-benefit analysis. Am J Public Health. 1988;78(4):450–4. Epub 1988/04/01.
28. Fischinger JM, Stephan B, Wasserscheid K, Eichler H, Gartner BC. A cost-benefit analysis of blood donor vaccination as an alternative to additional DNA testing for reducing transfusion transmission of hepatitis B virus. Vaccine. 2010;28(49.):7797-802. Epub 2010/09/30.):7797.
29. Gelles GM. Costs and benefits of HIV-1 antibody testing of donated blood. J Policy Anal Manage. 1993;12(3):512–31. Epub 1994/02/02.
30. Hornbrook MC, Dodd RY, Jacobs P, Friedman LI, Sherman KE. Reducing the incidence of non-A, non-B post-transfusion hepatitis by testing donor blood for alanine aminotransferase: economic considerations. N Engl J Med. 1982;307(21):1315–21. Epub 1982/11/18.
31. Cost-Effectiveness Analysis Registry. Catalog of Utility Weights. Boston, MA. Center for the Evaluation of Value and Risk in Health, Institute for Clincal Research and Health Policy Studies, Tufts Medical Center; 2013 [cited 2017 12/31/2017]; Available from: http://healtheconomics.tuftsmedicalcenter.org/cear4/SearchingtheCEARegistry/SearchtheCEARegistry.aspx.
32. Liljas B, Lindgren B. On individual preferences and aggregation in economic evaluation in healthcare. PharmacoEconomics. 2001;19(4):323–35. Epub 2001/06/01.
33. World Health Organization. Metrics: Disability-Adjusted Life Year (DALY) - Quantifying the Burden of Disease from mortality and morbidity; 2018 [cited 2018 1/2/2018]; Available from: http://www.who.int/healthinfo/global_burden_disease/metrics_daly/en/.
34. Sullivan SD, Mauskopf JA, Augustovski F, Jaime Caro J, Lee KM, Minchin M, et al. Budget impact analysis-principles of good practice: report of the ISPOR 2012 budget impact analysis good practice II task force. Value in Health: The Journal of the International Society for Pharmacoeconomics and Outcomes Research. 2014;17(1):5–14. Epub 2014/01/21.
35. Aledort LM, Broder M, Busch MP, Custer B, Fergusson DA, Goodnough LT, Hendler RS, Hofmann A, Klein HG, Louie JE, Page PL, Sazama K, Shander A, Shulman IA, Spence RK, Sullivan MT, Thurer RL. The cost of blood: multidisciplinary consensus conference for a standard methodology. Transfus Med Rev. 2005;19(1):66–78. Epub 2005/04/15.

36. Husereau D, Drummond M, Petrou S, Carswell C, Moher D, Greenberg D, et al. Consolidated health economic evaluation reporting standards (CHEERS)--explanation and elaboration: a report of the ISPOR health economic evaluation publication guidelines good reporting practices task force. Value in Health: The Journal of the International Society for Pharmacoeconomics and Outcomes Research. 2013;16(2):231–50. Epub 2013/03/30.
37. Drummond M, Tarricone R, Torbica A. Assessing the added value of health technologies: reconciling different perspectives. Value in Health: The Journal of the International Society for Pharmacoeconomics and Outcomes Research. 2013;16(1 Suppl):S7–13. Epub 2013/01/18.
38. Drummond MF, Sculpher MJ, Claxton K, Stoddart GL, Torrance GW. Methods for the economic evaluation of health care Programmes. 4th ed. Oxford: Oxford University Press; 2015.
39. Bai G, Anderson GF. Extreme markup: the fifty US hospitals with the highest charge-to-cost ratios. Health Aff (Millwood). 2015;34(6):922–8. Epub 2015/06/10.
40. Weinstein MC, Siegel JE, Gold MR, Kamlet MS, Russell LB. Recommendations of the panel on cost-effectiveness in health and medicine. JAMA. 1996;276(15):1253–8.
41. National Institute for Health and Care Excellence (NICE). Technology appraisal guidance. [cited 2017 12/31/2017]; Available from: https://www.nice.org.uk/about/what-we-do/our-programmes/nice-guidance/nice-technologyappraisal-guidance.
42. Parkinson B, de Abreu Lourenço R. Discounting in Economic Evaluations in Health Care: A Brief Review. Centre for Health Economics Research and Evaluation (CHERE) & Cancer Research Economics Support Team (CREST); 2015 [cited 2017 12/30/2017]. Available from: http://www.crest.uts.edu.au/pdfs/FactSheet_Discounting.pdf.
43. Klok RM, Postma MJ. Four quadrants of the cost-effectiveness plane: some considerations on the south-west quadrant. Expert Rev Pharmacoecon Outcomes Res. 2004;4(6):599–601. Epub 2004/12/01.
44. World Health Organization. CHOosing Interventions that are Cost Effective (WHO-CHOICE) 2007 [cited 2017 12/02/2017]; Available from: http://www.who.int/choice/country/pol/cost/en/index.html.
45. Bertram MY, Lauer JA, De Joncheere K, Edejer T, Hutubessy R, Kienya MP, et al. Cost–effectiveness thresholds: pros and cons. Bull World Health Organ. 2016;94:925.
46. Simoens S. Health economic assessment: a methodological primer. Int J Environ Res Public Health. 2009;6(12):2950–66. Epub 2010/01/06.
47. Shiroiwa T, Sung YK, Fukuda T, Lang HC, Bae SC, Tsutani K. International survey on willingness-to-pay (WTP) for one additional QALY gained: what is the threshold of cost effectiveness? Health Econ. 2010;19(4):422–37. Epub 2009/04/22.
48. Briggs AH, Weinstein MC, Fenwick EA, Karnon J, Sculpher MJ, Paltiel AD. Model parameter estimation and uncertainty analysis: a report of the ISPOR-SMDM modeling good research practices task force working Group-6. Med Decis Mak. 2012;32(5):722–32Epub 2012/09/20.
49. Briggs AH, Weinstein MC, Fenwick EA, Karnon J, Sculpher MJ, Paltiel AD. Model parameter estimation and uncertainty: a report of the ISPOR-SMDM modeling good research practices task force--6. Value in health: The Journal of the International Society for Pharmacoeconomics and Outcomes Research. 2012;15(6):835–42. Epub 2012/09/25.
50. Cost-Effectiveness Acceptability Curve (CEAC) [online]. (2016). York, England; York Health Economics Consortium; 2016 [cited 2018 1/5/2018]; Available from: http://www.yhec.co.uk/glossary/cost-effectiveness-acceptability-curve-ceac/.
51. Fenwick E, O'Brien BJ, Briggs A. Cost-effectiveness acceptability curves--facts, fallacies and frequently asked questions. Health Econ. 2004;13(5):405–15. Epub 2004/05/06.
52. Al MJ. Cost-effectiveness acceptability curves revisited. PharmacoEconomics. 2013;31(2.):Epub 2013/01/19.):93–100.
53. Husereau D, Drummond M, Petrou S, Carswell C, Moher D, Greenberg D, et al. Consolidated health economic evaluation reporting standards (CHEERS) statement. Int J Technol Assess Health Care. 2013;29(2):117–22. Epub 2013/04/17.

54. Eddy DM, Hollingworth W, Caro JJ, Tsevat J, McDonald KM, Wong JB. Model transparency and validation: a report of the ISPOR-SMDM modeling good research practices task Force-7. Med Decis Mak. 2012;32(5):733–43. Epub 2012/09/20.
55. Edgren G, Kamper-Jorgensen M, Eloranta S, Rostgaard K, Custer B, Ullum H, et al. Duration of red blood cell storage and survival of transfused patients (CME). Transfusion. 2010;50(6.):Epub 2010/02/18.):1185–95.
56. Borkent-Raven BA, Janssen MP, van der Poel CL, Schaasberg WP, Bonsel GJ, van Hout BA. Survival after transfusion in the Netherlands. Vox Sang. 2011;100(2):196–203. Epub 2010/08/24.
57. Kleinman S, Marshall D, AuBuchon J, Patton M. Survival after transfusion as assessed in a large multistate US cohort. Transfusion. 2004;44(3):386–90. Epub 2004/03/05.
58. Gauvin F, Champagne MA, Robillard P, Le Cruguel JP, Lapointe H, Hume H. Long-term survival rate of pediatric patients after blood transfusion. Transfusion. 2008;48(5):801–8. Epub 2008/01/23.
59. Vamvakas EC, Taswell HF. Long-term survival after blood transfusion. Transfusion. 1994;34(6):471–7.
60. Kamper-Jorgensen M, Ahlgren M, Rostgaard K, Melbye M, Edgren G, Nyren O, et al. Survival after blood transfusion. Transfusion. 2008;48(12):2577–84. Epub 2008/08/05.
61. Dorsey KA, Moritz ED. Notari EPt, Schonberger LB, Dodd RY. Survival of blood transfusion recipients identified by a look-back investigation. Blood transfusion = Trasfusione del sangue. 2014;12(1):67–72. Epub 2013/12/18.
62. Karafin MS, Bruhn R, Westlake M, Sullivan MT, Bialkowski W, Edgren G, et al. Demographic and epidemiologic characterization of transfusion recipients from four US regions: evidence from the REDS-III recipient database. Transfusion. 2017;57(12):2903–13. Epub 2017/10/27.
63. Seed CR, Kiely P, Hoad VC, Keller AJ. Refining the risk estimate for transfusion-transmission of occult hepatitis B virus. Vox Sang. 2017;112(1):3–8. Epub 2016/08/27.
64. Weusten JJ, van Drimmelen HA, Lelie PN. Mathematic modeling of the risk of HBV, HCV, and HIV transmission by window-phase donations not detected by NAT. Transfusion. 2002;42(5):537–48. Epub 2002/06/27.
65. Busch M, Walderhaug M, Custer B, Allain JP, Reddy R, McDonough B. Risk assessment and cost-effectiveness/utility analysis. Biologicals. 2009;37(2):78–87. Epub 2009/02/27.
66. Colon-Gonzalez FJ, Peres CA, Steiner Sao Bernardo C, Hunter PR, Lake IR. After the epidemic: Zika virus projections for Latin America and the Caribbean. PLoS Negl Trop Dis. 2017;11(11.):Epub 2017/11/02.):e0006007.
67. Lanteri MC, Kleinman SH, Glynn SA, Musso D, Keith Hoots W, Custer BS, et al. Zika virus: a new threat to the safety of the blood supply with worldwide impact and implications. Transfusion. 2016;56(7):1907–14. Epub 2016/06/11.
68. Lee BY, Alfaro-Murillo JA, Parpia AS, Asti L, Wedlock PT, Hotez PJ, et al. The potential economic burden of Zika in the continental United States. PLoS Negl Trop Dis. 2017;11(4.):Epub 2017/04/28.):e0005531.
69. Alfaro-Murillo JA, Parpia AS, Fitzpatrick MC, Tamagnan JA, Medlock J, Ndeffo-Mbah ML, et al. A cost-effectiveness tool for informing policies on Zika virus control. PLoS Negl Trop Dis. 2016;10(5.):Epub 2016/05/21.):e0004743.
70. Ellingson KD, Sapiano MRP, Haass KA, Savinkina AA, Baker ML, Henry RA, et al. Cost projections for implementation of safety interventions to prevent transfusion-transmitted Zika virus infection in the United States. Transfusion. 2017;57(Suppl 2):1625–33. Epub 2017/06/08.
71. Styles CE, Seed CR, Hoad VC, Gaudieri S, Keller AJ. Reconsideration of blood donation testing strategy for human T-cell lymphotropic virus in Australia. Vox Sang. 2017;112(8):723–32. Epub 2017/09/30.
72. Marano G, Vaglio S, Pupella S, Facco G, Catalano L, Piccinini V, et al. Human T-lymphotropic virus and transfusion safety: does one size fit all? Transfusion. 2016;56(1.):Epub 2015/09/22.):249–60.

73. Borkent-Raven BA, Janssen MP, van der Poel CL, Bonsel GJ, van Hout BA. Cost-effectiveness of additional blood screening tests in the Netherlands. Transfusion. 2012;52(3):478–88. Epub 2011/09/02.
74. Sailly JC, Lebrun T, Coudeville L. Cost-effective approach to the screening of HIV, HBV, HCV, HTLV in blood donors in France. Rev Epidemiol Sante Publique. 1997;45(2):131–41. Epub 1997/04/01. Approche cout-efficacite du depistage des virus VIH, VHB, VHC, HTLV chez les donneurs de sang en France.
75. Stigum H, Magnus P, Samdal HH, Nord E. Human T-cell lymphotropic virus testing of blood donors in Norway: a cost-effect model. Int J Epidemiol. 2000;29(6.):Epub 2000/12/02.):1076–84.
76. Levin AE, Krause PJ. Transfusion-transmitted babesiosis: is it time to screen the blood supply? Curr Opin Hematol. 2016;23(6):573–80. Epub 2016/10/18.
77. Stramer SL, Hollinger FB, Katz LM, Kleinman S, Metzel PS, Gregory KR, et al. Emerging infectious disease agents and their potential threat to transfusion safety. Transfusion. 2009;49(Suppl 2):1S–29S. Epub 2009/08/19.
78. Bloch EM, Herwaldt BL, Leiby DA, Shaieb A, Herron RM, Chervenak M, et al. The third described case of transfusion-transmitted Babesia duncani. Transfusion. 2012;52(7):1517–22. Epub 2011/12/16.
79. Herwaldt BL, Linden JV, Bosserman E, Young C, Olkowska D, Wilson M. Transfusion-associated babesiosis in the United States: a description of cases. Ann Intern Med. 2011;155(8):509–19. Epub 2011/09/07.
80. Leiby DA. Transfusion-transmitted Babesia spp.: bull's-eye on Babesia microti. Clin Microbiol Rev. 2011;24(1):14–28. Epub 2011/01/15.
81. Simon MS, Leff JA, Pandya A, Cushing M, Shaz BH, Calfee DP, et al. Cost-effectiveness of blood donor screening for Babesia microti in endemic regions of the United States. Transfusion. 2014;54(3 Pt 2):889–99. Epub 2013/11/21.
82. Goodell AJ, Bloch EM, Krause PJ, Custer B. Costs, consequences, and cost-effectiveness of strategies for Babesia microti donor screening of the US blood supply. Transfusion. 2014;54(9):2245–57. Epub 2014/08/12.
83. Bish EK, Moritz ED, El-Amine H, Bish DR, Stramer SL. Cost-effectiveness of Babesia microti antibody and nucleic acid blood donation screening using results from prospective investigational studies. Transfusion. 2015;55(9.):Epub 2015/05/23.):2256–71.
84. Criado-Fornelio A. A review of nucleic-acid-based diagnostic tests for Babesia and Theileria, with emphasis on bovine piroplasms. Parassitologia. 2007;49(Suppl 1):39–44. Epub 2007/08/19.
85. Moritz ED, Winton CS, Tonnetti L, Townsend RL, Berardi VP, Hewins ME, et al. Screening for Babesia microti in the U.S. blood supply. N Engl J Med. 2016;375(23):2236–45. Epub 2016/12/14.
86. Jajosky RP, Jajosky AN. Is babesiosis the most common transfusion transmitted infection in the United States of America? The answer is not simple! Transfusion and Apheresis Science: Official Journal of the World Apheresis Association: Official Journal of the European Society for Haemapheresis. 2017;56(4):609–10. Epub 2017/09/05.
87. Kleinman SH, Lelie N, Busch MP. Infectivity of human immunodeficiency virus-1, hepatitis C virus, and hepatitis B virus and risk of transmission by transfusion. Transfusion. 2009;49(11):2454–89. Epub 2009/08/18.
88. Zou S, Stramer SL, Dodd RY. Donor testing and risk: current prevalence, incidence, and residual risk of transfusion-transmissible agents in US allogeneic donations. Transfus Med Rev. 2012;26(2):119–28. Epub 2011/08/30.
89. Stramer SL, Krysztof DE, Brodsky JP, Fickett TA, Reynolds B, Dodd RY, et al. Comparative analysis of triplex nucleic acid test assays in United States blood donors. Transfusion. 2013;53(10 Pt 2):2525–37. Epub 2013/04/05.
90. Lelie N, Bruhn R, Busch M, Vermeulen M, Tsoi WC, Kleinman S, et al. Detection of different categories of hepatitis B virus (HBV) infection in a multi-regional study comparing

the clinical sensitivity of hepatitis B surface antigen and HBV-DNA testing. Transfusion. 2017;57(1):24–35. Epub 2016/09/28.
91. Bruhn R, Lelie N, Busch M, Kleinman S, International NATSG. Relative efficacy of nucleic acid amplification testing and serologic screening in preventing hepatitis C virus transmission risk in seven international regions. Transfusion. 2015;55(6):1195–205. Epub 2015/03/03.
92. Bruhn R, Lelie N, Custer B, Busch M, Kleinman S, International NATSG. Prevalence of human immunodeficiency virus RNA and antibody in first-time, lapsed, and repeat blood donations across five international regions and relative efficacy of alternative screening scenarios. Transfusion. 2013;53(10 Pt 2):2399–412. Epub 2013/06/21.
93. El Ekiaby M, Moftah F, Goubran H, van Drimmelen H, LaPerche S, Kleinman S, et al. Viremia levels in hepatitis C infection among Egyptian blood donors and implications for transmission risk with different screening scenarios. Transfusion. 2015;55(6):1186–94. Epub 2015/03/15.
94. van Hulst M, Hubben GA, Sagoe KW, Promwong C, Permpikul P, Fongsatitkul L, et al. Web interface-supported transmission risk assessment and cost-effectiveness analysis of postdonation screening: a global model applied to Ghana, Thailand. and the Netherlands Transfusion. 2009;49(12):2729–42.
95. Custer B, Janssen MP, Hubben G, Vermeulen M, van Hulst M. Development of a web-based application and multicountry analysis framework for assessing interdicted infections and cost-utility of screening donated blood for HIV. HCV and HBV Vox Sanguinis. 2017;112(6):526–34. Epub 2017/06/10.
96. Janssen MP, van Hulst M, Custer B, Economics ARH, Outcomes Working G. Collaborators. An assessment of differences in costs and health benefits of serology and NAT screening of donations for blood transfusion in different western countries. Vox Sang. 2017;112(6):518–25. Epub 2017/06/24.
97. Custer B, Busch MP, Marfin AA, Petersen LR. The cost-effectiveness of screening the U.S. blood supply for West Nile virus. Ann Intern Med. 2005;143(7):486–92. Epub 2005/10/06.
98. Kleinman S, Stassinopoulos A. Risks associated with red blood cell transfusions: potential benefits from application of pathogen inactivation. Transfusion. 2015;55(12.):Epub 2015/08/26.):2983–3000.
99. de Sousa G, Seghatchian J. Highlights of PBTI Coimbra conference on PRT of Plasma & Current Opinions on pathogen reduction treatment of blood components. Transfusion and Apheresis Science: Official Journal of the World Apheresis Association: Official Journal of the European Society for Haemapheresis. 2015;52(2):228–32. Epub 2015/03/15.
100. Seltsam A, Muller TH. Update on the use of pathogen-reduced human plasma and platelet concentrates. Br J Haematol. 2013;162(4):442–54. Epub 2013/05/29.
101. Solheim BG, Seghatchian J. Update on pathogen reduction technology for therapeutic plasma: an overview. Transfusion and Apheresis Science: Official Journal of the World Apheresis Association: Official Journal of the European Society for Haemapheresis. 2006;35(1):83–90. Epub 2006/08/29.
102. Prowse CV. Component pathogen inactivation: a critical review. Vox Sang. 2013;104(3):183–99. Epub 2012/11/09.
103. Schlenke P. Pathogen inactivation technologies for cellular blood components: an update. Transfus Med Hemother. 2014;41(4):309–25. Epub 2014/09/26.
104. Seltsam A. Pathogen inactivation of cellular blood products-an additional safety layer in transfusion medicine. Front Med. 2017;4:219. Epub 2017/12/20.
105. Di Minno G, Navarro D, Perno CF, Canaro M, Gurtler L, Ironside JW, et al. Pathogen reduction/inactivation of products for the treatment of bleeding disorders: what are the processes and what should we say to patients? Ann Hematol. 2017;96(8.):Epub 2017/06/19.):1253–70.
106. Yonemura S, Doane S, Keil S, Goodrich R, Pidcoke H, Cardoso M. Improving the safety of whole blood-derived transfusion products with a riboflavin-based pathogen reduction technology. Blood Transfusion = Trasfusione del sangue. 2017;15(4):357–64. Epub 2017/07/01.

107. Cancelas JA, Gottschall JL, Rugg N, Graminske S, Schott MA, North A, et al. Red blood cell concentrates treated with the amustaline (S-303) pathogen reduction system and stored for 35 days retain post-transfusion viability: results of a two-Centre study. Vox Sang. 2017;112(3):210–8. Epub 2017/02/22.
108. Drew VJ, Barro L, Seghatchian J, Burnouf T. Towards pathogen inactivation of red blood cells and whole blood targeting viral DNA/RNA: design, technologies, and future prospects for developing countries. Blood Transfusion = Trasfusione del sangue. 2017;15(6):512–21. Epub 2017/05/11.
109. Wiltshire M, Meli A, Schott MA, Erickson A, Mufti N, Thomas S, et al. Quality of red cells after combination of prion reduction and treatment with the intercept system for pathogen inactivation. Transfus Med (Oxford, England). 2016;26(3):208–14. Epub 2016/03/24.
110. Allain JP, Owusu-Ofori AK, Assennato SM, Marschner S, Goodrich RP, Owusu-Ofori S. Effect of Plasmodium inactivation in whole blood on the incidence of blood transfusion-transmitted malaria in endemic regions: the African investigation of the Mirasol system (AIMS) randomised controlled trial. Lancet. 2016;387(10029):1753–61. Epub 2016/04/27.
111. Cicchetti A, Berrino A, Casini M, Codella P, Facco G, Fiore A, et al. Health technology assessment of pathogen reduction technologies applied to plasma for clinical use. Blood Transfusion = Trasfusione del sangue. 2016;14(4):287–386. Epub 2016/07/13.
112. McCullough J, Goldfinger D, Gorlin J, Riley WJ, Sandhu H, Stowell C, et al. Cost implications of implementation of pathogen-inactivated platelets. Transfusion. 2015;55(10.):Epub 2015/05/20.):2312–20.
113. Girona-Llobera E, Jimenez-Marco T, Galmes-Trueba A, Muncunill J, Serret C, Serra N, et al. Reducing the financial impact of pathogen inactivation technology for platelet components: our experience. Transfusion. 2014;54(1):158–68. Epub 2013/05/10.
114. Pereira A. Health and economic impact of posttransfusion hepatitis B and cost-effectiveness analysis of expanded HBV testing protocols of blood donors: a study focused on the European Union. Transfusion. 2003;43(2):192–201. Epub 2003/02/01.
115. Huisman EL, van Eerd MC, Ouwens JN, de Peuter MA. Cost-effectiveness and budget impact study of solvent/detergent (SD) treated plasma (octaplasLG(R)) versus fresh-frozen plasma (FFP) in any patient receiving transfusion in Canada. Transfusion and Apheresis Science: Official Journal of the World Apheresis Association: Official Journal of the European Society for Haemapheresis. 2014;51(1):25–34. Epub 2013/05/28.
116. Membe SK, Coyle D, Husereau D, Cimon K, Tinmouth A, Normandin S. Octaplas compared with fresh frozen plasma to reduce the risk of transmitting lipid-enveloped viruses: an economic analysis and budget impact analysis. Ottawa: CADTH; 2011.
117. Huisman EL, de Silva SU, de Peuter MA. Economic evaluation of pooled solvent/detergent treated plasma versus single donor fresh-frozen plasma in patients receiving plasma transfusions in the United States. Transfusion and Apheresis Science: Official Journal of the World Apheresis Association: Official Journal of the European Society for Haemapheresis. 2014;51(1):17–24. Epub 2014/08/26.
118. Agapova M, Lachert E, Brojer E, Letowska M, Grabarczyk P, Custer B. Introducing pathogen reduction Technology in Poland: a cost-utility analysis. Transfus Med Hemother. 2015;42(3):158–65. Epub 2015/07/22.
119. Babigumira JB, Lubinga SJ, Castro E, Custer B. Cost-utility and budget impact of methylene blue-treated plasma compared to quarantine plasma. Blood Transfus. 2018;16(2):154–62. https://doi.org/10.2450/2016.0130-16. Epub 2016 Nov 16.
120. Custer B, Agapova M, Martinez RH. The cost-effectiveness of pathogen reduction technology as assessed using a multiple risk reduction model. Transfusion. 2010;50(11):2461–73. Epub 2010/05/26.
121. Bell CE, Botteman MF, Gao X, Weissfeld JL, Postma MJ, Pashos CL, et al. Cost-effectiveness of transfusion of platelet components prepared with pathogen inactivation treatment in the United States. Clin Ther. 2003;25(9):2464–86. Epub 2003/11/08.

122. Postma MJ, van Hulst M, De Wolf JT, Botteman M, Staginnus U. Cost-effectiveness of pathogen inactivation for platelet transfusions in the Netherlands. Transfus Med (Oxford, England). 2005;15(5):379–87. Epub 2005/10/06.
123. Janssen MP, van der Poel CL, Buskens E, Bonneux L, Bonsel GJ, van Hout BA. Costs and benefits of bacterial culturing and pathogen reduction in the Netherlands. Transfusion. 2006;46(6):956–65. Epub 2006/06/01.
124. Daniels N, van der Wilt GJ. Health technology assessment, deliberative process, and ethically contested issues. Int J Technol Assess Health Care. 2016;32(1–2):10–5. Epub 2016/07/30.
125. Briggs AH, Weinstein MC, Fenwick EA, Karnon J, Sculpher MJ, Paltiel AD, et al. Model parameter estimation and uncertainty analysis: a report of the ISPOR-SMDM modeling good research practices task force working Group-6. Med Decis Mak. 2012;32(5.):Epub 2012/09/20.):722–32.
126. Caro JJ, Briggs AH, Siebert U, Kuntz KM. Modeling good research practices--overview: a report of the ISPOR-SMDM modeling good research practices task Force-1. Med Decis Mak. 2012;32(5):667–77. Epub 2012/09/20.
127. Karnon J, Stahl J, Brennan A, Caro JJ, Mar J, Moller J. Modeling using discrete event simulation: a report of the ISPOR-SMDM modeling good research practices task Force-4. Med Decis Mak. 2012;32(5):701–11. Epub 2012/09/20.
128. Pitman R, Fisman D, Zaric GS, Postma M, Kretzschmar M, Edmunds J, et al. Dynamic transmission modeling: a report of the ISPOR-SMDM Modeling Good Research Practices Task Force Working Group-5. Med Decis Mak. 2012;32(5):712–21. Epub 2012/09/20.
129. Roberts M, Russell LB, Paltiel AD, Chambers M, McEwan P, Krahn M. Conceptualizing a model: a report of the ISPOR-SMDM modeling good research practices task force-2. Med Decis Mak. 2012;32(5):678–89. Epub 2012/09/20.
130. Siebert U, Alagoz O, Bayoumi AM, Jahn B, Owens DK, Cohen DJ, et al. State-transition modeling: a report of the ISPOR-SMDM modeling good research practices task Force-3. Med Decis Mak. 2012;32(5.):Epub 2012/09/20.):690–700.
131. Lee BY, Mueller LE, Tilchin CG. A systems approach to vaccine decision making. Vaccine. 2017;35(Supplement 1):A36–42.
132. Phelps C, Madhavan G, Rappuoli R, Colwell R, Fineberg H. Beyond cost-effectiveness: using systems analysis for infectious disease preparedness. Vaccine. 2017;35(Suppl 1):A46–A9. Epub 2016/12/27.
133. Bloom DE, Brenzel L, Cadarette D, Sullivan J. Moving beyond traditional valuation of vaccination: needs and opportunities. Vaccine. 2017;35(Supplement 1):A29–35.
134. Custer BS. Good evidence begets good policy: or so it should be. Transfusion. 2012;52(3):463–5. Epub 2012/03/13.

Chapter 5
Decision Systems

Philip Kiely

Introduction

Blood supplies internationally are as safe as they have ever been, and in most developed countries, the transfusion-transmission (TT) residual risks (RRs) for the major transfusion-relevant viruses, hepatitis B virus (HBV), human immunodeficiency virus types 1 and 2 (HIV-1/HIV-2) and hepatitis C virus (HCV), have been reduced to very low probabilities [1–3]. However, new threats to blood safety continue to arise, an important source of which are emerging and re-emerging infectious diseases (EIDs) [4–12]. While there is no precise and universally agreed definition of an EID, a widely accepted definition is "those whose incidence in humans has increased within the past 2 decades or threatens to increase in the near future" [8, 13]. The importance of monitoring new threats to blood safety from EIDs is indicated by expert opinion which, somewhat ominously, suggests we can continue to expect ongoing EID outbreaks [8, 11, 12, 14–17].

Monitoring and responding to new threats to blood safety from EIDs require a cross-disciplinary approach as indicated by the focus on developing consensus strategies or frameworks for identifying and managing these threats. Understandably, the growing awareness of the potential threat to blood safety from EIDs has renewed focus on the precautionary principle and its application to developing blood safety policies [18]. Broadly, the precautionary principle is an underlying philosophical approach to risk management that assumes a lack of scientific certainty about risk level is not a reason for postponing the implementation of risk

---

P. Kiely
Australian Red Cross Blood Service, Melbourne, Australia

Department of Epidemiology and Preventive Medicine, Monash University, Melbourne, Australia
e-mail: pkiely@redcrossblood.org.au

© Springer International Publishing AG, part of Springer Nature 2019
H. Shan, R. Y. Dodd (eds.), *Blood Safety*,
https://doi.org/10.1007/978-3-319-94436-4_5

mitigation strategies [19]. The precautionary principle is particularly relevant in the context of EIDs and blood safety as EID agents are often not well characterised, and therefore there is a need to make decisions about risk mitigation strategies on the basis of limited information. However, the precautionary principle has been criticised both at a broad philosophical level [20, 21] and in its application to managing potential threats to blood safety. Critics have argued that it can lead to unfeasible attempts to achieve zero risk, overly rigorous application can lead to very expensive but unnecessary interventions that may even compromise sufficiency of the blood supply and there is no agreed definition of the principle or how it should be applied [18, 22–24]. More recently, a detailed approach to risk assessment that takes into account the complexities of blood safety and the need for some level of risk tolerance has been developed under the auspices of the Alliance of Blood Operators (ABO) and referred to as Risk-based Decision-Making Framework for Blood Safety [25–27]. This framework is an ambitious attempt to provide "a structured and systematic process for considering all relevant factors in decisions on blood safety and for ensuring that finite resources are allocated to the most significant blood safety risks" [27]. In the USA, the AABB (formerly the American Association of Blood Banks) is developing a "toolkit" which will provide a systematic approach to EID risk assessment and the evaluation of proposed interventions [10].

Within the context of an overall risk-based decision-making framework, this chapter will focus on how *evidence-based* decision-making can be applied to assessing the potential threat posed by EIDs to blood safety and how such assessments can be used to inform decision-making about risk mitigation strategies. The evidence-based assessment process, as described in this chapter, can be defined in terms of three questions:

(i) Does an EID agent represent a risk, actual or potential, to blood safety?
(ii) If an agent does represent an actual or potential risk to blood safety, what is the level of that risk?
(iii) How can risk assessment outcomes be interpreted and applied in a local context?

The first two questions relate directly to the assessment process itself. The third question recognises that risk assessments are performed within a local jurisdictional context, taking into account the local epidemiology, resource availability, risk perceptions and collaboration of relevant local authorities.

Prior to discussing the risk assessment of EID agents, it is important to understand how they differ from the major or "classical" transfusion-relevant viruses noted above. The major transfusion-relevant viruses are now relatively well characterised, transmitted human to human without vectors or host reservoirs, and have an endemic worldwide distribution; tests suitable for universal donor screening are available and have been implemented in most countries, and TT risks can be estimated by risk models [28–35]. In contrast, EID agents are typically less well characterised; many that are known to be transfusion-transmissible are primarily vector-borne including dengue virus (DENV), West Nile virus (WNV), Zika virus

(ZIKV), *Plasmodium* spp. (malaria) and *Trypanosoma cruzi* (Chagas disease) and have a defined geographical distribution [8]. Additionally, tests suitable for blood donor screening have not been developed or approved for most agents. However, even when screening tests are available, universal donor screening may not be feasible due to inadequate resources, or not considered cost-effective if the level of risk is perceived to be relatively low. Therefore EID outbreaks are typically unpredictable, and risk assessments often have a high degree of uncertainty.

Unless otherwise specified, in this chapter the term "transfusion-transmission (TT) risk" refers to the risk of transmitting an EID agent by transfusion, regardless of clinical outcome, while the term "threat to blood safety" refers to the risk of transmitting a clinical disease to a recipient.

Qualitative Assessment: When Do EID Agents Represent a Potential Threat to Blood Safety?

To determine whether an EID agent represents a potential threat to blood safety requires an assessment against a number of well-defined criteria [8, 11, 15] which are summarised in Fig. 5.1. However, as will be discussed in this section, the lack of information about EID agents can create uncertainty in determining the extent to which they meet these criteria and the potential impact of this uncertainty for risk-based decision-making.

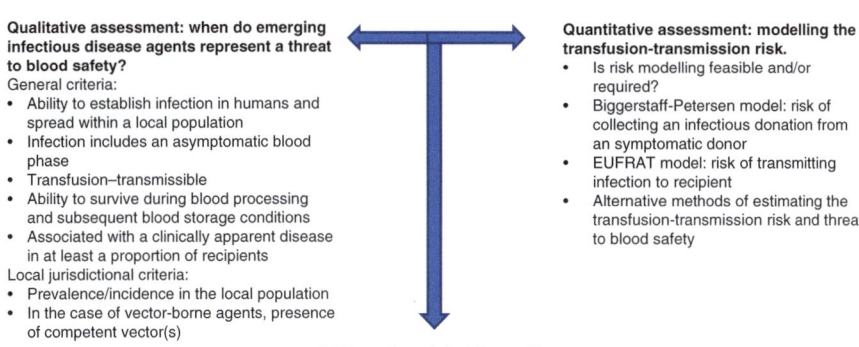

Fig. 5.1 Risk assessment and evidence-based decision-making

Ability to Establish Infection in Humans and Spread Within Human Populations

The first indication that a newly identified EID agent is able to establish infection in humans and spread within populations is typically a result of symptomatic cases seeking health care with subsequent clinical diagnosis and laboratory confirmation. Once reported to health authorities, surveillance systems can then be initiated [36, 37]. However, in some circumstances, detection of an EID agent within a population may be delayed if it has a high rate of asymptomatic infection (assuming asymptomatic cases would not seek health care and would therefore not be diagnosed or reported) or a long incubation period prior to symptom onset. In low-income countries, laboratory testing may not be available due to a lack of resources, or for very recently identified agents, test may not be available to confirm diagnosis. Additionally, symptomatic infections may be clinically misdiagnosed when a number of EID agents with similar clinical symptoms are co-circulating, e.g. co-circulation of chikungunya virus (CHIKV), DENV and ZIKV [38, 39]. In the case of a number of important transfusion-transmissible flaviviruses, there is the added difficulty of cross-reactivity in immunoglobulin M (IgM) assays, complicating the laboratory confirmation of recent infection [40].

Regional Presence of the Agent and Competent Vector(s)

If an EID agent has been demonstrated to infect humans, to represent a threat within a specific region obviously requires the presence of the agent and local transmission. Additionally, for vector-borne agents, local transmission requires the presence of competent vectors. Even within a country, the agent and/or vectors may not be present in all regions. For example, in Australia, the mosquito vector *Aedes aegypti* is primarily restricted to northern Queensland [41] giving rise to geographically restricted outbreaks of locally transmitted DENV [42–45]. As a consequence, the risk posed by DENV to blood safety in Australia is managed by restricting blood collections in regions experiencing a current outbreak to fractionated plasma products for the duration of the outbreak period. In the case of vector-borne agents, it is also important to consider the potential for nonvector modes of transmission. For example, while ZIKV is primarily transmitted to humans by infected mosquitoes, sexual transmission has been reported [46–50] giving rise to the potential for local human-to-human transmission even in the absence of competent vectors.

Infection Includes an Asymptomatic Blood Phase

In the context of blood safety, it is generally assumed that infected donors who have developed clinical symptoms will either not present to donate (self-defer due to feeling unwell) or will be prevented from donating by a pre-donation interview and health check. In contrast, infected donors without clinical symptoms would typically be unaware of their infection and not self-defer. Such donors would not be interdicted by a pre-donation questionnaire and could therefore proceed to give an infectious donation. This includes donors who do not develop symptoms over the entire course of the infection (subclinical infection) and those who do develop symptoms following an incubation period. The level of risk posed by these donors is related to the length of the asymptomatic blood phase – the total blood phase period for subclinical infections and the presymptomatic blood phase for those who do develop symptoms. The durations of these asymptomatic but infectious periods are important parameters for risk modelling and will be further discussed in the following section.

Transfusion-Transmissible

To represent a potential threat to blood safety, an EID agent must not only be present in the donation but also transmissible by the intravenous route. However, even if TT is suspected based on an asymptomatic blood phase and/or demonstrated TT of related agents, confirming TT can be difficult. The absence of reported transfusion-transmitted cases may reflect underreporting due to a high proportion of asymptomatic cases, misdiagnosis of infection or inadequate reporting systems. Definitively establishing TT as the source of infection requires phylogenetic comparison of isolates from both the implicated donor and recipient which may not be possible due to a lack of laboratory infrastructure (which may sometimes be the case in low-income countries) or the absence of detectable agent in the blood by the time TT is suspected and follow-up testing is performed. In the absence of definitively proven TT, probable TT can be assigned if the diagnosis of infection in the implicated donor and associated recipient(s) is consistent with transmission at the time of transfusion and/or the absence of infection in the recipient prior to transfusion.

However, some caution is required in outbreak/endemic areas where infection is relatively common in the general population as it may not be possible to exclude other modes of transmission. For example, prior to the outbreak in the Americas, ZIKV was suspected to be transfusion-transmissible as infection included an asymptomatic blood phase [51] and the related flaviviruses, DENV [52–59] and WNV [60–67], had been shown to be transfusion-transmissible. However, TT of ZIKV was not reported until 2015 in the current outbreak in Brazil [68–72].

If an agent is suspected of being transfusion-transmissible, a number of factors can affect the TT efficiency. For example, a lookback study performed in Brazil during a DENV outbreak estimated the TT efficiency of DENV from RNA-positive components to susceptible recipients was 37.5% [73]. Factors that may contribute to the reduction of the transfusion-transmissibility of DENV include the need for mosquito saliva to enhance DENV replication and virulence, the presence of protective immunity in recipients in endemic areas and the frequent co-transfusion of antibody-positive units which may neutralise the infectivity of viraemic donations [56, 57]. TT efficiency will also be affected by the duration of the infectious blood phase and the level of the agent in the blood. For example, human parvovirus B19 (B19V) (primate erythroparvovirus 1) has been demonstrated to be present in blood donors [74–80], but very few TT cases have been reported. This may in part be due to the fact that a high proportion of infections are either asymptomatic or accompanied by non-specific symptoms and therefore not recognised. Other potentially contributing factors include a brief period of high-level viraemia followed by persistent infection characterised by low-level viraemia with concomitant neutralising anti-B19V IgG and the high prevalence of neutralising anti-B19V in recipients [75, 81–84]. Both the *European Pharmacopoeia* and FDA specify a B19V limit of 10^4 IU/mL for manufacturing pools destined for plasma products based on a lack of documented cases of transmission from pooled plasma products with less than 10^4 IU/mL.

Ability to Survive During Blood Processing and Subsequent Blood Storage Conditions

Even if present in a donation and potentially transfusion-transmissible, an agent must also be able to survive the blood processing procedures and storage conditions. For example, *Treponema pallidum*, the infectious agent for syphilis, is inactivated by storage for several days at temperatures <20°C. [85, 86]. Additionally, leucoreduction of blood components can substantially reduce, if not completely remove, the TT risk of agents associated with leucocytes such as human T cell lymphotropic virus types 1 and 2 (HTLV-1/HTLV-2) [87–89] and some members of the Herpesviridae family including cytomegalovirus (CMV) [90–95], possibly human herpes virus 8 (HHV-8) [96] and Epstein-Barr virus (EBV) [97, 98]. Additionally, the TT risk of EID agents associated with manufactured plasma-derived products is substantially reduced by the inclusion of a number of steps that inactivate or remove EID agents including pasteurisation, low pH treatment, solvent/detergent viral inactivation, and nanofiltration [99–103]. As a consequence, the TT risk of EID agents is primarily associated with fresh blood components.

Associated with a Clinically Apparent Disease in At Least a Proportion of Recipients

If an EID agent has been demonstrated to be, or is potentially, transfusion-transmissible, it is only considered a threat to blood safety if it causes a clinically significant disease in recipients. However, determining the disease association of EID agents can be problematic. Firstly, when an agent is newly identified in humans, it may take some time to accumulate the epidemiological data to establish a disease association. This is particularly true if infections have a high asymptomatic rate and/or there is underreporting due to misdiagnosis or inadequate reporting systems.

Secondly, agent virulence may vary over time and in different locations due to strain variation. Thirdly, as agents spread geographically, different human populations may show differences in disease susceptibility.

An example of the complexity in determining disease association is WNV, first isolated in 1937 in a woman in the West Nile district in Uganda. Prior to the 1990s, there were outbreaks in sub-Saharan Africa and the Middle East which were characterised by a mild and self-limited febrile illness [104]. However, by the late 1990s, there were more frequent reports of epidemics in urban areas of Europe and the Middle East, followed by New York in 1999, and these strains were associated with a notable increase in reported cases of human neuroinvasive disease [64, 104, 105]. This potential for increased virulence associated with strain variation has also been demonstrated in Australia. In that country the indigenous WNV strain (Kunjin virus or WNV_{KUN}) was responsible for an unprecedented outbreak of equine encephalitis in 2011, attributed to a newly emerged strain [106]. A similar phenomenon has also been observed with ZIKV, first isolated in 1947 from the blood of a sentinel rhesus monkey in the Zika Forest, near Lake Victoria in Uganda. The first reported case of ZIKV isolated from a human was in Nigeria in 1954 [107]. Subsequently, very few cases of ZIKV were reported prior to the first major outbreak on Yap Island in 2007, and most were considered to be asymptomatic with a minority characterised by mild self-limiting symptoms. However, during a second major outbreak in 2013–2014 in the Western Pacific, an association between ZIKV infection and Guillain-Barre syndrome (GBS) was reported in French Polynesia [108–110]. This was followed, in the subsequent outbreak in the Americas (2015–2016), by a reported association of ZIKV with neurological disorders, including microcephaly, in newborns [111–114].

A contrasting example is human pegivirus (HPgV), formerly known as GBV-C/HGV and identified in 1995 [115, 116]. The virus was demonstrated to be transfusion-transmissible and initially thought to be hepatotropic and a cause of hepatitis in humans – hence the original name of hepatitis G virus (HGV) [117, 118]. However, numerous studies since the late 1990s have failed to demonstrate that HPgV is a cause of acute, chronic or fulminant hepatitis, and the virus is now considered not to be associated with disease in humans and therefore not a threat to blood safety [117, 119–121].

Quantitative Assessment: Estimating the Transfusion-Transmission Risk of EID Agents

In addition to assessing whether an EID agent represents a potential threat to blood safety, risk modelling can be used to quantitatively estimate the level of risk (Fig. 5.1). Since the 1990s a number of models have been developed to estimate TT risk associated with the major transfusion-transmissible viruses [28–33, 35, 122]. Risk modelling for these agents is based on two key parameters, the detectable incidence of infection in the donor population (which is known due to universal donor screening) and the infectious window period (the period during which an acutely infected asymptomatic donor may be infectious but not detectable by the screening assay). In contrast, in the case of EID agents for which donor screening has not been implemented, the incidence of infection in the donor population is not known, and a screening assay window period is not applicable. Therefore the incidence-window period methodology is not applicable to EID agents for which donor screening has not been implemented. As a consequence, risk models have been developed for EID agents based on the reported incidence of infection in the general population, from which an estimate of the incidence in the blood donor population can be derived. Two formal risk models and a number of less formal approaches have been published. However, to apply these risk models and interpret their outcomes in a local jurisdictional context, it is important to understand their conceptual basis and the way in which risk is reported [123]. Additionally, as EID risk modelling is typically based on limited information, a number of necessary assumptions are required, and risk estimates will have a measure of uncertainty. The assumptions of two important models, the Biggerstaff-Petersen (BP) and EUFRAT models, are summarised in Table 5.1. In addition, a number of EID agents that are currently considered a high priority [8, 10, 58, 128, 129] as actual or potential threats to blood safety are listed in Table 5.2, along with a summary of the key parameters that are critical for risk modelling.

Table 5.1 Assumptions and limitations of the Biggerstaff-Petersen and EUFRAT models [123–127]

	Assumptions common to both models	Additional assumptions for the BP model	Additional assumptions for EUFRAT
Assumptions related to reported case numbers	*Reported* incident infections represent all symptomatic infections	Symptom onset dates for reported (symptomatic) cases are similar to asymptomatic infections	
Assumptions related to blood donor characteristics	Donation frequency is constant throughout the period of observation All donors have the same risk of infection, which is constant during the period of observation Asymptomatic infection does not affect the donation behaviour of donors Likelihood of detection of infectious donors by the pre-donation questionnaire is constant throughout the infectious period	Donors have the same risk of infection as the general population Blood components from viraemic blood donors transmit infection with 100% efficiency Donors with symptomatic infections would either not present to donate or would be excluded from donating	

Table 5.1 (continued)

	Assumptions common to both models	Additional assumptions for the BP model	Additional assumptions for EUFRAT
Assumptions related to infection	Historically estimated ratio of total infections/symptomatic infections and viraemic periods are applicable to the study population and remain constant during period of observation Relative timing and duration of viraemia is independent of symptom onset time Duration of viraemia is the same for both symptomatic and asymptomatic cases		Risk from travelling donors is based on the duration of visit to outbreak/endemic area and time from departure to donating Travelling donors have the same risk of infection as local inhabitants in outbreak/endemic area The proportion of donors that develop chronic infections is constant during period of observation
Limitations	Input parameters required for both models are often not well defined and contribute to the inherent uncertainty of the models	To perform the statistical resampling in the BP model, the dates of symptom onset for reported incident cases are required The BP model assumes 100% efficiency of transmission by transfusion, and the entire general population is susceptible to infection and does not take into account pathogen reduction/inactivation due to blood processing and storage	A number of parameters in the EUFRAT model, including the difference in risk of infection between donors and the general population, the proportion of symptomatic cases in the general population that do not seek health care or are misdiagnosed, the transfusion-transmission efficiency of infected end products and the level of immunity in the general population, are typically unknown for EID agents

Biggerstaff-Petersen Model: The Risk of Asymptomatic Viraemic Infections in Blood Donors

The first reported model for estimating the TT risk associated with an EID agent was developed by Biggerstaff and Petersen (BP model) [124, 125] in response to West Nile virus (WNV) outbreaks in the USA, first reported in Queens, New York City, in 1999 [67, 217]. WNV is a mosquito-borne virus within the *Flavivirus* genus, and TT has been well documented [60–67, 217]. The model was used to

Table 5.2 Some EID agents considered to represent a threat to blood safety and important input parameters for risk modelling

Agent	Vector/host	Geographical distribution	Incubation period	Estimated duration of presymptomatic and total viraemic periods	Percentage of asymptomatic infections	Transfusion-transmissible?
Viruses						
Chikungunya virus (CHIKV)	Aedes species mosquitoes, particularly A. aegypti and A. albopictus [130, 131]	Widespread in Africa, Asia, Oceania (except Australia), Central/South America and Caribbean from 2013 [132]	1–12 days (average 2–4 days) [131, 133]	Presymptomatic, up to 2.5 days [134]; total, 7–17 days [133–136]	75–95%; may vary with age and viral genotype [130, 137, 138]	Not reported but suspected based on asymptomatic viraemic period, high level of viraemia and high incidence during outbreaks [139]
Dengue virus (DENV)	Several Aedes species mosquitoes, particularly A. aegypti and A. albopictus [140, 141]	Endemic in more than 100 countries in tropical and subtropical Southeast Asia, the Americas, the Western Pacific, Africa and the eastern Mediterranean regions; incidence has increased 30-fold in the past 50 years [141]	3–14 days (average 4–7 days) [142, 143]	Presymptomatic, 1–2 days [142, 144]; total, 9.1 days (95% CI, 4.4–13.9 days) [145]	50–85% [146–148]	A number of transfusion-transmission cases have been reported [52–56, 59, 68, 73, 149–152]
West Nile virus (WNV)	Primarily Culex species mosquitoes [153]	Almost worldwide distribution since the 1990s [64, 153, 154]	2–15 days [64, 105, 153]	Presymptomatic, 1–2 days less than incubation period [124, 155, 156]; total, 20–24 days [67, 157]	80%, most symptomatic infections are mild and self-limiting; up to 1% of infections develop neurological complications [64, 153, 154]	A number of transfusion-transmission cases have been reported [60–63, 65, 66, 158]

Zika virus (ZIKV)	*Aedes* species mosquitoes, primarily *A. aegypti* and *A. africanus* (Africa) [107, 159]	A number of African countries, India, Pakistan, Southeast Asia; recent outbreaks on Yap Island (2007), French Polynesia and the Western Pacific Islands (2014–2015) and the Americas (from 2015) [159–161]	Estimated range, 3–14 days [107, 161, 162]; systematic reviews estimated a median incubation period of 5.9 days (95% CI, 4.4–7.6) [163] and 6.2 days (95% CI, 5.7–6.6) [164].	Presymptomatic: 3–10 days [51]; systematic review modelling estimated a mean detectable viraemic period of 9.9 days (95% CI, 6.9–21.4) [163]; small number of cases with extended viraemia in plasma (between 37 and 50 days) [165] and whole blood (between 100 and 150 days) have been reported [165–167]	Estimated 82% (95% CI, 73–90%) [168]	4 cases were reported in Brazil in 2015–2016 [68,69,72]
Hepatitis E virus (HEV)	In developing countries, associated with faecal-contaminated drinking water; in developed countries, typically zoonotic transmission due to undercooked pork or game and contact with pigs [169]	Global distribution [169–172]	Typically 4–6 weeks, can extend from 9 days to 2 months [169, 173]	In acute infection, typically brief viraemic period during prodromal phase, clearing at onset of clinical symptoms, may last up to 6–8 weeks [170, 174, 175]	Estimated 67–98% in developed countries, varies with genotype and recipient-related factors [169, 172, 176–178]	A number of confirmed and suspected transfusion-transmitted cases have been reported [179–188]

(continued)

Table 5.2 (continued)

Agent	Vector/host	Geographical distribution	Incubation period	Estimated duration of presymptomatic and total viraemic periods	Percentage of asymptomatic infections	Transfusion-transmissible?
Protozoan parasites						
Babesia species	Tick species of the *Ixodes* genus, primarily *Ixodes scapularis* in the USA and *I. ricinus* in Europe [189]	Most cases of human babesiosis have been reported in the north-eastern and upper Midwestern USA (*B. microti*); most other cases have been reported in Europe, predominantly France, the UK and Ireland (*B. divergens*) with cases sporadically reported in Asia, Africa, Australia, Europe and South America [189, 190]	1–4 weeks after the bite of a *B. microti*-infected tick and 11 to 176 days after transfusion of contaminated blood products [189, 191]	Following an initial period of parasitaemia and clearance, a proportion of cases will have persistent, low-level, intermittently detectable parasitaemia which may persist from several months to >12 months [192, 193]	Most infections in immunocompetent individuals are either subclinical (19% in adults and 40% in children) or mild to moderate symptoms; severe disease may occur in at-risk individuals [190, 194, 195]	159 transfusion-transmitted cases reported in the USA between 1979 and 2009 [191]
Leishmania species	Female phlebotomine sandflies of the *Phlebotomus* (Old World) and *Lutzomyia* (New World) genera [196]	Endemic in at least 98 countries, primarily Indian subcontinent, East Africa, Mediterranean basin, the Middle East, Central Asia and the Americas [197, 198]	Incubation period varies with form of leishmaniasis: 2 weeks to 18 months for visceral leishmaniasis [199, 200] and 2 weeks to several months for cutaneous leishmaniasis [196, 201]	Asymptomatic parasitaemia duration varies with *Leishmania* spp. and virulence, probably low level and episodic, from a few weeks to >12 months	In immunocompetent individuals infection is typically asymptomatic, up to 80–95% depending on species, virulence and host-related factors [200, 202]	14 suspected cases of transfusion-transmitted *Leishmania* spp. infections have been reported; considered to be underreported [203]

Plasmodium species (malaria)	Mosquito species of the *Anopheles* genus [204]	In 2015, malaria transmission was reported in 91 countries in tropical and subtropical Africa (90% of cases), the Middle East, Asia and Central and South America [205]	7–30 days, depending on *Plasmodium* spp. [206]	Infection with *Plasmodium* spp. can result in asymptomatic parasitaemia or "semi-immunity" which may last >12 months [207]	Asymptomatic parasitaemia is common, rate varies with endemicity and *Plasmodium* spp. [208, 209]	*Plasmodium* species are readily transfusion-transmissible and one of the most common transfusion-transmitted infections [210, 211]
Trypanosoma cruzi (Chagas disease)	Several insect species of the Triatomine subfamily [212]	Endemic throughout Mexico, Central America and South America [213, 214]	Acute infection: symptoms appear 1–2 weeks after infection; progresses to chronic asymptomatic phase [213, 214]	In acute infection, parasitaemia is detectable within 1–2 weeks of infection and lasts for 6–8 weeks; chronic infection is characterised by low or undetectable parasitaemia	Most acute infections are asymptomatic; intermittent or low level parasitaemia in asymptomatic chronic infection [213]	Transfusion-transmitted *T. cruzi* infections have been reported; probably underreported due to inadequate reporting systems in a number of endemic countries [215, 216]

retrospectively estimate the TT risk of WNV in the USA prior to the implementation of donor screening in 2003.

As the incidence of WNV infection in US blood donors was not known prior to donor screening, the BP model used the reported incidence of WNV neurologic disease (WNND) in the general population to derive an estimate of the incidence of asymptomatic infection which in turn was used to estimate the proportion of viraemic but asymptomatic donors. This estimated proportion of viraemic but asymptomatic donors was equated to the risk of an infected donation entering the blood supply, which in turn was interpreted as the risk of transmitting WNV by transfusion. The BP model included a statistical resampling methodology (Monte Carlo simulation) for estimating the proportion of donors who were asymptomatically viraemic *at any point in time* and a methodologically simpler formula for estimating *the average proportion of asymptomatically infected donors over a specified time period*.

In order to derive an estimate of the proportion of asymptomatically infected donors from the prevalence of WNND in the general population, the statistical resampling methodology requires a number of input variables. Based on data from the local outbreak, the dates of symptom onset for each reported case and the population of the outbreak area were required. Additionally, a number of variables derived from published historical data were also required: the time course of WNV viraemia, ratio of WNND cases to total number of WNV infections and the ratio of asymptomatic/symptomatic infections (most symptomatic infections result in West Nile fever and do not develop neurological symptoms). Based on the symptom onset dates for the reported WNND cases, the statistical resampling simulated the number of symptomatic viraemic cases at time t using the range of possible viraemic periods prior and subsequent to symptom onset. Further, based on the size of the general population, the ratio of total WNV infections/reported WNND cases and the assumption that infected donors who develop symptoms are only at risk of donating prior to symptom onset, the model derived a risk curve that represented the estimated proportion of asymptomatic cases in the population which was assumed to be the same for the donor population and this was equated to the TT risk of WNV.

The BP formula for estimating the average TT risk can be expressed as

$$\text{Average TT risk} = \left(\frac{(R * P_{asym} * D_{asym}) + (R * P_{sym} * D_{sym})}{L} \right) * I$$

where R is the ratio of total infections/reported cases of WNND, P_{asym} is the proportion of asymptomatic (subclinical) infections and P_{sym} is the proportion of symptomatic infections, D_{asym} is the duration of viraemia in cases that do not develop symptoms and D_{sym} is the duration of viraemia prior to symptom onset for cases that develop symptoms (presymptomatic viraemic period), L is the length of the period of observation and I is the incidence of WNND cases (typically expressed as cases per 10^4 population).

To help understand the conceptual basis of this formula, it can be rearranged as

$$\text{Average TT risk} = \left(\frac{\left(P_{asym} * D_{asym} \right) + \left(P_{sym} * D_{sym} \right)}{L} \right) * R * I$$

The term $[(P_{asym} * D_{asym}) + (P_{sym} * D_{sym})]$ is the average asymptomatic viraemic period, taking into account that the asymptomatic viraemic period in the proportion of cases that do not develop clinical symptoms is the entire viraemic period, and for the proportion that does develop clinical symptoms, it is restricted to the presymptomatic viraemic period.

Therefore, $\left(\dfrac{\left(P_{asym} * D_{asym} \right) + \left(P_{sym} * D_{sym} \right)}{L} \right)$ is the average proportion of time an infected individual is asymptomatically viraemic during the period of observation, which is the average risk that an infected donor will donate blood while asymptomatically viraemic; this is then multiplied by (R*I) which represents the incidence of all infections (both subclinical and those that develop symptoms). Therefore, the BP formula can be expressed as

$$\text{Average risk} = \Pr \begin{pmatrix} \text{collecting viraemic} \\ \text{donation} \\ \text{from each asympomatitically} \\ \text{infected donor} \end{pmatrix} * (\text{incidence of infection})$$

It can now be seen that the BP formula for average risk is actually an estimate of *the risk of collecting an infectious donation from an asymptomatically infected donor during the period of observation.*

Since its original application to WNV outbreaks in the USA, the principles of the BP model have been used to estimate the TT risk of DENV in Australia during outbreaks in 2004 and 2008–2009 [43, 45]; CHIKV on La Reunion island in 2005–2007 [218], Thailand in 2009 [219] and Italy in 2007 [220]; hepatitis A virus (HAV) in Latvia in 2008 [221]; Ross River virus (RRV) in Australia in 2013–2014 [222, 223]; and the potential TT risk of WNV in Switzerland if autochthonous cases were to be reported in that country [224]. In most of these studies, the BP formula for average risk for a defined time period was used rather than the statistical resampling approach. Presumably this is due, at least in part, to the former being computationally simpler and not requiring the exact dates of symptom onset for reported cases. A worked example of the BP formula is provided in Box 5.1. These studies show that the BP model can be applied to a range of EID agents and demonstrate that regular risk modelling across regions can provide an indicator of changing risk levels over time and geographically, thereby informing decisions regarding the implementation of risk mitigation strategies.

> **Box 5.1 Application of the Biggerstaff-Petersen model: chikungunya fever on Reunion Island, 2005 [218]**
> A retrospective estimate of collecting a viraemic blood donation on Reunion Island during an outbreak period: 28 March–18 December 2005
> The Biggerstaff-Petersen formula is
>
> $$\text{Average TT risk} = \left(\frac{(P_{asym} * D_{asym}) + (P_{sym} * D_{sym})}{L} \right) * R * I$$
>
> D_{asym} = total viraemic period = 7.5 days
> P_{asym} = proportion of asymptomatic infections = 0.15
> L = length of observation period = 266 days
> R = ratio of total infections/symptomatic (reported) cases
>
> D_{sym} = presymptomatic viraemic period = 1.5 days
> P_{sym} = proportion of symptomatic infections = 0.85
>
> I = incidence of symptomatic (reported) cases/10^5 population
>
> $(R \times I)$ = Incidence of (symptomatic and asymptomatic) chikungunya virus infections/100,000 population = 1,067
> Estimated number of symptomatic cases = 6,864
> Total number of cases = 6864/P_{sym} = 6864/0.85 = 8,075
> Average TT risk = risk of collecting a viraemic blood donation/100,000 donations = [((0.15 × 7.5) + (0.85 x 1.5))/L] × 1067 = 9.6 (95% CI, 9.4 – 9.8)
> Estimated number of infectious blood donations = 1.2/12,800 donations (95% CI, 1.2 – 1.3)
>
> Population of Reunion Island = 756,745

The EUFRAT: The Risk of Transmitting Infection

The European Centre for Disease Prevention and Control (ECDC) has developed a TT risk model referred to as the European Up-Front Risk Assessment Tool (EUFRAT) [126, 127]. The EUFRAT has a web-based interface, and its stated aims are to assess and quantify the TT risk of an EID during an ongoing outbreak.

The EUFRAT differs in a number of important ways from the BP model. EUFRAT provides an estimate of the risk of transmitting an EID agent to a recipient by estimating a series of risks that begin with the risk of blood donors becoming infected. Methodologically the EUFRAT can be divided into a logical sequence of four or five steps, each with an associated risk. Based on the EUFRAT User Manual, the EUFRAT is summarised below as a four-step process [127].

The first step estimates the risk of a donor being infectious at the time of donation, which is assumed to be proportional to the prevalence of infection in the general population. This risk is a function of the duration of the infectious blood phase and includes correction factors for the difference between the risk of donors becoming infected compared to the general population (if known) and the proportion of undetected cases. The second step estimates the number of donations derived from infectious donors and incorporates the prevalence of infection in the donor population (from step 1), the mean donation frequency and the probability that an infected donor will be interdicted by a pre-donation assessment procedure. The third step estimates the number of infected donations released for processing into blood components and infected end products based on pathogen removal or inactivation due to the blood processing procedures and, if implemented, the effectiveness of donor screening and pathogen reduction technology. The final step is an estimate of the risk of recipients becoming infected following transfusion which will depend on the TT efficiency of the agent and the proportion of recipients who are immune to the agent. Additionally, the EUFRAT has the option for defining input parameters as either fixed values or a distribution of values. The latter allows for parameter uncertainty by using Monte Carlo simulation which determines the value of a parameter by repeat random sampling from a triangular distribution defined by a plausible range entered by the user.

Similar to the BP model, the EUFRAT has been used in a number of reported studies to estimate the TT risk for CHIKV [126, 225], DENV [226], *Coxiella burnetii* [225, 227] and RRV [223] (Table 5.1). The EUFRAT has also been used in a non-outbreak area to estimate the TT risk associated with donors returning from an outbreak area [226] and extended to retrospectively estimate the TT risk during an outbreak period *and* the subsequent (future) risk associated with donors who potentially remain infectious for some time following the end of the outbreak or period of observation [225].

Alternative Approaches to Estimating Transfusion-Transmission Risk

In addition to the BP and EUFRAT models, a number of other approaches have been used to estimate TT risk, three of which are briefly described below with worked examples for each in Box 5.2. These approaches may be appropriate where there is insufficient information to use the BP or EUFRAT models or when formal risk modelling is not required.

Box 5.2 Examples of alternative approaches to estimating transfusion-transmission risk

Force of infection: DENV in Singapore 2005

Assumptions: (i) 80% of population are eligible to donate; (ii) ratio of total infections/symptomatic infections = 3

Study data: (i) population of Singapore = 4,000,000, (ii) number of reported (symptomatic) cases = 14,209 and (iii) annual number of donations in Singapore = 80,000

Risk modelling:

Total number (symptomatic and asymptomatic) cases in adults eligible to donate = 14,209 × 0.80 × 3 = 34,101 cases in 12 months
Average of number of cases/week = 34,101/52
Force of infection (proportion of population infected per week = 656/4,000,000 = 0.00016
Annual number of viraemic donations during 2005 = (number of donations) × (force of infection) = 80,000 × 0.00016 = 13 or 1.6 viraemic donations/10,000 donations

DENV IgM detection and incident infections in donors: DENV in Cairns, Australia, 2008–2009.

Assumptions: (i) all IgM+ donors were infected during the period of observation, i.e. they are incident infections; (ii) due to donor eligibility criteria, risk is primarily due to donors who do not develop symptoms; (iii) duration of viraemic period = 7 days; (iv) IgM−/RNA+ asymptomatic period = 5 days; (v) duration of IgM = 182 days (6 months) and (vi) duration of (IgM−/RNA+) + (IgM+) periods = 187 days

Study data: (i) IgM seroprevalence in donations = 0.18% (most probable value), (ii) number of donations during outbreak period = 5,753, (iii) number of donors during outbreak period = 2,770 and (iv) donation frequency = (number of donations/number of donors) = 5,753/2,770 = 2.0769

Risk modelling:

Probability of collecting infectious donation = [(duration of viraemic period period)/(IgM−/RNA+) + (IgM+) periods] × (IgM donation seroprevalence) x (donation frequency) = (7/187) × 0.0018 × 2.0769 = 0.00014
Number of infectious donations = (Probability of collecting infectious donation) × (number of donations) = 0.00014 × 5,753 = 0.80508
Risk collecting an infectious donation = (1/number of infectious donations) x (number of donations) = (1/0.80508) × (5,735) = 1 in 7,146 donations

Pilot study – viraemic blood donors: HEV in Australia, 2016

Assumptions: (i) HEV RNA prevalence in fresh components is the same as whole blood donors; (ii) proportion of HEV RNA-positive donations resulting in a TT infection = 0.42; (iii) proportion of TT infections resulting in an adverse or severe outcome = 0.05 or 0.01, respectively; and (iv) background immunity in the recipient population = 0.

Study data: (i) number of donors = 74,131, (ii) number of HEV RNA-positive donors = 1 and (iii) rate of HEV RNA detection in blood donors = 1/74131 = 0.001349% (95% CI, 0.000238-0.007641%)

Risk estimate (all components):

Number of donations issued in 2016 = 986,224
Number of donations transfused in 2016 = 827,397 (83.4%)
Number of viraemic components transfused/year = (number of donations transfused x rate of HEV RNA detection in blood donors) = 827,397 × 1.349×10^{-5} = 11.16
Number of transfusions resulting in HEV infection = (number of viraemic components transfused/year) × (proportion of HEV RNA-positive donations resulting in a TT-infection) = 11.2 × 0.42 = 4.69
Number of transfusion resulting in a symptomatic infection = (number of transfusions resulting in HEV infection) × (proportion of TT-infections resulting in an adverse outcome) = 4.69 × 0.05 = 0.23
Number of transfusions resulting in a severe outcome = (number of transfusions resulting in HEV infection) × (proportion of TT-infections resulting in a severe outcome) = 4.69 × 0.01 = 0.047
Risk of a symptomatic infection per component transfused = 1 in 3,530,048 (95% CI 1 in 70,557,190 to 1 in 715,753) or 1 infection every 4.3 years (95% CI 1 in every 85 years to 1 in every 0.9 year
Risk of a severe infection per component transfused = 1 in 17,650,238 (95% CI 1 in 352,785,951 to 1 in 3,578,765) or 1 infection every 21.3 years (95% CI 1 in every 462 years to 1 in every 4.34 years

Force of Infection: DENV in Singapore, 2005 The TT risk of DENV in Singapore in 2005 was estimated based on the force of infection, i.e. the rate at which susceptible individuals become infected per unit of time [228]. In this approach, the number of infectious donors was estimated, and this was equated to the number of infectious transfusions. TT risk was expressed as the estimated number of infected blood transfusions per 10,000 transfusions.

IgM Detection and Incident Infections in Donors: DENV in Cairns, Australia, 2008–2009 During an outbreak of dengue in Queensland, Australia, in 2008–2009, the TT risk of DENV was estimated using the IgM seroprevalence in blood donors [43]. The probability of collecting an infectious donation was estimated based on the seroprevalence of IgM in blood donors (assumed to represent recent infections), the duration of IgM and the duration of the infectious viraemic period. TT risk was expressed as the risk of collecting an infectious unit per total donations collected. A similar methodology was used in the mid-1990s to estimate the TT risk of RRV in Queensland [229].

Pilot Study – Viraemic Blood Donors: HEV in Australia, 2016 The TT risk of HEV in Australia has been modelled based on a pilot study of Australian blood donors [230]. A large sample of blood donors was screened for HEV RNA to provide an estimate of the prevalence of HEV viraemia in the donor population. Based on the proportion of donations from which blood components are actually transfused and the TT efficiency of HEV, the number of transfusion-transmitted HEV infections was estimated. Further, based on the estimated number of symptomatic and severe infections, the corresponding risks were expressed as the number of symptomatic or severe infections per component transfused, respectively.

While these approaches for estimating TT risk have several limitations, they highlight the diversity of possible methods to model and express TT risk. In addition, the DENV and HEV examples have the advantage that they are based on infection rates in the donor population under observation.

Interpreting Risk Assessments

The Local Context

Although blood safety has been the subject of considerable debate, there is no universally accepted agreement on what constitutes an acceptable risk level (risk tolerance) or appropriate risk mitigation strategies [18, 23, 231–236]. Therefore, it is important that each jurisdiction performs its own risk assessment, based on local epidemiological data, and determines acceptable risk levels in collaboration with the relevant local authorities – blood services, governments and health departments, regulators and end users. It is also important to consider the risk perception within the local community and the need to maintain public confidence in the safety of the blood supply as this can affect the likelihood of patients being prepared to accept a transfusion and the willingness of donors to provide blood [237]. This is particularly important in the age of the Internet and social media. The general public increasingly uses online sources to obtain information, which may not necessarily be accurate but nonetheless can inform the public's perception of risk. This has been clearly demonstrated in the ZIKV outbreak in the Americas where the general public has used social media and online sources for information on ZIKV [238–241].

The Threat to Blood Safety: Qualitative Assessment

Determining whether an EID agent represents a threat to blood safety in terms of the criteria described above will primarily require a qualitative assessment. A useful approach is to prioritise the criteria based on local epidemiological data and how well the agent and its associated disease are characterised. For example, in an expert elicitation study, a group of experts were asked to rank a set of hypothetical diseases with varying degrees of uncertainty associated with the disease characteristics [242, 243]. The characteristics considered were transfusion-transmissibility, asymptomatic blood phase, prevalence of infection and disease impact. The results showed that for scenarios where there was a lack of data concerning disease characteristics, it was the uncertainty concerning the asymptomatic phase and the disease impact that were the most important drivers of perceived risk. However, for scenarios where the disease characteristics were well established, the prevalence of infection and transfusion-transmissibility were the key drivers of perceived risk.

Estimating Transfusion-Transmission Risk: Quantitative Assessment

Prior to quantitatively estimating TT risk, each jurisdiction should consider two important questions: (i) Is it required, and (ii) is it feasible based on what is known about the agent? Blood services and regulatory authorities may take the view that if an EID agent is present in a population and is considered potentially transfusion-transmissible, risk mitigation strategies should be implemented without, or regardless of, risk modelling. For example, as a precautionary measure, the FDA mandated universal donor screening for ZIKV in the USA without formal modelling of the TT risk [244, 245]. The extent to which risk modelling can provide a meaningful estimate of TT risk will depend on how well characterised the agent and its associated disease are. If the use of the BP and EUFRAT models is not feasible, there are, as noted, a number of alternative approaches to estimating TT risk. Finally, when determining an acceptable level of risk, it is important to understand how different models express risk. For example, as noted, the BP model expresses risk as the risk of an infectious but asymptomatic donor presenting to donate, while the EUFRAT allows for risk to be expressed as the actual risk of transmitting infection to recipients. Additionally, based on the alternative approaches noted above, risk can also be expressed as the number of infected donations collected, or the number of symptomatic infections transmitted, per unit of time.

Case Study: Ross River Virus and Blood Safety in Australia

To illustrate how the qualitative and quantitative aspects of assessing TT risk can be applied to a specific agent in a local jurisdiction, and inform decisions regarding risk mitigation strategies, the example of Ross River virus (RRV) in Australia is described below.

Background

RRV is an arthropod-borne virus of the *Alphavirus* genus [246] and is the most common and widespread arboviral disease in Australia, being endemic in many regions and epidemic in nonendemic regions. It is also endemic in Papua New Guinea (PNG), and epidemics have been previously reported throughout the late 1970s to early 1980s in Fiji, American Samoa, the Cook Islands and New Caledonia [247]. A recent report has provided evidence that RRV has been circulating in American Samoa since 1980 [248] and there has been ongoing "silent" circulation in French Polynesia [249]. A number of mosquito species have been implicated as possible RRV vectors, but those most strongly associated with the transmission cycle are *Aedes vigilax* and *Aedes camptorhynchus* (northern and southern Australian coastlines), *Culex annulirostris* (throughout all of Australia except Tasmania) and *Aedes notoscriptus* [247, 250].

RRV: Meeting the Criteria as a Potential Threat to Blood Safety

The ability of RRV to establish infection in humans and spread within populations, and its presence in Australia, has been well established. Previous outbreaks in the Western Pacific region are believed to have been caused by a viraemic traveller from Australia [248, 251]. In Australia, RRV infection is notifiable, and reported case numbers are monitored and published [251]. During the 10-year period between 2007 and 2016, the reported annual case numbers of RRV in Australia varied between 3,337 and 4,661 with the exception of 2015 when 9,554 cases were reported, the highest reported annual total. In December 2016 there was another increase in reported cases with highest ever reported case numbers nationally for a December–February period (3,661) [251].

The duration of RRV viraemia in humans has not been well characterised, and estimates are primarily based on animal models which suggest a presymptomatic infectious period of 1 day (plausible range 0.5 to 2) and for subclinical cases, an infectious period of 5 days (plausible range 2 to 9 days) [222, 247, 252]. These estimates are consistent with the related alphavirus, CHIKV, which can be detected approximately 2.3 to 2.5 days prior to symptom onset and can persist from 6 to 13 days [134, 135].

While transfusion-transmission of RRV has been suspected for several years, the first probable case was not reported until 2014 (in Australia) and remains the only reported case [252, 253]. Therefore, while RRV is considered to be potentially transfusion-transmissible, this may not be an efficient mode of transmission. This would also appear to be consistent with the related CHIKV. Although reported case numbers worldwide for CHIKV are several orders of magnitude higher than RRV [130, 254], infection includes an asymptomatic viraemic period, and viraemia has been reported in blood donors [134, 136, 218, 219], no confirmed cases of transfusion-transmitted CHIKV have been reported.

Specific data regarding the ability of RRV to survive blood processing and storage has not been reported. However, in the absence of evidence to the contrary, it should be assumed that the virus can survive blood processing. This is supported by comparison with WNV, ZIKV and DENV which are also enveloped RNA arboviruses and have been demonstrated to be transfusion-transmissible and therefore able to survive blood processing and storage.

RRV can cause a nonfatal disease known as epidemic polyarthritis or RRV disease. The incubation period for the onset of symptoms can vary from 2 to 21 days with an average of 7–9 days. The most common symptoms are fever, polyarthralgia and rash; other symptoms may include lymphadenopathy, lethargy, headache, myalgias, photophobia and glomerulonephritis. The typical period of incapacity is 1 to 2 weeks, with fever, nausea and skin rash usually disappearing within the first 2 weeks of symptom onset. In cases with protracted illness, the prognosis is good with most patients experiencing progressive resolution of symptoms, such as joint pain and tiredness, over a period of 3–6 months. The estimated ratio of asymptomatic/symptomatic infections for RRV varies between 1:2 and 3:1 [247].

Estimating the TT Risk of RRV in Australia

Both the BP and EUFRAT models have been used to estimate the TT risk of RR in Australia [223]. Risk modelling was performed both nationally and for the state of Western Australia (WA) for the period 1 June 2013 to 31 May 2014; additionally, modelling was performed for WA for the period 1 January 2014 to 31 March 2014, a period of high reported incidence. The PB model was used to estimate the risk of collecting a viraemic donation, while the EUFRAT was used to estimate the risk of infection in donors. For the period 1 June 2013 to 31 May 2014, the national TT risk was estimated as 1 in 166,486 (minimum/maximum range, 1 in 659,078 to 149,158) donations for the PB model and 1 in 95,039 (95% CI, 311,328 to 32,399) for the EUFRAT, this compared to 1 in 58,657 (232,208 to 17,320) and 1 in 33,481 (95% CI, 106,695 to 11,415), respectively, for WA. For the high incidence period in WA, the estimated risks were 1 in 26,177 (103,628 to 7,729) for the PB model and 1 in 14,943 (95% CI, 48, 593 to 5,094) for EUFRAT. While the two models give different risk estimates, this difference does not appear to be statistically significant as the most plausible BP estimates were within the 95% CI of the EUFRAT estimates.

This example of modelling the TT risk of RRV highlights two important aspects of risk modelling. Firstly, due to the uncertainty associated with the key input variables (duration of viraemic periods and ratio of asymptomatic/symptomatic infections), the modelled risk estimates have wide upper and lower limits. Secondly, the focal and seasonal nature of the RRV incidence and corresponding TT risk is evident.

Evidence-Based Decision-Making

Based on the qualitative assessment of whether RRV represents a potential threat to blood safety and the quantitative estimates of TT risk provided by formal modelling, there are a number of other factors that were incorporated into the risk assessment:

- There is some evidence that blood collections are underrepresented in areas at high risk of RRV transmission, and therefore the risk modelling would overestimate the TT risk.
- Background levels of immunity in the community will vary on a regional basis [255]; therefore, regions with higher incidence of RRV in the past will have higher levels of background immunity, thereby reducing the risk of infection in the donor population and transmission to recipients.
- RRV infection does not result in life-threatening disease, and the typical period of incapacity is 1–2 weeks, even protracted illness has a good prognosis.
- RRV viraemia in Australian blood donors appears to be low. This is based on a recent study of approximately 7,500 at-risk donors which did not detect any viraemic donors [256].
- In Australia, donors are asked if they are feeling healthy and well, whether they have been unwell or seen a doctor or any other health-care practitioner. These questions would be expected to interdict donors who have or recently had a symptomatic RRV infection. Additionally, donors reporting a history of RRV infection are deferred for 4 weeks from date of recovery.
- Following donation, donors are advised to notify the blood service of post-donation illness.

Given that there are no approved assays for RRV screening of blood donor, the following risk mitigation strategies were considered:

- There is no suitable or approved screening test for blood donor screening.
- Geographically based fresh component restrictions during high transmission periods: considered not practicable given scope and duration of RRV outbreaks, significant cost and loss of product.
- Pathogen inactivation: not considered feasible in Australia at present and arguably not cost-effective.
- Enhanced donor education, particularly relating to reporting post-donation illness and strengthening existing messages and advising donors to notify the blood

service within a week of donating if they develop a cough, cold, diarrhoea or other infection and within 2 months if they are diagnosed or hospitalised with a serious infectious disease. The reported TT-RRV case was associated with a late post-donation notification.

Based on this assessment of the threat to blood safety, risk modelling and the additional local jurisdictional considerations, the option to enhance donor education and strengthen existing message about reporting post-donation illness was assessed as the most appropriate risk mitigation strategy.

Summary and Conclusions

With the increased threat to blood safety posed by EID agents, it is important that in addition to ongoing surveillance, local jurisdictions perform evidence-based risk assessments to inform decisions regarding risk mitigation strategies. This chapter has described a three-way approach to evidence-based risk assessment and decision-making: (i) qualitatively assessing whether an EID agent represents a potential threat to blood safety, (ii) quantitatively estimating the TT risk and (iii) decision-making at the local jurisdictional level. This approach will help ensure that risk mitigation strategies are proportionate to the level of risk, feasible and cost-effective that sufficiency of supply is not unnecessarily compromised and confidence in the safety of the blood supply is maintained.

References

1. Shander A, Lobel GP, Javidroozi M. Transfusion practices and infectious risks. Expert Rev Hematol. 2016;9(6):597–605. PubMed PMID: 26959944. Epub 2016/03/10. Eng.
2. Dodd R. Transfusion-transmitted infections: testing strategies and residual risk. ISTB Sci Ser. 2014;9:1–5.
3. Seed CR, Kiely P, Keller AJ. Residual risk of transfusion transmitted human immunodeficiency virus, hepatitis B virus, hepatitis C virus and human T lymphotrophic virus. Intern Med J. 2005;35(10):592–8. PubMed PMID: 16207258.
4. Chamberland ME, Epstein J, Dodd RY, Persing D, Will RG, DeMaria A Jr, et al. Blood safety. Emerg Infect Dis. 1998;4(3):410–1. PubMed PMID: 9716958. PMCID: PMC2640272. Epub 1998/08/26. eng.
5. Chamberland ME. Emerging infectious agents: do they pose a risk to the safety of transfused blood and blood products? Clin Infect Dis. 2002;34(6):797–805. PubMed PMID: 11850862. Epub 2002/02/19. eng.
6. Chamberland ME, Alter HJ, Busch MP, Nemo G, Ricketts M. Emerging infectious disease issues in blood safety. Emerg Infect Dis. 2001;7(3 Suppl):552–3. PubMed PMID: 11485669. PMCID: PMC2631858. Epub 2001/08/04. eng.
7. Dodd RY, Leiby DA. Emerging infectious threats to the blood supply. Annu Rev Med. 2004;55:191–207. PubMed PMID: 14746517. Epub 2004/01/30. eng.
8. Stramer SL, Hollinger FB, Katz LM, Kleinman S, Metzel PS, Gregory KR, et al. Emerging infectious disease agents and their potential threat to transfusion safety. Transfusion. 2009;49(Suppl 2):1S–29S. PubMed PMID: 19686562. Epub 2009/08/19. eng.

9. Atreya C, Nakhasi H, Mied P, Epstein J, Hughes J, Gwinn M, et al. FDA workshop on emerging infectious diseases: evaluating emerging infectious diseases (EIDs) for transfusion safety. Transfusion. 2011;51(8):1855–71. PubMed PMID: 21392016. Epub 2011/03/12. eng.
10. Stramer SL, Dodd RY. Transfusion-transmitted emerging infectious diseases: 30 years of challenges and progress. Transfusion. 2013;53(10 Pt 2):2375–83. PubMed PMID: 23926897. Epub 2013/08/10. eng.
11. Stramer SL. Current perspectives in transfusion-transmitted infectious diseases: emerging and re-emerging infections. ISBT Sci Ser. 2014;9(1):30–6. PubMed PMID: 25210533. PMCID: PMC4142007. Epub 2014/09/12. Eng.
12. Walsh GM, Shih AW, Solh Z, Golder M, Schubert P, Fearon M, et al. Blood-Borne Pathogens: A Canadian Blood Services Centre for Innovation Symposium. Transfus Med Rev. 2016;30(2):53–68. PubMed PMID: 26962008. Epub 2016/03/11. eng.
13. US Centers for Disease Control and Prevention. Emerging Infectious Diseases. EID Journal Background and Goals. https://wwwnc.cdc.gov/eid/page/background-goals [12 February, 2017]. Available from: https://wwwnc.cdc.gov/eid/page/background-goals.
14. van Doorn HR. Emerging infectious diseases. Medicine. 2014;42(1):60–3. PubMed PMID: 24563608. PMCID: PMC3929004. Epub 2014/02/25. Eng.
15. Heymann DL, Dar OA. Prevention is better than cure for emerging infectious diseases. BMJ. 2014;348:g1499. PubMed PMID: 24563451. Epub 2014/02/25. eng.
16. Howard CR, Fletcher NF. Emerging virus diseases: can we ever expect the unexpected? Emerg Microbes Infect. 2012;1(12):e46. PubMed PMID: 26038413. PMCID: 3630908. Epub 2012/12/01. eng.
17. University of Minnesota. Centre for Disease Research and Policy. Available from: http://www.cidrap.umn.edu/infectious-disease-topics/tularemia#overview&1-3.
18. Wilson K. A framework for applying the precautionary principle to transfusion safety. Transfus Med Rev. 2011;25(3):177–83. PubMed PMID: 21429704. Epub 2011/03/25. eng.
19. Hergon E, Moutel G, Duchange N, Bellier L, Rouger P, Herve C. Risk management in transfusion after the HIV blood contamination crisis in France: the impact of the precautionary principle. Transfus Med Rev. 2005;19(4):273–80. PubMed PMID: 16214016. Epub 2005/10/11. eng.
20. Boyer-Kassem T. Is the precautionary principle really incoherent? Risk Anal. 2017;37(11):2026-34. Epub 2017/03/01. eng.
21. Peterson M. Yes, the precautionary principle is incoherent. Risk Anal. 2017;37(11):2035–8. PubMed PMID: 28230256. Epub 2017/02/24.eng.
22. Germain M, Ghibu S, Delage G. The precautionary principle in blood safety: not quite the same as aiming for zero risk. Transfus Med Rev. 2012;26(2):181–4. reply pg 4–6. PubMed PMID: 22153563. Epub 2011/12/14. eng.
23. Kramer K, Zaaijer HL, Verweij MF. The precautionary principle and the tolerability of blood transfusion risks. The American Journal of Bioethics : AJOB. 2017;17(3):32–43. PubMed PMID: 28207362. Epub 2017/02/17. eng.
24. Watkins NA, Dobra S, Bennett P, Cairns J, Turner ML. The management of blood safety in the presence of uncertain risk: a United Kingdom perspective. Transfus Med Rev. 2012;26(3):238–51. PubMed PMID: 22126710. Epub 2011/12/01. eng.
25. Stein J, Besley J, Brook C, Hamill M, Klein E, Krewski D, et al. Risk-based decision-making for blood safety: preliminary report of a consensus conference. Vox Sang. 2011;101(4):277–81. PubMed PMID: 21781125. Epub 2011/07/26. eng.
26. Leach Bennett J, Blajchman MA, Delage G, Fearon M, Devine D. Proceedings of a Consensus Conference: Risk-Based Decision Making for Blood Safety. Transfus Med Rev. 2011;25(4):267–92.
27. Alliance of Blood Operators. Risk-based decision-making framework for blood safety. v1.1, 2 April 2015. Available from: https://allianceofbloodoperators.org/media/115522/rbdm-framework-2-april-2015-v11-for-website.pdf.
28. Kleinman S, Busch MP, Korelitz JJ, Schreiber GB. The incidence/window period model and its use to assess the risk of transfusion-transmitted human immunodeficiency virus and

hepatitis C virus infection. Transfus Med Rev. 1997;11(3):155–72. PubMed PMID: 9243769. Epub 1997/07/01. eng.
29. Weusten J, Vermeulen M, van Drimmelen H, Lelie N. Refinement of a viral transmission risk model for blood donations in seroconversion window phase screened by nucleic acid testing in different pool sizes and repeat test algorithms. Transfusion. 2011;51(1):203–15. PubMed PMID: 20707858. Epub 2010/08/17. eng.
30. Weusten JJ, van Drimmelen HA, Lelie PN. Mathematic modeling of the risk of HBV, HCV, and HIV transmission by window-phase donations not detected by NAT. Transfusion. 2002;42(5):537–48. PubMed PMID: 12084161. Epub 2002/06/27. eng.
31. Yasui Y, Yanai H, Sawanpanyalert P. Tanaka H. A statistical method for the estimation of window-period risk of transfusion-transmitted HIV in donor screening under non-steady state. Biostatistics. 2002;3(1):133–43. PubMed PMID: 12933629. Epub 2003/08/23. eng.
32. Busch MP, Glynn SA, Stramer SL, Strong DM, Caglioti S, Wright DJ, et al. A new strategy for estimating risks of transfusion-transmitted viral infections based on rates of detection of recently infected donors. Transfusion. 2005;45(2):254–64. PubMed PMID: 15660836. Epub 2005/01/22. eng.
33. Custer B. Risk modelling in blood safety – review of methods, strengths and limitations. ISBT Sci Ser. 2010;5(n1):294–9.
34. Bish EK, Ragavan PK, Bish DR, Slonim AD, Stramer SL. A probabilistic method for the estimation of residual risk in donated blood. Biostatistics. 2014;15(4):620–35. PubMed PMID: 24784858. Epub 2014/05/03. eng.
35. van der Heiden M, Ritter S, Hamouda O, Offergeld R. Estimating the residual risk for HIV, HCV and HBV in different types of platelet concentrates in Germany. Vox Sang. 2015;108(2):123–30. PubMed PMID: 25335096. Epub 2014/10/22. eng.
36. Kluberg SA, Mekaru SR, McIver DJ, Madoff LC, Crawley AW, Smolinski MS, et al. Global Capacity for Emerging Infectious Disease Detection, 1996-2014. Emerg Infect Dis. 2016;22(10):E1–6. PubMed PMID: 27649306. PMCID: PMC5038396. Epub 2016/09/21. eng.
37. Scarpino SV, Meyers LA, Johansson MA. Design Strategies for Efficient Arbovirus Surveillance. Emerg Infect Dis. 2017;23(4):642–4. PubMed PMID: 28322711. Epub 2017/03/23. eng.
38. Mayer SV, Tesh RB, Vasilakis N. The emergence of arthropod-borne viral diseases: A global prospective on dengue, chikungunya and zika fevers. Acta Trop. 2017;166:155–63. PubMed PMID: 27876643. PMCID: PMC5203945. Epub 2016/11/24. eng.
39. Patterson J, Sammon M, Dengue GM. Zika and Chikungunya: Emerging Arboviruses in the New World. West J Emerg Med. 2016;17(6):671–9. PubMed PMID: 27833670. Epub 2016/11/12. eng.
40. Chua A, Prat I, Nuebling CM, Wood D, Moussy F. Update on Zika Diagnostic Tests and WHO's Related Activities. PLoS Negl Trop Dis. 2017;11(2):e0005269. PubMed PMID: 28151953. PMCID: PMC5289415. Epub 2017/02/06. eng.
41. Hanna JN, Ritchie SA, Richards AR, Humphreys JL, Montgomery BL, Ehlers GJ, et al. Dengue in north Queensland, 2005-2008. Commun Dis Intel Quart Rep. 2009;33(2):198–203. PubMed PMID: 19877538. Epub 2009/11/03. eng.
42. Ritchie SA, Pyke AT, Hall-Mendelin S, Day A, Mores CN, Christofferson RC, et al. An explosive epidemic of DENV-3 in Cairns, Australia. PLoS One. 2013;8(7):e68137. PubMed PMID: 23874522. PMCID: PMC3712959. Epub 2013/07/23. eng.
43. Faddy HM, Seed CR, Fryk JJ, Hyland CA, Ritchie SA, Taylor CT, et al. Implications of dengue outbreaks for blood supply, Australia. Emerg Infect Dis. 2013;19(5):787–9. PubMed PMID: 23648012. PMCID: PMC3647514. Epub 2013/05/08. eng.
44. Warrilow D, Northill JA, Pyke AT. Sources of dengue viruses imported into Queensland, Australia, 2002-2010. Emerg Infect Dis. 2012;18(11):1850–7. PubMed PMID: 23092682. PMCID: PMC3559152. Epub 2012/10/25. eng.
45. Seed CR, Kiely P, Hyland CA, Keller AJ. The risk of dengue transmission by blood during a 2004 outbreak in Cairns, Australia. Transfusion. 2009;49(7):1482–7. PubMed PMID: 19389025.

46. Venturi G, Zammarchi L, Fortuna C, Remoli M, Benedetti E, Fiorentini C, et al. An autochthonous case of Zika due to possible sexual transmission, Florence, Italy, 2014. Euro Surveill. 2016;21(8):pii=30148.
47. Hills SL, Russell K, Hennessey M, Williams C, Oster AM, Fischer M, et al. Transmission of Zika Virus Through Sexual Contact with Travelers to Areas of Ongoing Transmission - Continental United States, 2016. MMWR Morb Mortal Wkly Rep. 2016;65(8):215–6. PubMed PMID: 26937739. Epub 2016/03/05. eng.
48. D'Ortenzio E, Matheron S, Yazdanpanah Y, de Lamballerie X, Hubert B, Piorkowski G, et al. Evidence of Sexual Transmission of Zika Virus. N Engl J Med. 2016;374(22):2195–8. PubMed PMID: 27074370. Epub 2016/04/14. eng.
49. Deckard DT, Chung WM, Brooks JT, Smith JC, Woldai S, Hennessey M, et al. Male-to-male sexual transmission of Zika virus – Texas, January 2016. MMWR Morb Mortal Wkly Rep. 2016;65(14):372–4. PubMed PMID: 27078057. Epub 2016/04/15. eng.
50. Davidson A, Slavinski S, Komoto K, Rakeman J, Weiss D. Suspected female-to-male sexual transmission of Zika Virus — New York City, 2016. Morb Mortal Wkly Rep. 2016;65:716–7.
51. Musso D, Nhan T, Robin E, Roche C, Bierlaire D, Zisou K, et al. Potential for Zika virus transmission through blood transfusion demonstrated during an outbreak in French Polynesia, November 2013 to February 2014. Euro Surveill. 2014;19(14):pii:20761. PubMed PMID: 24739982. Epub 2014/04/18. eng.
52. Chuang V, Wong TY, Leung YH, Ma E, Law YL, Tsang O, et al. Review of dengue fever cases in Hong Kong during 1998 to 2005. Hong Kong Med J. 2008;14(3):170–7. PubMed PMID: 18525084. Epub 2008/06/06. eng.
53. Tambyah PA, Koay ES, Poon ML, Lin RV, Ong BK. Dengue hemorrhagic fever transmitted by blood transfusion. N Engl J Med. 2008;359(14):1526–7. PubMed PMID: 18832256. Epub 2008/10/04. eng.
54. Linnen JM, Vinelli E, Sabino EC, Tobler LH, Hyland C, Lee TH, et al. Dengue viremia in blood donors from Honduras, Brazil, and Australia. Transfusion. 2008;48(7):1355–62. PubMed PMID: 18503610. Epub 2008/05/28. eng.
55. Mohammed H, Linnen JM, Munoz-Jordan JL, Tomashek K, Foster G, Broulik AS, et al. Dengue virus in blood donations, Puerto Rico, 2005. Transfusion. 2008;48(7):1348–54. PubMed PMID: 18503611. Epub 2008/05/28. eng.
56. Teo D, Ng LC, Lam S. Is dengue a threat to the blood supply? Transfus Med. 2009;19(2):66–77. PubMed PMID: 19392949. PMCID: PMC2713854. Epub 2009/04/28. eng.
57. Lanteri MC, Busch MP. Dengue in the context of "safe blood" and global epidemiology: to screen or not to screen? Transfusion. 2012;52(8):1634–9. PubMed PMID: 22882092. PMCID: PMC3509801. Epub 2012/08/14. eng.
58. Lanteri MC, Kleinman SH, Glynn SA, Musso D, Keith Hoots W, Custer BS, et al. Zika virus: a new threat to the safety of the blood supply with worldwide impact and implications. Transfusion. 2016;56(7):1907–14. PubMed PMID: 27282638. Epub 2016/06/11. Eng.
59. Stramer S, Linnen M, Carrick M, Bentsen C, Krysztof P, Hunsperger E, et al. Dengue donor viremia determined by RNA and NS1 antigen, and detection of dengue transfusion transmission during the 2007 dengue outbreak in Puerto Rico (abstract). Vox Sang. 2010;99(Supplement 1):32.
60. Transfusion-associated transmission of West Nile virus—Arizona, 2004. MMWR Morb Mortal Wkly Rep. 2004;53(36):842–4. PubMed PMID: 15371966. Epub 2004/09/17. eng.
61. West Nile virus transmission through blood transfusion--South Dakota, 2006. MMWR Morb Mortal Wkly Rep. 2007;56(4):76–9. PubMed PMID: 17268405. Epub 2007/02/03. eng.
62. Montgomery SP, Brown JA, Kuehnert M, Smith TL, Crall N, Lanciotti RS, et al. Transfusion-associated transmission of West Nile virus, United States 2003 through 2005. Transfusion. 2006;46(12):2038–46. PubMed PMID: 17176314. Epub 2006/12/21. eng.
63. West Nile virus transmission via organ transplantation and blood transfusion - Louisiana, 2008. MMWR Morb Mortal Wkly Rep. 2009;58(45):1263–7. PubMed PMID: 19940831. Epub 2009/11/27. eng.

64. Marka A, Diamantidis A, Papa A, Valiakos G, Chaintoutis SC, Doukas D, et al. West Nile virus state of the art report of MALWEST Project. Int J Environ Res Public Health. 2013;10(12):6534–610. PubMed PMID: 24317379. PMCID: PMC3881129. Epub 2013/12/10. eng.
65. Fatal West Nile virus infection after probable transfusion-associated transmission--Colorado, 2012. MMWR Morb Mortal Wkly Rep. 2013;62(31):622–4. PubMed PMID: 23925171. Epub 2013/08/09. eng.
66. Groves JA, Shafi H, Nomura JH, Herron RM, Baez D, Dodd RY, et al. A probable case of West Nile virus transfusion transmission. Transfusion. 2017;57(3pt2):850–6. PubMed PMID: 28164314. Epub 2017/02/07. eng.
67. Dodd RY, Foster GA, Stramer SL. Keeping Blood Transfusion Safe From West Nile Virus: American Red Cross Experience, 2003 to 2012. Transfus Med Rev. 2015;29(3):153–61. PubMed PMID: 25841631. Epub 2015/04/07. eng.
68. Barjas-Castro ML, Angerami RN, Cunha MS, Suzuki A, Nogueira JS, Rocco IM, et al. Probable transfusion-transmitted Zika virus in Brazil. Transfusion. 2016;56(7):1684–8. PubMed PMID: 27329551. Epub 2016/06/23. eng.
69. Reuters. Brazil reports Zika infection from blood transfusions. 4 February, 2016. 2016. Available from: http://www.reuters.com/article/us-health-zika-brazil-blood-idUSKC-N0VD22N.
70. Musso D, Aubry M, Broult J, Stassinopoulos A, Green J. Zika virus: new emergencies, potential for severe complications, and prevention of transfusion-transmitted Zika fever in the context of co-circulation of arboviruses. Blood Transfus. 2017;15(3):272–3. PubMed PMID: 27177409. Epub 2016/05/14. Eng.
71. Outbreak News Today. Transfusion-associated Zika virus reported in Brazil. Posted by Robert Herriman on December 18, 2015. Available from: http://outbreaknewstoday.com/transfusion-associated-zika-virus-reported-in-brazil-76935/.
72. Motta IJ, Spencer BR, Cordeiro da Silva SG, Arruda MB, Dobbin JA, Gonzaga YB, et al. Evidence for transmission of Zika virus by platelet transfusion. N Engl J Med. 2016;375(11):1101–3. PubMed PMID: 27532622. Epub 2016/08/18. Eng.
73. Sabino EC, Loureiro P, Lopes ME, Capuani L, McClure C, Chowdhury D, et al. Transfusion-Transmitted Dengue and Associated Clinical Symptoms During the 2012 Epidemic in Brazil. J Infect Dis. 2016;213(5):694–702. PubMed PMID: 26908780. PMCID: PMC4747611. Epub 2016/02/26. eng.
74. Candotti D, Etiz N, Parsyan A, Allain JP. Identification and characterization of persistent human erythrovirus infection in blood donor samples. J Virol. 2004;78(22):12169–78. PubMed PMID: 15507603. PMCID: PMC525065. Epub 2004/10/28. eng.
75. Kleinman SH, Glynn SA, Lee TH, Tobler L, Montalvo L, Todd D, et al. Prevalence and quantitation of parvovirus B19 DNA levels in blood donors with a sensitive polymerase chain reaction screening assay. Transfusion. 2007;47(10):1756–64. PubMed PMID: 17880600. Epub 2007/09/21. eng.
76. Kooistra K, Mesman HJ, de Waal M, Koppelman MH, Zaaijer HL. Epidemiology of high-level parvovirus B19 viraemia among Dutch blood donors, 2003-2009. Vox Sang. 2011;100(3):261–6. PubMed PMID: 20946549. Epub 2010/10/16. eng.
77. Lee TH, Kleinman SH, Wen L, Montalvo L, Todd DS, Wright DJ, et al. Distribution of parvovirus B19 DNA in blood compartments and persistence of virus in blood donors. Transfusion. 2011;51(9):1896–908. PubMed PMID: 21303368. PMCID: PMC3591477. Epub 2011/02/10. eng.
78. Matsukura H, Shibata S, Tani Y, Shibata H, Furuta RA. Persistent infection by human parvovirus B19 in qualified blood donors. Transfusion. 2008;48(5):1036–7. PubMed PMID: 18454740. Epub 2008/05/06. eng.
79. Schmidt M, Themann A, Drexler C, Bayer M, Lanzer G, Menichetti E, et al. Blood donor screening for parvovirus B19 in Germany and Austria. Transfusion. 2007;47(10):1775–82. PubMed PMID: 17714425. Epub 2007/08/24. eng.

80. Thomas I, Di Giambattista M, Gerard C, Mathys E, Hougardy V, Latour B, et al. Prevalence of human erythrovirus B19 DNA in healthy Belgian blood donors and correlation with specific antibodies against structural and non-structural viral proteins. Vox Sang. 2003;84(4):300–7. PubMed PMID: 12757504. Epub 2003/05/22. eng.
81. Soucie JM, De Staercke C, Monahan PE, Recht M, Chitlur MB, Gruppo R, et al. Evidence for the transmission of parvovirus B19 in patients with bleeding disorders treated with plasma-derived factor concentrates in the era of nucleic acid test screening. Transfusion. 2013;53(6):1217–25. PubMed PMID: 22998193. PMCID: PMC4519820. Epub 2012/09/25. eng.
82. Hourfar MK, Mayr-Wohlfart U, Themann A, Sireis W, Seifried E, Schrezenmeier H, et al. Recipients potentially infected with parvovirus B19 by red blood cell products. Transfusion. 2011;51(1):129–36. PubMed PMID: 20663115. Epub 2010/07/29. eng.
83. Satake M, Hoshi Y, Taira R, Momose SY, Hino S, Tadokoro K. Symptomatic parvovirus B19 infection caused by blood component transfusion. Transfusion. 2011;51(9):1887–95. PubMed PMID: 21332725. Epub 2011/02/22. eng.
84. US Food and Drug Administration. Guidance for Industry: Nucleic Acid Testing (NAT) to Reduce the Possible Risk of Parvovirus B19V Transmission by Plasma-Derived Products. July 2009. http://www.fda.gov/BiologicsBloodVaccines/GuidanceComplianceRegulatoryInformation/Guidances/Blood/ucm071592.htm.
85. World Health Organisation. Screening donated blood for transfusion transmissible infections. Recommedations. 2010. Available from: http://apps.who.int/iris/bitstream/10665/44202/1/9789241547888_eng.pdf.
86. Adegoke AO, Akanni OE. Survival of Treponema pallidum in banked blood for prevention of Syphilis transmission. N Am J Med Sci. 2011;3(7):329–32. PubMed PMID: 22540107. PMCID: PMC3336882. Epub 2012/04/28. eng.
87. Hewitt PE, Davison K, Howell DR, Taylor GP. Human T-lymphotropic virus lookback in NHS Blood and Transplant (England) reveals the efficacy of leukoreduction. Transfusion. 2013;53(10):2168–75. PubMed PMID: 23384161. Epub 2013/02/07. eng.
88. Marano G, Vaglio S, Pupella S, Facco G, Catalano L, Piccinini V, et al. Human T-lymphotropic virus and transfusion safety: does one size fit all? Transfusion. 2016;56(1):249–60. PubMed PMID: 26388300. Epub 2015/09/22. eng.
89. Murphy EL. Infection with human T-lymphotropic virus types-1 and -2 (HTLV-1 and -2): Implications for blood transfusion safety. Transfus Clin Biol. 2016;23(1):13–9. PubMed PMID: 26778839. PMCID: PMC5042452. Epub 2016/01/19. eng.
90. Adler SP, Nigro G. Prevention of maternal-fetal transmission of cytomegalovirus. Clin Infect Dis. 2013;57(Suppl 4):S189–92. PubMed PMID: 24257425. Epub 2013/12/07. eng.
91. Ljungman P. Risk of cytomegalovirus transmission by blood products to immunocompromised patients and means for reduction. Br J Haematol. 2004;125(2):107–16. PubMed PMID: 15059132. Epub 2004/04/03. eng.
92. Vamvakas EC. Is white blood cell reduction equivalent to antibody screening in preventing transmission of cytomegalovirus by transfusion? A review of the literature and meta-analysis. Transfus Med Rev. 2005;19(3):181–99. PubMed PMID: 16010649. Epub 2005/07/13. eng.
93. Roback JD, Josephson CD. New insights for preventing transfusion-transmitted cytomegalovirus and other white blood cell–associated viral infections. Transfusion. 2013;53(10):2112–6.
94. Ziemann M, Hennig H. Prevention of Transfusion-Transmitted Cytomegalovirus Infections: Which is the Optimal Strategy? Transfus Med Hemother. 2014;41(1):40–4. PubMed PMID: 24659946. PMCID: PMC3949610. Epub 2014/03/25. eng.
95. Seed CR, Wong J, Polizzotto MN, Faddy H, Keller AJ, Pink J. The residual risk of transfusion-transmitted cytomegalovirus infection associated with leucodepleted blood components. Vox Sang. 2015;109(1):11–7. PubMed PMID: 25854287.
96. Operskalski EA. HHV-8, transfusion, and mortality. J Infect Dis. 2012;206(10):1485–7. PubMed PMID: 22949305. Epub 2012/09/06. eng.
97. Qu L, Triulzi DJ, Rowe DT, Griffin DL, Donnenberg AD. Stability of lymphocytes and Epstein-Barr virus during red blood cell storage. Vox Sang. 2007;92(2):125–9. PubMed PMID: 17298574. Epub 2007/02/15. eng.

98. Qu L, Rowe DT, Donnenberg AD, Griffin DL, Triulzi DJ. Effects of storage and leukoreduction on lymphocytes and Epstein-Barr virus genomes in platelet concentrates. Transfusion. 2009;49(8):1580–3. PubMed PMID: 19413731. PMCID: PMC4165079. Epub 2009/05/06. eng.
99. Di Minno G, Perno CF, Tiede A, Navarro D, Canaro M, Guertler L, et al. Current concepts in the prevention of pathogen transmission via blood/plasma-derived products for bleeding disorders. Blood Rev. 2016;30(1):35–48. PubMed PMID: 26381318. Epub 2015/09/19. eng.
100. Burnouf T. Plasma fractionation. ISBT Science Series. 2012;7(1):62–7.
101. Burnouf T. Current status and new developments in the production of plasma derivatives. ISBT Science Series. 2016;11(S2):18–25.
102. Burnouf T, Radosevich M. Reducing the risk of infection from plasma products: specific preventative strategies. Blood Rev. 2000;14(2):94–110. PubMed PMID: 11012252. Epub 2000/09/30. eng.
103. CSL Behring. Virus inactivation/removal & prion removal. Available from: http://www.cslbehring.com/quality-safety/integrated-safety-system/virus-inactivation.htm.
104. Gray TJ, Webb CE. A review of the epidemiological and clinical aspects of West Nile virus. Int J Gen Med. 2014;7:193–203. PubMed PMID: 24748813. PMCID: PMC3990373. Epub 2014/04/22. eng.
105. Sejvar JJ. Clinical manifestations and outcomes of West Nile virus infection. Viruses. 2014;6(2):606–23. PubMed PMID: 24509812. PMCID: PMC3939474. Epub 2014/02/11. eng.
106. Prow NA, Edmonds JH, Williams DT, Setoh YX, Bielefeldt-Ohmann H, Suen WW, et al. Virulence and Evolution of West Nile Virus, Australia, 1960-2012. Emerg Infect Dis. 2016;22(8):1353–62. PubMed PMID: 27433830. PMCID: PMC4982165. Epub 2016/07/21. eng.
107. Musso D, Gubler DJ. Zika virus. Clin Microbiol Rev. 2016;29(3):487–524. PubMed PMID: 27029595. Epub 2016/04/01. eng.
108. Cao-Lormeau VM, Blake A, Mons S, Lastere S, Roche C, Vanhomwegen J, et al. Guillain-Barre Syndrome outbreak associated with Zika virus infection in French Polynesia: a case-control study. Lancet. 2016;387(10027):1531–9. PubMed PMID: 26948433. Epub 2016/03/08. eng.
109. Ladhani SN, O'Connor C, Kirkbride H, Brooks T, Morgan D. Outbreak of Zika virus disease in the Americas and the association with microcephaly, congenital malformations and Guillain-Barre syndrome. Arch Dis Child. 2016;101(7):600–2. PubMed PMID: 26998633. Epub 2016/03/22. eng.
110. Dirlikov E, Major CG, Mayshack M, Medina N, Matos D, Ryff KR, et al. Guillain-Barre Syndrome During Ongoing Zika Virus Transmission - Puerto Rico, January 1-July 31, 2016. MMWR Morb Mortal Wkly Rep. 2016;65(34):910–4. PubMed PMID: 27584942. Epub 2016/09/02. Eng.
111. Pacheco O, Beltran M, Nelson CA, Valencia D, Tolosa N, Farr SL, et al. Zika Virus Disease in Colombia - Preliminary Report. N Engl J Med. 2016. 10.1056/NEJMoa1604037 Jun 15. PubMed PMID: 27305043. Epub 2016/06/16. Eng.
112. de Araujo TV, Rodrigues LC, de Alencar Ximenes RA, de Barros Miranda-Filho D, Montarroyos UR, de Melo AP, et al. Association between Zika virus infection and microcephaly in Brazil, January to May, 2016: preliminary report of a case-control study. Lancet Infect Dis. 2016;16(12):1356–63. https://doi.org/10.1016/S1473-3099. Sep 15. PubMed PMID: 27641777. Epub 2016/09/20. Eng.
113. Watrin L, Ghawche F, Larre P, Neau JP, Mathis S, Fournier E. Guillain-Barre Syndrome (42 Cases) Occurring During a Zika Virus Outbreak in French Polynesia. Medicine (Baltimore). 2016;95(14):e3257. PubMed PMID: 27057874. Epub 2016/04/09. eng.
114. Magalhaes-Barbosa MC, Prata-Barbosa A, Robaina JR, Raymundo CE, Lima-Setta F, Cunha AJ. Trends of the microcephaly and Zika virus outbreak in Brazil, January-July 2016. Travel Med Infect Dis. 2016;14(5):458–63. PubMed PMID: 27057874. Epub 2016/10/25. Eng.

115. Heuft HG, Berg T, Schreier E, Kunkel U, Tacke M, Schwella N, et al. Epidemiological and clinical aspects of hepatitis G virus infection in blood donors and immunocompromised recipients of HGV-contaminated blood. Vox Sang. 1998;74(3):161–7. PubMed PMID: 9595643. Epub 1998/05/22. eng.
116. Bernardin F, Operskalski E, Busch M, Delwart E. Transfusion transmission of highly prevalent commensal human viruses. Transfusion. 2010;50(11):2474–83. PubMed PMID: 20497515. Epub 2010/05/26. eng.
117. Theze J, Lowes S, Parker J, Pybus OG. Evolutionary and phylogenetic analysis of the hepaciviruses and pegiviruses. Genome Biol Evol. 2015;7(11):2996–3008. PubMed PMID: 26494702. Epub 2015/10/24. eng.
118. Leary TP, Muerhoff AS, Simons JN, Pilot-Matias TJ, Erker JC, Chalmers ML, et al. Sequence and genomic organization of GBV-C: a novel member of the flaviviridae associated with human non-A-E hepatitis. J Med Virol. 1996;48(1):60–7. PubMed PMID: 8825712. Epub 1996/01/01. eng.
119. Chivero ET, Stapleton JT. Tropism of human pegivirus (formerly known as GB virus C/hepatitis G virus) and host immunomodulation: insights into a highly successful viral infection. J Gen Virol. 2015;96(Pt 7):1521–32. PubMed PMID: 25667328. Epub 2015/02/11. eng.
120. Kleinman S. Hepatitis G virus biology, epidemiology, and clinical manifestations: Implications for blood safety. Transfus Med Rev. 2001;15(3):201–12. PubMed PMID: 11471122. Epub 2001/07/27. eng.
121. Stapleton JT, Foung S, Muerhoff AS, Bukh J, Simmonds P. The GB viruses: a review and proposed classification of GBV-A, GBV-C (HGV), and GBV-D in genus Pegivirus within the family Flaviviridae. J Gen Virol. 2011;92(Pt 2):233–46. PubMed PMID: 21084497. PMCID: PMC3081076. Epub 2010/11/19. eng.
122. Bruhn R, Lelie N, Busch M, Kleinman S. Relative efficacy of nucleic acid amplification testing and serologic screening in preventing hepatitis C virus transmission risk in seven international regions. Transfusion. 2015;55(6):1195–205. PubMed PMID: 25727549. Epub 2015/03/03. eng.
123. Kiely P, Gambhir M, Cheng AC, McQuilten ZK, Seed CR, Wood EM. Emerging infectious diseases and blood safety: modeling the transfusion-transmission risk. Transfus Med Rev. 2017;31(3):154–64. PubMed PMID: 28545882. Epub 2017/05/27. eng.
124. Biggerstaff BJ, Petersen LR. Estimated risk of West Nile virus transmission through blood transfusion during an epidemic in Queens, New York City. Transfusion. 2002;42(8):1019–26. PubMed PMID: 12385413. Epub 2002/10/19. eng.
125. Biggerstaff BJ, Petersen LR. Estimated risk of transmission of the West Nile virus through blood transfusion in the US, 2002. Transfusion. 2003;43(8):1007–17. PubMed PMID: 12869104. Epub 2003/07/19. eng.
126. Oei W, Janssen MP, van der Poel CL, van Steenbergen JE, Rehmet S, Kretzschmar ME. Modeling the transmission risk of emerging infectious diseases through blood transfusion. Transfusion. 2013;53(7):1421–8. PubMed PMID: 23113823. Epub 2012/11/02. eng.
127. European Up-Front Risk Assessment Tool (EUFRAT) User Manual. Document TTA20151215EUM. Available from: http://eufrattool.ecdc.europa.eu/docs/EUFRAT_User_Manual.pdf.
128. Custer B. Assessing the risk of transfusion-transmitted emerging infectious diseases. ISBT Sci Ser. 2016;11(S2):79–85.
129. Teo D. Emerging and imported infections in the region – what's bothering us today? ISBT Sci Ser. 2014;9(1):141–7.
130. Petersen LR, Powers AM. Chikungunya: epidemiology. F1000 Research. 2016;5. PubMed PMID: 26918158. PMCID: PMC4754000. Epub 2016/02/27. eng.
131. Thiboutot MM, Kannan S, Kawalekar OU, Shedlock DJ, Khan AS, Sarangan G, et al. Chikungunya: a potentially emerging epidemic? PLoS Negl Trop Dis. 2010;4(4):e623. PubMed PMID: 20436958. PMCID: PMC2860491. Epub 2010/05/04. eng.

132. Nsoesie EO, Kraemer MU, Golding N, Pigott DM, Brady OJ, Moyes CL, et al. Global distribution and environmental suitability for chikungunya virus, 1952 to 2015. Euro Surveill. 2016;21(20). PubMed PMID: 27239817. PMCID: PMC4902126. Epub 2016/05/31. eng.
133. Simon F, Javelle E, Oliver M, Leparc-Goffart I, Marimoutou C. Chikungunya virus infection. Curr Infect Dis Rep. 2011;13(3):218–28. PubMed PMID: 21465340. PMCID: PMC3085104. Epub 2011/04/06. eng.
134. Gallian P, Leparc-Goffart I, Richard P, Maire F, Flusin O, Djoudi R, et al. Epidemiology of Chikungunya virus outbreaks in Guadeloupe and Martinique, 2014: An observational study in volunteer blood donors. PLoS Negl Trop Dis. 2017;11(1):e0005254. PubMed PMID: 28081120. PMCID: PMC5230756. Epub 2017/01/13. eng.
135. Riswari SF, Ma'roef CN, Djauhari H, Kosasih H, Perkasa A, Yudhaputri FA, et al. Study of viremic profile in febrile specimens of chikungunya in Bandung, Indonesia. J Clin Virol. 2016;74:61–5. PubMed PMID: 26679829. Epub 2015/12/19. eng.
136. Appassakij H, Khuntikij P, Kemapunmanus M, Wutthanarungsan R, Silpapojakul K. Viremic profiles in asymptomatic and symptomatic chikungunya fever: a blood transfusion threat? Transfusion. 2013;53(10 Pt 2):2567–74. PubMed PMID: 23176378. Epub 2012/11/28. eng.
137. Burt FJ, Chen W, Miner JJ, Lenschow DJ, Merits A, Schnettler E, et al. Chikungunya virus: an update on the biology and pathogenesis of this emerging pathogen. Lancet Infect Dis. 2017;17(4):e107–e17. PubMed PMID: 28159534. Epub 2017/02/06. eng.
138. Yoon I-K, Alera MT, Lago CB, Tac-An IA, Villa D, Fernandez S, et al. High rate of subclinical chikungunya virus infection and association of neutralizing antibody with protection in a prospective cohort in the Philippines. PLoS Negl Trop Dis. 2015;9(5):e0003764.
139. Petersen LR, Epstein JS. Chikungunya virus: new risk to transfusion safety in the Americas. Transfusion. 2014;54(8):1911–5. PubMed PMID: 25130331. Epub 2014/08/19. eng.
140. Whitehorn J, Kien DT, Nguyen NM, Nguyen HL, Kyrylos PP, Carrington LB, et al. Comparative Susceptibility of Aedes albopictus and Aedes aegypti to Dengue Virus Infection After Feeding on Blood of Viremic Humans: Implications for Public Health. J Infect Dis. 2015;212(8):1182–90. PubMed PMID: 25784733. PMCID: PMC4577038. Epub 2015/03/19. eng.
141. Messina JP, Brady OJ, Scott TW, Zou C, Pigott DM, Duda KA, et al. Global spread of dengue virus types: mapping the 70 year history. Trends Microbiol. 2014;22(3):138–46. PubMed PMID: 24468533. PMCID: PMC3946041. Epub 2014/01/29. eng.
142. Murgue B, Roche C, Chungue E, Deparis X. Prospective study of the duration and magnitude of viraemia in children hospitalised during the 1996-1997 dengue-2 outbreak in French Polynesia. J Med Virol. 2000;60(4):432–8. PubMed PMID: 10686027. Epub 2000/02/24. eng.
143. Guzman MG, Gubler DJ, Izquierdo A, Martinez E, Halstead SB. Dengue infection. Nat Rev Dis Primers. 2016;2:16055. PubMed PMID: 27534439. Epub 2016/08/19. eng.
144. Gubler DJ. Dengue and dengue hemorrhagic fever. Clin Microbiol Rev. 1998;11(3):480–96. PubMed PMID: 9665979. PMCID: PMC88892. Epub 1998/07/17. eng.
145. Busch MP, Sabino EC, Brambilla D, Lopes ME, Capuani L, Chowdhury D, et al. Duration of Dengue Viremia in Blood Donors and Relationships Between Donor Viremia, Infection Incidence and Clinical Case Reports During a Large Epidemic. J Infect Dis. 2016;214(1):49–54. PubMed PMID: 27302934. PMCID: PMC4907419. Epub 2016/06/16. eng.
146. Rodriguez-Figueroa L, Rigau-Perez JG, Suarez EL, Reiter P. Risk factors for dengue infection during an outbreak in Yanes, Puerto Rico in 1991. Am J Trop Med Hyg. 1995;52(6):496–502. PubMed PMID: 7611553. Epub 1995/06/01. eng.
147. Endy TP, Anderson KB, Nisalak A, Yoon IK, Green S, Rothman AL, et al. Determinants of inapparent and symptomatic dengue infection in a prospective study of primary school children in Kamphaeng Phet. Thailand PLoS Negl Trop Dis. 2011;5(3):e975. PubMed PMID: 21390158. PMCID: PMC3046956. Epub 2011/03/11. eng.
148. Burke DS, Nisalak A, Johnson DE, Scott RM. A prospective study of dengue infections in Bangkok. The American Journal of Tropical Medicine and Hygiene. 1988;38(1):172–80.

149. Stramer SL, Linnen JM, Carrick JM, Foster GA, Krysztof DE, Zou S, et al. Dengue viremia in blood donors identified by RNA and detection of dengue transfusion transmission during the 2007 dengue outbreak in Puerto Rico. Transfusion. 2012;52(8):1657–66. PubMed PMID: 22339201. Epub 2012/02/22. eng.
150. Levi JE, Nishiya A, Felix AC, Salles NA, Sampaio LR, Hangai F, et al. Real-time symptomatic case of transfusion-transmitted dengue. Transfusion. 2015;55(5):961–4. PubMed PMID: 25605570. Epub 2015/01/22. eng.
151. Oh HB, Muthu V, Daruwalla ZJ, Lee SY, Koay ES, Tambyah PA. Bitten by a bug or a bag? Transfusion-transmitted dengue: a rare complication in the bleeding surgical patient. Transfusion. 2015;55(7):1655–61. PubMed PMID: 25728040. Epub 2015/03/03. eng.
152. Matos D, Tomashek KM, Perez-Padilla J, Munoz-Jordan J, Hunsperger E, Horiuchi K, et al. Probable and possible transfusion-transmitted dengue associated with NS1 antigen-negative but RNA confirmed-positive red blood cells. Transfusion. 2016;56(1):215–22. PubMed PMID: 26469514. Epub 2015/10/16. eng.
153. David S, Abraham AM. Epidemiological and clinical aspects on West Nile virus, a globally emerging pathogen. Infect Dis. 2016;48(8):571–86. PubMed PMID: 27207312. Epub 2016/05/22. eng.
154. Chancey C, Grinev A, Volkova E, Rios M. The global ecology and epidemiology of West Nile virus. Biomed Res Int. 2015;2015:376230. PubMed PMID: 25866777. PMCID: PMC4383390. Epub 2015/04/14. eng.
155. Goldblum N, Sterk VV, Jasinskaklingberg W. The natural history of West Nile fever. II. Virological findings and the development of homologous and heterologous antibodies in West Nile infection in man. Am J Hyg. 1957;66(3):363–80. PubMed PMID: 13478585. Epub 1957/11/01. eng.
156. Southam CM, Moore AE. Induced virus infections in man by the Egypt isolates of West Nile virus. Am J Trop Med Hyg. 1954;3(1):19–50. PubMed PMID: 13114588. Epub 1954/01/01. eng.
157. Busch MP, Kleinman SH, Tobler LH, Kamel HT, Norris PJ, Walsh I, et al. Virus and antibody dynamics in acute west nile virus infection. J Infect Dis. 2008;198(7):984–93. PubMed PMID: 18729783. Epub 2008/08/30. eng.
158. Meny GM, Santos-Zabala L, Szallasi A, Stramer SL. West Nile virus infection transmitted by granulocyte transfusion. Blood. 2011;117(21):5778–9. PubMed PMID: 21617013. Epub 2011/05/28. eng.
159. Vorou R. Zika virus, vectors, reservoirs, amplifying hosts, and their potential to spread worldwide: what we know and what we should investigate urgently. Int J Infect Dis. 2016;48:85–90. PubMed PMID: 27208633. Epub 2016/05/22. eng.
160. Aziz H, Zia A, Anwer A, Aziz M, Fatima S, Faheem M. Zika virus: Global health challenge, threat and current situation. J Med Virol. 2017;89(6):943–51. PubMed PMID: 27862008. Epub 2016/11/20. eng.
161. Song BH, Yun SI, Woolley M, Lee YM. Zika virus: History, epidemiology, transmission, and clinical presentation. J Neuroimmunol. 2017;308:50–64. PubMed PMID: 28285789. Epub 2017/03/14. eng.
162. Plourde AR, Bloch EMA. Literature Review of Zika Virus. Emerg Infect Dis. 2016;22(7):1185–92. PubMed PMID: 27070380. Epub 2016/04/14. eng.
163. Lessler J, Ott CT, Carcelen AC, Konikoff JM, Williamson J, Bi Q, et al. Times to key events in Zika virus infection and implications for blood donation: a systematic review. Bull World Health Organ. 2016;94(11):841–9. PubMed PMID: 27821887. PMCID: PMC5096355. Epub 2016/11/09. Eng.
164. Krow-Lucal ER, Biggerstaff BJ, Staples JE. Estimated incubation period for Zika Virus disease. Emerg Infect Dis. 2017;23(5):841–5. PubMed PMID: 28277198. Epub 2017/03/10. eng.
165. Jean Michel M, Catherine M, Christophe P, Sabine C-R, Pierre D, Guillaume M-B, et al. Zika virus infection and prolonged viremia in wholeblood specimens. Emerg Infect Dis J. 2017;23(5):863–5.

166. Lustig Y, Mendelson E, Paran N, Melamed S, Schwartz E. Detection of Zika virus RNA in whole blood of imported Zika virus disease cases up to 2 months after symptom onset, Israel, December 2015 to April 2016. Euro Surveill. 2016;21(26). PubMed PMID: 27386894. Epub 2016/07/09. eng.
167. Froeschl G, Huber K, von Sonnenburg F, Nothdurft HD, Bretzel G, Hoelscher M, et al. Long-term kinetics of Zika virus RNA and antibodies in body fluids of a vasectomized traveller returning from Martinique: a case report. BMC Infect Dis. 2017;17(1):55. PubMed PMID: 28068904. PMCID: PMC5223480. Epub 2017/01/11. eng.
168. Duffy MR, Chen TH, Hancock WT, Powers AM, Kool JL, Lanciotti RS, et al. Zika virus outbreak on Yap Island, Federated States of Micronesia. N Engl J Med. 2009;360(24):2536–43. PubMed PMID: 19516034. Epub 2009/06/12. eng.
169. Khuroo MS, Khuroo MS, Hepatitis E. an emerging global disease - from discovery towards control and cure. J Viral Hepat. 2016;23(2):68–79. PubMed PMID: 26344932. Epub 2015/09/08. eng.
170. Perez-Gracia MT, Mateos Lindemann ML. Caridad Montalvo Villalba M. Hepatitis E: current status. Rev Med Virol. 2013;23(6):384–98. PubMed PMID: 24038432. Epub 2013/09/17. eng.
171. Dalton HR, Seghatchian J. Hepatitis E virus: Emerging from the shadows in developed countries. Transfus Apher Sci. 2016;55(3):271–4. PubMed PMID: 27843081. Epub 2016/11/16. eng.
172. Khuroo MS, Khuroo MS, Khuroo NS. Transmission of hepatitis E virus in developing countries. Viruses. 2016;8(9). PubMed PMID: 27657112. PMCID: PMC5035967. Epub 2016/09/23. eng.
173. Sayed IM, Vercouter AS, Abdelwahab SF, Vercauteren K, Meuleman P. Is hepatitis E virus an emerging problem in industrialized countries? Hepatology. 2015;62(6):1883–92. PubMed PMID: 26175182. Epub 2015/07/16. eng.
174. Marano G, Vaglio S, Pupella S, Facco G, Bianchi M, Calizzani G, et al. Hepatitis E: an old infection with new implications. Blood Transfus. 2015;13(1):6–17. PubMed PMID: 25369613. PMCID: PMC4317085. Epub 2014/11/05. eng.
175. Vollmer T, Diekmann J, Eberhardt M, Knabbe C, Dreier J. Hepatitis E in blood donors: investigation of the natural course of asymptomatic infection, Germany, 2011. Euro Surveill. 2016;21(35). PubMed PMID: 27608433. PMCID: PMC5015460. Epub 2016/09/09. eng.
176. Scobie L, Dalton HR, Hepatitis E. source and route of infection, clinical manifestations and new developments. J Viral Hepat. 2013;20(1):1–11. PubMed PMID: 23231079. Epub 2012/12/13. eng.
177. Guillois Y, Abravanel F, Miura T, Pavio N, Vaillant V, Lhomme S, et al. High Proportion of Asymptomatic Infections in an Outbreak of Hepatitis E Associated With a Spit-Roasted Piglet, France, 2013. Clin Infect Dis. 2016;62(3):351–7. PubMed PMID: 26429341. Epub 2015/10/03. eng.
178. Said B, Ijaz S, Kafatos G, Booth L, Thomas HL, Walsh A, et al. Hepatitis E outbreak on cruise ship. Emerg Infect Dis. 2009;15(11):1738–44. PubMed PMID: 19891860. PMCID: PMC2857258. Epub 2009/11/07. eng.
179. Matsubayashi K, Nagaoka Y, Sakata H, Sato S, Fukai K, Kato T, et al. Transfusion-transmitted hepatitis E caused by apparently indigenous hepatitis E virus strain in Hokkaido. Japan Transfusion. 2004;44(6):934–40. PubMed PMID: 15157263. Epub 2004/05/26. eng.
180. Khuroo MS, Kamili S, Yattoo GN. Hepatitis E virus infection may be transmitted through blood transfusions in an endemic area. J Gastroenterol Hepatol. 2004;19(7):778–84. PubMed PMID: 15209625. Epub 2004/06/24. eng.
181. Fukuda S, Sunaga J, Saito N, Fujimura K, Itoh Y, Sasaki M, et al. Prevalence of antibodies to hepatitis E virus among Japanese blood donors: identification of three blood donors infected with a genotype 3 hepatitis E virus. J Med Virol. 2004;73(4):554–61. PubMed PMID: 15221899. Epub 2004/06/29. eng.

182. Boxall E, Herborn A, Kochethu G, Pratt G, Adams D, Ijaz S, et al. Transfusion-transmitted hepatitis E in a 'nonhyperendemic' country. Transfus Med. 2006;16(2):79–83. PubMed PMID: 16623913. Epub 2006/04/21. eng.
183. Colson P, Coze C, Gallian P, Henry M, De Micco P, Tamalet C. Transfusion-associated hepatitis E, France. Emerg Infect Dis. 2007;13(4):648–9. PubMed PMID: 17561564. PMCID: PMC2725983. Epub 2007/06/15. eng.
184. Matsubayashi K, Kang JH, Sakata H, Takahashi K, Shindo M, Kato M, et al. A case of transfusion-transmitted hepatitis E caused by blood from a donor infected with hepatitis E virus via zoonotic food-borne route. Transfusion. 2008;48(7):1368–75. PubMed PMID: 18651907. Epub 2008/07/25. eng.
185. Mallet V, Sberro-Soussan R, Vallet-Pichard A, Roque-Afonso AM, Pol S. Transmission of hepatitis E virus by plasma exchange: a case report. Ann Intern Med. 2016;164(12):851–2. PubMed PMID: 26926359. Epub 2016/03/02. eng.
186. Riveiro-Barciela M, Sauleda S, Quer J, Salvador F, Gregori J, Piron M, et al. Red blood cell transfusion-transmitted acute hepatitis E in an immunocompetent subject in Europe: a case report. Transfusion. 2017;57(2):244–7. PubMed PMID: 27785789. Epub 2016/10/28. eng.
187. Loyrion E, Trouve-Buisson T, Pouzol P, Larrat S, Decaens T, Payen JF. Hepatitis E virus infection after platelet transfusion in an immunocompetent trauma patient. Emerg Infect Dis. 2017;23(1):146–7. PubMed PMID: 27983485. PMCID: PMC5176217. Epub 2016/12/17. eng.
188. Hoad VC, Gibbs T, Ravikumara M, Nash M, Levy A, Tracy SL, et al. First confirmed case of transfusion-transmitted hepatitis E in Australia. Med J Aust. 2017;206(7):289–90. PubMed PMID: 28403756. Epub 2017/04/14. eng.
189. Vannier E, Krause PJ. Human babesiosis. N Engl J Med. 2012;366(25):2397–407. PubMed PMID: 22716978. Epub 2012/06/22. eng.
190. Vannier EG, Diuk-Wasser MA, Ben Mamoun C, Babesiosis KPJ. Infect Dis Clin N Am. 2015;29(2):357–70. PubMed PMID: 25999229. PMCID: PMC4458703. Epub 2015/05/23. eng.
191. Herwaldt BL, Linden JV, Bosserman E, Young C, Olkowska D, Wilson M. Transfusion-associated babesiosis in the United States: a description of cases. Ann Intern Med. 2011;155(8):509–19. PubMed PMID: 21893613. Epub 2011/09/07. eng.
192. Leiby DA, Johnson ST, Won KY, Nace EK, Slemenda SB, Pieniazek NJ, et al. A longitudinal study of Babesia microti infection in seropositive blood donors. Transfusion. 2014;54(9):2217–25. PubMed PMID: 24673297. PMCID: PMC4772885. Epub 2014/03/29. eng.
193. Bloch EM, Levin AE, Williamson PC, Cyrus S, Shaz BH, Kessler D, et al. A prospective evaluation of chronic Babesia microti infection in seroreactive blood donors. Transfusion. 2016;56(7):1875–82. PubMed PMID: 27184253. Epub 2016/05/18. eng.
194. Krause PJ, McKay K, Gadbaw J, Christianson D, Closter L, Lepore T, et al. Increasing health burden of human babesiosis in endemic sites. Am J Trop Med Hyg. 2003;68(4):431–6. PubMed PMID: 12875292. Epub 2003/07/24. eng.
195. Vannier E, Gewurz BE, Krause PJ. Human babesiosis. Infect Dis Clin N Am. 2008;22(3):469–88. viii-ix. PubMed PMID: 18755385. PMCID: PMC3998201. Epub 2008/08/30. eng.
196. Pace D. Leishmaniasis. J Inf Secur. 2014;69(Suppl 1):S10–8. PubMed PMID: 25238669. Epub 2014/09/23. eng.
197. Alvar J, Velez ID, Bern C, Herrero M, Desjeux P, Cano J, et al. Leishmaniasis worldwide and global estimates of its incidence. PLoS One. 2012;7(5):e35671. PubMed PMID: 22693548. PMCID: PMC3365071. Epub 2012/06/14. eng.
198. Pigott DM, Bhatt S, Golding N, Duda KA, Battle KE, Brady OJ, et al. Global distribution maps of the leishmaniases. eLife, vol. 3; 2014. PubMed PMID: 24972829. PMCID: PMC4103681. Epub 2014/06/29. eng.
199. Ready PD. Epidemiology of visceral leishmaniasis. Clin Epidemiol. 2014;6:147–54. PubMed PMID: 24833919. PMCID: PMC4014360. Epub 2014/05/17. eng.

200. Saporito L, Giammanco GM, De Grazia S, Colomba C. Visceral leishmaniasis: host-parasite interactions and clinical presentation in the immunocompetent and in the immunocompromised host. Int J Infect Dis. 2013;17(8):e572–6. PubMed PMID: 23380419. Epub 2013/02/06. eng.
201. Ameen M. Cutaneous leishmaniasis: advances in disease pathogenesis, diagnostics and therapeutics. Clin Exp Dermatol. 2010;35(7):699–705. PubMed PMID: 20831602. Epub 2010/09/14. eng.
202. Mansueto P, Seidita A, Vitale G, Cascio A. Transfusion transmitted leishmaniasis. What to do with blood donors from endemic areas? Travel Med Infect Dis. 2014;12(6 Pt A):617–27. PubMed PMID: 25459431. Epub 2014/12/03. eng.
203. Jimenez-Marco T, Fisa R, Girona-Llobera E, Cancino-Faure B, Tomas-Perez M, Berenguer D, et al. Transfusion-transmitted leishmaniasis: a practical review. Transfusion (Paris). 2016;56(Suppl 1):S45–51. PubMed PMID: 27001361. Epub 2016/03/24. eng.
204. White NJ, Pukrittayakamee S, Hien TT, Faiz MA, Mokuolu OA, Dondorp AM. Malaria. Lancet. 2014;383(9918):723–35. PubMed PMID: 23953767. Epub 2013/08/21. eng.
205. World Malaria Report 2016. Geneva: World Health Organization; 2016. Licence: CC BY-NC-SA 3.0 IGO. Available from: http://apps.who.int/iris/bitstream/10665/252038/1/9789241511711-eng.pdf?ua=1.
206. Centers for Disease Control and Prevention. Malaria. Available from: https://www.cdc.gov/malaria/about/disease.html.
207. Lindblade KA, Steinhardt L, Samuels A, Kachur SP, Slutsker L. The silent threat: asymptomatic parasitemia and malaria transmission. Expert Rev Anti-Infect Ther. 2013;11(6):623–39. PubMed PMID: 23750733. Epub 2013/06/12. eng.
208. Bousema T, Okell L, Felger I, Drakeley C. Asymptomatic malaria infections: detectability, transmissibility and public health relevance. Nat Rev Microbiol. 2014;12(12):833–40. PubMed PMID: 25329408. Epub 2014/10/21. eng.
209. Galatas B, Bassat Q, Mayor A. Malaria Parasites in the Asymptomatic: Looking for the Hay in the Haystack. Trends Parasitol. 2016;32(4):296–308. PubMed PMID: 26708404. Epub 2015/12/29. eng.
210. Nansseu JR, Noubiap JJ, Ndoula ST, Zeh AF, Monamele CG. What is the best strategy for the prevention of transfusion-transmitted malaria in sub-Saharan African countries where malaria is endemic? Malar J. 2013;12:465. PubMed PMID: 24373501. PMCID: PMC3877868. Epub 2014/01/01. eng.
211. Kitchen AD, Chiodini PL. Malaria and blood transfusion. Vox Sang. 2006;90(2):77–84. PubMed PMID: 16430664. Epub 2006/01/25. eng.
212. Justi SA, Galvao C. The Evolutionary Origin of Diversity in Chagas Disease Vectors. Trends Parasitol. 2017;33(1):42–52. PubMed PMID: 27986547. Epub 2016/12/18. eng.
213. Bern C. Chagas' Disease. N Engl J Med. 2015;373(19):1882. PubMed PMID: 26535522. Epub 2015/11/05. eng.
214. Centers for Disease Control. Parasites - American Trypanosomiasis (also known as Chagas Disease). Available from: https://www.cdc.gov/parasites/chagas/epi.html.
215. Benjamin RJ, Stramer SL, Leiby DA, Dodd RY, Fearon M, Castro E. Trypanosoma cruzi infection in North America and Spain: evidence in support of transfusion transmission. Transfusion. 2012;52(9):1913–21. quiz 2. PubMed PMID: 22321142. Epub 2012/02/11. eng.
216. Castro E. Chagas' disease: lessons from routine donation testing. Transfus Med. 2009;19(1):16–23. PubMed PMID: 19302451. Epub 2009/03/24. eng.
217. Murray KO, Mertens E, Despres P. West Nile virus and its emergence in the United States of America. Vet Res. 2010;41(6):67. PubMed PMID: 21188801. PMCID: PMC2913730. Epub 2010/12/29. eng.
218. Brouard C, Bernillon P, Quatresous I, Pillonel J, Assal A, De Valk H, et al. Estimated risk of Chikungunya viremic blood donation during an epidemic on Reunion Island in the Indian Ocean, 2005 to 2007. Transfusion. 2008;48(7):1333–41. PubMed PMID: 18298600. Epub 2008/02/27. eng.

219. Appassakij H, Promwong C, Rujirojindakul P, Wutthanarungsan R, Silpapojakul K. The risk of blood transfusion-associated Chikungunya fever during the 2009 epidemic in Songkhla Province, Thailand. Transfusion. 2014;54(8):1945–52. PubMed PMID: 24527811. Epub 2014/02/18. eng.
220. Liumbruno GM, Calteri D, Petropulacos K, Mattivi A, Po C, Macini P, et al. The Chikungunya epidemic in Italy and its repercussion on the blood system. Blood Transfus. 2008;6(4):199–210. PubMed PMID: 19112735. PMCID: PMC2626913. Epub 2008/12/31. eng.
221. Perevoscikovs J, Lenglet A, Lucenko I, Steinerte A, Payne Hallstrom L, Coulombier D. Assessing the risk of a community outbreak of hepatitis A on blood safety in Latvia, 2008. Euro Surveill. 2010;15(33):19640. PubMed PMID: 20739001. Epub 2010/08/27. eng.
222. Shang G, Seed CR, Gahan ME, Rolph MS, Mahalingam S. Duration of Ross River viraemia in a mouse model--implications for transfusion transmission. Vox Sang. 2012;102(3):185–92. PubMed PMID: 21923861. Epub 2011/09/20. eng.
223. Seed CR, Hoad VC, Faddy HM, Kiely P, Keller AJ, Pink J. Re-evaluating the residual risk of transfusion-transmitted Ross River virus infection. Vox Sang. 2016;110(4):317–23. PubMed PMID: 26748600. Epub 2016/01/11. eng.
224. Niederhauser C, Fontana S, Glauser A, Steinemann C, Koller A. West Nile Virus preparedness plan to ensure safe blood components in Switzerland: a risk-based approach. ISBT Sci Ser. 2017;12(2):314–21.
225. Mapako T, Oei W, van Hulst M, Kretzschmar ME, Janssen MP. Modelling the risk of transfusion transmission from travelling donors. BMC Infect Dis. 2016;16:143. PubMed PMID: 27038919. PMCID: PMC4818889. Epub 2016/04/04. eng.
226. Oei W, Lieshout-Krikke RW, Kretzschmar ME, Zaaijer HL, Coutinho RA, Eersel M, et al. Estimating the risk of dengue transmission from Dutch blood donors travelling to Suriname and the Dutch Caribbean. Vox Sang. 2016;110(4):301–9. PubMed PMID: 26765798. Epub 2016/01/15. eng.
227. Oei W, Kretzschmar ME, Zaaijer HL, Coutinho R, van der Poel CL, Janssen MP. Estimating the transfusion transmission risk of Q fever. Transfusion. 2014;54(7):1705–11. PubMed PMID: 24456030. Epub 2014/01/25. eng.
228. Wilder-Smith A, Chen LH, Massad E, Wilson ME. Threat of dengue to blood safety in dengue-endemic countries. Emerg Infect Dis. 2009;15(1):8–11. PubMed PMID: 19116042. PMCID: PMC2660677. Epub 2009/01/01. eng.
229. Weinstein P, Weinstein SR, Rowe RJ. Transfusions: how many cases of Ross River virus infection do we cause? Med J Aust. 1995;163(5):276. PubMed PMID: 7565220. Epub 1995/09/04. eng.
230. Hoad VC, Seed C, Fryk JJ, Harley R, Flower R, Hogema B, et al. Hepatitis E virus RNA in Australian blood donors: prevalence and risk assessment. Vox Sang. 2017;112(7):614–21.
231. Custer B, Hoch JS. Cost-effectiveness analysis: what it really means for transfusion medicine decision making. Transfus Med Rev. 2009;23(1):1–12. PubMed PMID: 19056030. Epub 2008/12/06. eng.
232. Menitove JE, Leach Bennett J, Tomasulo P, Katz LM. How safe is safe enough, who decides and how? From a zero-risk paradigm to risk-based decision making. Transfusion. 2014;54(3 Pt 2):753–7. PubMed PMID: 24617628. Epub 2014/03/13. eng.
233. Kramer K, Verweij MF, Zaaijer HL. An inventory of concerns behind blood safety policies in five Western countries. Transfusion. 2015;55(12):2816–25. PubMed PMID: 26331441. Epub 2015/09/04. eng.
234. Kiely P. Screening blood donors for hepatitis C virus: the challenge to consider cost-effectiveness. Transfusion. 2015;55(6):1143–6. PubMed PMID: 26074174. Epub 2015/06/16. eng.
235. Kramer K, Verweij MF, Zaaijer HL. Are there ethical differences between stopping and not starting blood safety measures?. Vox Sang. 2017;112(5):417–24. PubMed PMID: 28466467. Epub 2017/05/04. eng.

236. Verweij M, Kramer K. Donor blood screening and moral responsibility: how safe should blood be?. J Med Ethics. 2016; 44(3):187–91. PubMed PMID: 26868666. Epub 2016/02/13. eng.
237. Lee D. Perception of blood transfusion risk. Transfus Med Rev. 2006;20(2):141–8. PubMed PMID: 16565026. Epub 2006/03/28. eng.
238. Fu KW, Liang H, Saroha N, Tse ZT, Ip P, Fung IC. How people react to Zika virus outbreaks on Twitter? A computational content analysis. Am J Infect Control. 2016;44(12):1700–2. PubMed PMID: 27566874. Epub 2016/08/28. eng.
239. Sharma M, Yadav K, Yadav N, Ferdinand KC. Zika virus pandemic-analysis of Facebook as a social media health information platform. Am J Infect Control. 2017;45(3):301–2. PubMed PMID: 27776823. Epub 2016/10/26. eng.
240. Southwell BG, Dolina S, Jimenez-Magdaleno K, Squiers LB, Kelly BJ. Zika Virus-related news coverage and online behavior, United States, Guatemala, and Brazil. Emerg Infect Dis. 2016;22(7):1320–1. PubMed PMID: 27100826. PMCID: PMC4918164. Epub 2016/04/22. eng.
241. Venkatraman A, Mukhija D, Kumar N, Nagpal SJ. Zika virus misinformation on the internet. Travel Med Infect Dis. 2016;14(4):421–2. PubMed PMID: 27267799. Epub 2016/06/09. Eng.
242. Neslo RE, Oei W, Janssen MP. Insight into "Calculated Risk": an application to the prioritization of emerging infectious diseases for blood transfusion safety. Risk Anal. 2017;37(9):1783–95. PubMed PMID: 28229466. Epub 2017/02/24. eng.
243. Oei W, Neslo R, Janssen MP. A consensus-based tool for ranking the risk of blood-transmissible infections. Transfusion. 2016;56(8):2108–14. PubMed PMID: 27217225. Epub 2016/05/25. eng.
244. U.S. Food and Drug Administration (FDA). Revised Recommendations for Reducing the Risk of Zika Virus Transmission by Blood and Blood Components. Guidance for Industry. August 2016. Available from: http://www.fda.gov/ucm/groups/fdagov-public/@fdagov-biogen/documents/document/ucm518213.pdf.
245. Katz LM, Rossmann SN. Zika and the Blood Supply: A Work in Progress. Arch Pathol Lab Med. 2017;141(1):85–92. PubMed PMID: 27788336. Epub 2016/10/28. Eng.
246. International Committee on Taxonomy of Viruses. Available from: http://www.ictvonline.org/virusTaxonomy.asp?bhcp=1.
247. Harley D, Sleigh A, Ritchie S. Ross River virus transmission, infection, and disease: a cross-disciplinary review. Clin Microbiol Rev. 2001;14(4):909–32. table of contents. PubMed PMID: 11585790. PMCID: PMC89008. Epub 2001/10/05. eng.
248. Lau C, Aubry M, Musso D, Teissier A, Paulous S, Despres P, et al. New evidence for endemic circulation of Ross River virus in the Pacific Islands and the potential for emergence. Int J Infect Dis. 2017;57:73–6. PubMed PMID: 28188934. Epub 2017/02/12. eng.
249. Aubry M, Finke J, Teissier A, Roche C, Broult J, Paulous S, et al. Silent circulation of Ross River virus in French Polynesia. Int J Infect Dis. 2015;37:19–24. PubMed PMID: 26086687. Epub 2015/06/19. eng.
250. Victoria State Government - Health.Vic. Ross River virus disease. Available from: https://www2.health.vic.gov.au/public-health/infectious-diseases/disease-information-advice/ross-river-virus.
251. Australian Government. Department of Health. Notifiable Diseases Surveillance System. Available from: http://www9.health.gov.au/cda/source/cda-index.cfm.
252. Seed CR, Kiely P, Hoad VC, Keller AJ. Refining the risk estimate for transfusion-transmission of occult hepatitis B virus. Vox Sang. 2017;112(1):3–8. PubMed PMID: 27564651. Epub 2016/08/27. eng.
253. Hoad VC, Speers DJ, Keller AJ, Dowse GK, Seed CR, Lindsay MD, et al. First reported case of transfusion-transmitted Ross River virus infection. Med J Aust. 2015;202(5):267–70. PubMed PMID: 25758699. Epub 2015/03/12. eng.

254. Pan American Health Organisation. Number of Reported Cases of Chikungunya Fever in the Americas, by Country or Territory 2017 (to week noted). Epidemiological Week / EW 21 (Updated as of 26 May 2017). Available from: http://www.paho.org/hq/index.php?option=com_docman&task=doc_view&Itemid=270&gid=40264&lang=en.
255. Faddy H, Dunford M, Seed C, Olds A, Harley D, Dean M, et al. Seroprevalence of Antibodies to Ross River and Barmah Forest Viruses: Possible Implications for Blood Transfusion Safety After Extreme Weather Events. EcoHealth. 2015;12(2):347–53. PubMed PMID: 25537629. Epub 2014/12/30. eng.
256. Faddy HM, Tran T, Seed C, Hoad VC, Chan HT, Harley R, et al. Ross River virus in 'at-risk' Australian blood donors: implications for blood supply safety. Vox Sang. 2016;111. (Suppl. 1:75.

Part II
Case Studies

Chapter 6
HIV and Blood Safety

Mrigender Virk and Hua Shan

Introduction

On June 5, 1981, the Centers for Disease Control and Prevention (CDC) reported five cases of pneumocystis pneumonia in young homosexual males living in Los Angeles. This report, printed in *Morbidity and Mortality Weekly Report* (MMWR), was the first publication of patients with acquired immune deficiency syndrome (AIDS) in the USA [1]. Although nearly 2 years would pass before the cause, human immunodeficiency virus (HIV), was discovered, a string of infections would reach national spotlight and mark the beginning of an epidemic.

History of HIV

Molecular phylogenetics has demonstrated that HIV infections in humans likely resulted from a zoonotic transfer and mutation of a related retrovirus found in non-human primates, simian immunodeficiency virus (SIV) [2]. This transfer occurred in equatorial Africa in the late nineteenth or early twentieth centuries and is due to a multitude of factors affecting the region at that time. Humans may have been exposed to SIV in the distant past through "bushmeat" hunting practices, but colonization, urbanization, and changing social practices in the 1900s created an avenue for rapid transmission and evolution of the virus in human hosts. Other theories suggest that an increase in unsterile needle use occurred in this timeframe due to

---

M. Virk
Department of Pathology, Stanford Hospital, Stanford, CA, USA

H. Shan (✉)
Department of Pathology, Stanford University, Stanford, CA, USA
e-mail: hshan@stanfordhealthcare.org

© Springer International Publishing AG, part of Springer Nature 2019
H. Shan, R. Y. Dodd (eds.), *Blood Safety*,
https://doi.org/10.1007/978-3-319-94436-4_6

new vaccination campaigns, and all of these events collectively may have allowed SIV to reach an infectivity threshold and transform into the virus responsible for AIDS.

Analyses of preserved blood samples show that the earliest documented HIV infection occurred in the city of Leopoldville in the Belgian Congo and spread along the Congo River, western coast of Africa, and along Belgian railways. Geographic mapping of the spread of HIV outside of Africa demonstrates an arrival and epidemic in Haiti around 1966 and spread to the USA in or around 1969 [3]. Due to the long incubation period for HIV, which can be a decade or longer, the virus spread without detection until the 1980s. Soon after the initial CDC report in MMWR, major newspapers published the story, and physicians across the nation began reporting similar cases. By the end of 1981, there were 270 reports of opportunistic infections and immune deficiency in homosexual males in the USA, and nearly 50% had died.

With continued reporting of otherwise healthy homosexual males developing opportunistic infections, it was theorized that this syndrome had a basis in sexual transmission and was initially termed gay-related immunodeficiency, or GRID, by federal epidemiologists [4]. No infectious agent had yet been identified as the cause, but cluster studies of individuals with the syndrome pointed the CDC in that direction. Along with opportunistic infections, physicians began finding the syndrome to be associated with Kaposi sarcoma, anemia, immune thrombocytopenia, and various additional malignancies [5–7]. It was soon realized that this disease was not just occurring in homosexual males and the term acquired immune deficiency syndrome was adopted. Dr. Bruce Chabner of the National Cancer Institute (NCI) said that the problem had grown and was now "of concern to all Americans."

The "4H Disease"

Homosexuality and IV drug use soon became apparent risk factors in patients with AIDS, but a new group, Haitians, would be the next to fall under scientific scrutiny [8–11]. In another CDC MMWR, a report of 35 cases of AIDS was described in Haitian immigrants, of which none were homosexual and only one reported IV drug use [12]. Although there was likely a higher prevalence of HIV in Haitians at the time due to the migration pattern of the virus, this report made physicians and the public hyperaware of the group and contributed to widespread discrimination. Haiti responded to these reports by forming the Haitian Group for the Study of Kaposi's Sarcoma and Opportunistic Infections (GHESKIO) and published the first case series on the epidemic. The researchers retrospectively examined 61 cases of AIDS and found that the risk factors for these patients were identical to those in the USA. The majority were male and lived in a suburb of Port-au-Prince where prostitution was widespread [13]. The prevalence of HIV in Haiti continued to rise over the decades, reaching 8% in the country's capital, but heterosexual intercourse was the dominant mode of transmission, and so the demographics of those infected trended more toward females instead of males as the years passed [14, 15].

In July of 1982, the CDC released a report of three cases of *Pneumocystis carinii* pneumonia in patients with hemophilia A [16]. The editorial note from this report stated that the

> clinical and immunologic features these three patients share are strikingly similar to those recently observed among certain individuals from the following groups: homosexual males, heterosexuals who abuse IV drugs, and Haitians who recently entered the United States. Although the cause of the severe immune dysfunction is unknown, the occurrence among the three hemophiliac cases suggests the possible transmission of an agent through blood products.

This report would have a lasting impact on the patient populations identified as being at risk for AIDS and initiating the discussion of the involvement of blood products in disease transmission. AIDS soon carried a label as the "4H disease" and with it the social stigma for homosexuals, Haitians, hemophiliacs, and heroin addicts.

Transfusion-Transmissible Disease

Early in the epidemic, it was estimated that approximately 5% of patients with symptoms consistent with AIDS did not fit within any of the recognized risk groups. It wasn't until an infant with erythroblastosis fetalis developed the disease that a blood-borne infectious agent with the ability to be transmitted by transfusion was given credence [17]. The infant showed laboratory evidence of hypergammaglobulinemia, T-cell depletion and dysfunction, and autoimmune thrombocytopenia. These findings were not characteristic of any known congenital syndromes at the time, and a retrospective review of the patient's exchange transfusions was initiated [18]. One unit of platelets was identified that came from a male donor who was asymptomatic at the time of donation but subsequently was diagnosed with AIDS. This report was a pivotal moment in the epidemic because it not only identified the possibility of a transfusion-transmitted etiology but also suggested that the incubation period for the infectious agent may be relatively long. There was general consensus that AIDS was caused by an infectious agent and was tentatively referred to as the "AIDS agent." There was enough anecdotal evidence at this point for the Assistant Secretary for Health to gather an advisory committee to discuss the situation at hand. The Blood Product Advisory Committee (BPAC) would meet for the first time in 1982 and continue to monitor events through the epidemic.

This epidemic could not have occurred at a more inopportune time. President Ronald Reagan and his administration were brought into office due to their campaigns for reducing government regulations, and major public health organizations were undergoing changes in leadership. The country had lost confidence in the CDC after the swine flu epidemic in 1976, during which time the federal government initiated a mass immunization campaign for an infection that failed to be substantial. The effort was successful in immunizing 40 million Americans against swine flu, but the disease never spread, and links to Guillain-Barré cast a shadow on public health officials, with a loss of credibility that would spill over into the emergence of HIV [19].

The CDC held its first public meeting in Atlanta on January 4, 1983. The meeting was attended by the National Institute of Health (NIH); the Food and Drug Administration (FDA); blood bank organizations including the American Association of Blood Banks (AABB), the American Red Cross (ARC), and the Council of Community Blood Centers (CCBC); the National Hemophilia Foundation (NHF); the American Blood Resources Association (ABRA); and the National Gay Task Force. Dr. Donald Francis from the CDC, one of the first scientists to suggest an infectious etiology for AIDS, presented the epidemiology of the disease and suggested that blood banks question donors about their sexual history and defer those who fall into high-risk groups. He also suggested implementation of a test for hepatitis B core antibody (anti-HBc) as a surrogate marker for AIDS. It had been suggested that hepatitis B core antibody had a 90% correlation with patients who had AIDS, demonstrating a possible screening tool until the "AIDS agent" could be identified [20]. Unfortunately, this correlation did not mean the test would be specific, and this was one of many points from the meeting that were met with resistance. Additionally, this claim from the CDC was not presented with published data, which led to further skepticism from other committees. The meeting laid the groundwork for the future of HIV screening, and there was agreement that it would be desirable to eliminate high-risk donors, but there was no consensus on how this would be achieved.

Each of the strategies postulated by the workgroup had pros and cons. Education and voluntary donor deferral allowed high-risk groups to play an active role in protecting the blood supply and was inexpensive, but could not ensure compliance. Questioning donors as a part of the health history could be easily implemented in the current process but was seen as insensitive and unethical. Homosexual activist groups strongly opposed this proposal and felt that this would institutionalize the discrimination they were already facing at the time. The blood bank community was also opposed to this strategy, as they had transitioned from paid to volunteer donors in the 1970s and such an intrusive health history questionnaire could destroy relationships with donors and lead to blood shortages [21]. The third strategy, testing units for anti-HBc, faced the strongest resistance from the blood bank community. It was presented as a surrogate screening tool with a high sensitivity, but this added costs and deferral of many acceptable donors without strong evidence to warrant implementation. In attempts to prevent a new epidemic with donor deferrals and increased testing, there was significant controversy over the rights of the individual and judicious use of resources versus overall public health concerns.

Statements and Recommendations

Soon after this meeting, the AABB, ARC, and CCBC released a joint statement with their perspective:

The possibility of blood borne transmission, still unproven, has been raised. This latter impression is reinforced by eight confirmed cases in hemophiliacs treated with antihemophilic factor (AHF) concentrate, by a case in a newborn infant who received 19 units of blood components, one of which was from a donor who later died of AIDS, and by fewer than 10 unconfirmed case reports in other transfusion recipients. No agent has been isolated and there is no test for the disease or for potential carriers. Evidence of transmission by blood transfusion is inconclusive.

Although the statement opened with a sense of uncertainty regarding AIDS being acquired from transfusions, there was adequate acknowledgment of the possibility and suggested measures to be taken by public health authorities and blood banks [22]. These measures focused on risk/benefit assessment in the use of blood products and reasonable attempts to decrease blood donations from individuals in high-risk groups. This statement did not propose direct questioning of donors about their sexual history but instead suggested evaluating for the earliest symptoms of AIDS, such as night sweats, unexplained fevers, lymphadenopathy, and unexpected weight loss. Additionally, the statement did not advise routine testing by surrogate markers but did support allocation of federal funds to further research the cause of AIDS and how it is transmitted.

The community of blood banks faced a major dilemma in this moment, balancing patient safety based on limited medical evidence while dealing with political, legal, and ethical issues. Blood banks were confronted with immense federal and public pressure to deliver the safest product possible but risked alienation of certain groups and a shortage of blood products. It was estimated that homosexual males constituted up to 15% of the donor population, and further risk stratification within the group may be necessary to reduce the toll on the donor population [23].

The NHF followed up soon after with their recommendations and outlined patient groups in which cryoprecipitate should be used for treatment instead of antihemophilic factor (AHF). These groups included children less than 4 years of age, newly diagnosed patients, and those with mild hemophilia [24]. This recommendation was based on the smaller donor pool contributing to cryoprecipitate transfusions as opposed to AHF. The group also made recommendations for concentrate manufacturers to make serious efforts to reduce exposure from high-risk donor groups and for blood banks to adjust processing to accommodate for the increased demands for cryoprecipitate.

Finally, on March 4, 1983, the CDC released their report of inter-agency recommendations to prevent the spread of AIDS [25]. This report outlined the current data on the disease, described the parallel to hepatitis B, and highlighted the long latency period of the suspected infection. The report acknowledged the fact that the cause remained unknown and that this compromised the ability to take preventative measures but made the following recommendations based on available evidence:

1. Sexual contact should be avoided with persons known or suspected to have AIDS.
2. Members of groups at increased risk for AIDS should refrain from donating plasma and/or blood.
3. Studies should be conducted to evaluate screening procedures for their effectiveness in identifying and excluding plasma and blood with a high probability of transmitting AIDS.

4. Physicians should adhere strictly to medical indications for transfusions, and autologous blood transfusions are encouraged.
5. Work should continue toward development of safer blood products for use by hemophilia patients.

Later that month, Dr. Petricciani, Director of the FDA, published letters to establishments collecting blood and source plasma and manufacturers of plasma derivatives [26–28]. These letters stressed the implementation of education for donors from high-risk groups, standard procedures for donor evaluation, and quarantining of products collected from individuals suspected to have AIDS. Many public health officials were disappointed with the limited strength and scale of the recommendations from the above groups, but this was consistent with the limited knowledge and evidence on AIDS at the time.

By June of 1983, 1601 cases of AIDS had been reported to the CDC, of which 94% occurred in patients belonging to the 4 previously identified risk groups [29]. Over the course of the epidemic to that point, more than ten million patients had been transfused blood products, but only 15 cases of possible transfusion-associated AIDS had been reported. This was recognized in a second joint statement from the blood bank community, which stated that "the risk of possible transfusion-associated AIDS is on the order of one case per million patients transfused" [29]. The statement was issued primarily to combat a growing public perception of the association between all blood transfused and AIDS, but this quoted statistic would create a long-lasting controversy due to the true risk of transmission which was not apparent at the time. Although the apparent rate of transfusion-associated AIDS appeared to be very low in 1983, many scientists and physicians worried that the latency period was causing serious underestimation of the actual risk level.

Surrogate Screening Tests

Authorities encouraged studies to evaluate screening methodologies and other procedures to eliminate high-risk donations, but during the early years of the epidemic, all federal funding was allocated for epidemiologic research and surveillance [30]. Many blood centers were more concerned about the blood supply than the stance taken by the joint statement and initiated their own pilot studies. The New York Blood Center implemented confidential unit deferral by the donor, Irwin Memorial Blood Bank studied anti-HBc as a surrogate marker, and Stanford University Blood Bank tested CD4/CD8 ratios to eliminate patients with AIDS.

Several immunologic studies of AIDS patients in the early 1980s identified particular immune profiles that were suggested as early indicators of the disease [32–34]. These included low total lymphocyte count (<1500 cells/cmm), decreased CD4/CD8 ratios (<0.9), and positive circulating immune complexes. The Stanford University Blood Bank was already conducting immunology research unrelated to AIDS in 1983, so this study was easily implemented. The study ran for 2 years, between July 1983 and June 1985, during which time a total of 33,831 blood donations were screened for T-lymphocyte ratios. This led to discarding of 586 donations with CD4/CD8 ratios less than or equal to 0.85 [35]. Only a fraction of this data was available for review during national meetings in 1983, but Dr. Edgar Engleman, the Director of the Stanford University Blood Bank, strongly encouraged the blood bank community to adopt similar testing. Unfortunately, wide-scale implementation would have required costly equipment, and many were not convinced by the benefits. Serum samples from the discarded donations were retained for testing after discovery of HIV, and 1.9% of those were found to be positive. This translates into approximately 11 infected donations which would have been split into 3 components each, potentially preventing transmission of HIV in 33 patients [35].

The CDC's initial claims that 90% of patients with AIDS would test positive with anti-HBc soon came under scrutiny as different groups showed varying results. Irwin Memorial Blood Bank ran their pilot study for 3 months and found that 6% of all donors tested positive for anti-HBc. The frequency of anti-HBc was higher in males than females, but the frequency was more correlated to ethnic origin than sexual preference [31]. Dr. Herbert Perkins, Director of the Irwin Memorial Blood Bank, concluded that the test did not have a clear benefit in preventing transmission of AIDS and exclusion of 6% of donors would have a substantial negative impact on the donor pool.

The BPAC would meet again in December of 1983 to review available data and discuss possibilities of surrogate tests to prevent the spread of AIDS from blood donations. This meeting largely concentrated on the results of anti-HBc testing and ultimately resulted in the majority being opposed to the implementation. CDC data showed that 84% of homosexual males tested positive for anti-HBc and that 96% of IV drug users were also positive. This reflected a high sensitivity, but the test was not very specific [31]. Representatives at the meeting who opposed the testing cited the variability in positive tests based on region and ethnicity and the inability of the test to distinguish high-risk homosexuals who had multiple partners from those who were low risk. There was also speculation that centers that had implemented anti-HBc screening were attracting high-risk individuals who were seeking test results. Therefore, prevalence statistics may be biased, and the blood donor centers may be inherently increasing the risk of transfusion-transmitted diseases. Also, the elimination of certain immigrant ethnic groups based on previous hepatitis B infection and anti-HBc seropositivity would reduce availability of rare blood types needed to treat that patient population.

The committee would form a task force specifically dedicated to the evaluation of surrogate testing, but this may have been more beneficial and effective if created after the initial meeting almost a year earlier. The task force examined all additional data on the subject, including a large study out of the University of New Mexico that looked at various surrogate tests including total lymphocyte count, T-lymphocyte ratios, anti-HBc, cytomegalovirus (CMV), herpes, and circulating immune complexes [36]. This study concluded that none of the tests showed significant correlation and that surrogate tests for AIDS were nonspecific and not helpful in screening blood donor units. The task force was unable to support the use of any surrogate markers, but the discussion would soon become obsolete as researchers were on the verge of characterizing HIV. Later (1986), anti-HBc was implemented in donor screening as a surrogate screening test for non-A and non-B hepatitis.

Discovery of HIV

Isolation of the virus that causes AIDS was marked by innovative research, worldwide interest, and significant controversy surrounding key roles in the discovery. On May 20, 1983, Dr. Luc Montagnier's lab at the Pasteur Institute in France published a report in *Science* describing a new retrovirus that was isolated from a lymph node of a patient with signs of AIDS [37]. They described the virus as belonging to a recently classified group of T-lymphotropic viruses but distinct from HTLV-I that had been isolated by Dr. Robert Gallo's lab just a few years earlier [38]. Lymphocytes containing the new virus did not react with p19 and p24 antibodies (donated by Dr. Gallo's lab), whereas lymphocytes harboring HTLV-I as a control were strongly reactive. Dr. Montagnier's lab called this virus the lymphadenopathy-associated virus (LAV) and suggested that it may be the cause of AIDS.

Dr. Gallo and his associates made significant contributions to the study of T lymphocytes, identifying T-cell growth factor (TCGF, later renamed interleukin-2) and making it possible to grow the cells in culture [39]. Almost a year after the report was published from the Pasteur Institute, Dr. Gallo published an article describing their work in isolating a retrovirus and determining its association with patients diagnosed with AIDS [40]. They were able to produce large amounts of the virus by growing it in an immortalized T-cell clone which allowed for more accurate characterization. Dr. Gallo called this virus HTLV-III but acknowledged in the report that LAV had not been grown in enough quantity to be isolated and compared. Additional research from Dr. Gallo's lab that was published at the same time grew peripheral blood lymphocytes from patients with AIDS and detected HTLV-III in a significant number of cases [41]. Serum samples from these patients also detected antibodies to HTLV-III at a rate significantly higher than normal controls. This work established that HTLV-III was the primary cause of AIDS and identified a method to produce large amounts of the virus for further investigation.

Dr. Jay Levy at the University of California, San Francisco, would also isolate the virus in 1984 and named it AIDS-associated retrovirus [42]. Gene sequencing of the various isolates would come to show that these were all variants of the same virus, showing up to 6% divergence in nucleotides [43]. These differences were all found to be located in the *env* gene which codes for the exterior proteins of the virus and still proves to be the greatest obstacle in creating a vaccine. The International Committee on Taxonomy of Viruses would later conclude that none of the initially proposed names would be kept and the new retrovirus would be called HIV.

HIV Screening Tests

Due to the isolation of the virus responsible for AIDS, the blood bank community and plasma manufacturers had more reason to resist implementation of testing surrogate markers and await a more specific screening test. By June of 1984, the NIH had developed a screening test that detected antibodies to HIV and selected companies that would make it commercially available. The FDA received an application for licensing this test in December of 1984, but it wasn't until March of 1985 that the licenses were granted and the test could be made available to blood banks (Fig. 6.1). Nearly 2 years had passed since the initial report of discovery of the virus to the implementation of a screening test.

The first licensed test was an enzyme-linked immunosorbent assay (ELISA). It is an antibody detection test that has a high sensitivity (97%) but was known to give false-positive results in 0.1–1.0% of patients [44]. This posed a problem to blood banks, and a confirmatory test, the Western blot, was later added as a confirmation for screening results. This greatly reduced the risk of HIV transmission from blood products, but because these tests were detecting antibodies, there was still a window period of up to 2 months after an individual was infected and subsequently tested seropositive. In 1996 the HIV p24 antigen test was implemented and marked the first step in transitioning from detection of antibody formation to detection of the virus itself. In 1999 a duplex nucleic acid test (NAT) for HIV and hepatitis C virus (HCV) RNA detection was introduced, and window periods dramatically dropped to under 15 days. Because all HIV p24 antigen-positive samples were also identified as positive by NAT, the p24 test was discontinued.

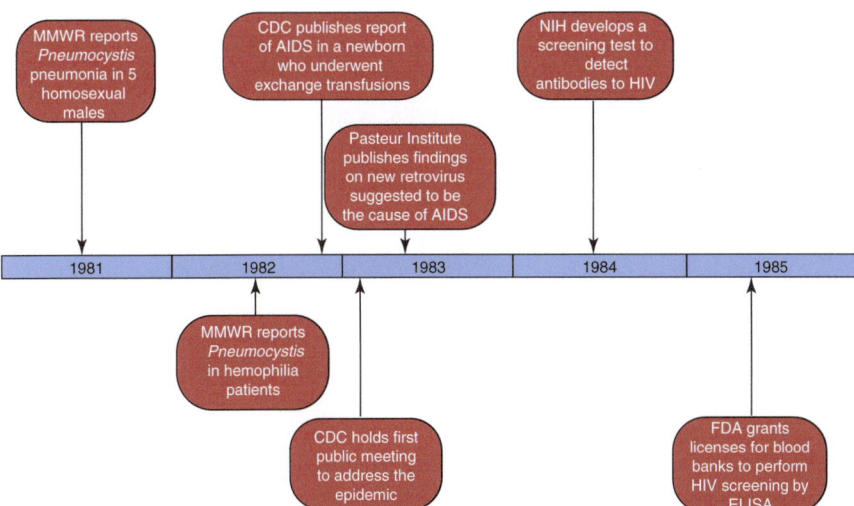

Fig. 6.1 Timeline of early major events in AIDS epidemic, from the first report by the CDC in 1981 to the licensing of a HIV screening test by the FDA in 1985

A study of homosexual and bisexual males who were being treated for sexually transmitted diseases in San Francisco demonstrated a prevalence of infection much higher than the apparent presence of symptomatic AIDS, correctly suggesting that the syndrome would affect the country for long after the spread of the virus was controlled [45]. Testing became increasingly sensitive and specific for HIV as the years passed, but reports of HIV transmission continued to grow early in the epidemic, and significant damage had already been done.

Transmission Data

The CDC estimated that 12,000–25,000 cases of transfusion-transmitted HIV infection occurred prior to antibody screening [46]. Using data from this time, it was estimated that 90% of patients receiving a blood component infected with HIV would seroconvert, and this was independent of age, sex, underlying condition, or type of component transfused [47, 48]. Upon CDC investigation of all AIDS case reports suspected to be caused by blood transfusions, investigators estimated that five cases of transfusion-associated AIDS occurred per year after implementation of antibody screening and prior to NAT testing [54]. Presentations to the NIH consensus conference in 1995 estimated that the risk of HIV transmission from blood products after screening dropped to 1 in 420,000 units but several other studies had differing results, with ranges of 1 in 36,000 to 1 in 225,000 [49–53]. The residual risk of transfusion-transmitted HIV dropped to 1 in 1.5 to two million units after national implementation of NAT in donor screening in 1999 [55–57].

The most detrimental effects of the HIV epidemic in a single group occurred in the hemophilia population using plasma-derived clotting factors. These products are made by pooling plasma from thousands of donors into a single lot and precipitating out fractions with cold ethanol [58]. Approximately 80% of the hemophilia A population and 50% of the hemophilia B population were infected with HIV due to clotting factor products between 1978 and 1986, with peak seroconversion occurring between 1982 and 1983 [59, 60]. According to a 10-year study from 1982 to 1991, the incidence of hemophilia was approximately 1 in 5032 live male births, and 79% of those were hemophilia A [61]. The US Census of 1980 counted a male population of 110 million, which translates to an estimated 22,000 living with hemophilia at the time (17,500 with hemophilia A and 4500 with hemophilia B) [62]. Extrapolation of the exact numbers in each population acquiring the disease is difficult because of multiple variables, including severity of disease, year of onset and initiation of therapy, and type of therapy received. It appears that hemophilia B patients were less affected because of the increased concentration of cold ethanol required to fractionate factor IX concentrates. Early efforts to reduce the risk for hemophilia patients included replacing factor concentrate with cryoprecipitate and using heat-treated concentrates. Implementation of donor screening and eventual availability of pathogen-reduced concentrates (e.g., solvent-detergent-treated concentrate) and recombinant factor products further greatly reduced HIV risk for this population.

Funding and Politics

One of the major criticisms in handling the emergence of HIV was less than optimal federal funding and resource allocation. Public health officials arranged national meetings and developed recommendations for action, but did not propose sources to support these actions early in the epidemic. This left private plasma fractionators and blood banks to fund their own studies and added to the resistance to implementing testing that was not supported by strong scientific evidence. One of the major factors in this problem is the lengthy process of forming a federal budget. When considering AIDS funding, this required a working group of scientists, public health organizations, policymakers, and congress. HIV was spreading at a rate that was faster than perceived by all of the above groups, and therefore there was not an extreme sense of urgency. Additionally, the timeframe for building a federal budget occurs nearly 2 years in advance of the proposed fiscal year, and there were minimal mechanisms for rapid response to emerging issues.

Because of these problems, the presidential budget allocation for medical research was nearly always outdated and insufficient. For the years 1982 and 1983, at the peak of the HIV crisis, the presidential budget had no funds set to be distributed for AIDS research [63]. The president's budget proposal is not the final budget that determines funding, and in 1982, the first year that AIDS research was funded, $5.6 million were marked for the NIH and CDC. This criticism is not just from reviewers looking at the epidemic retrospectively, but was an active complaint in the midst of the epidemic. On December 6, 1983, a congressional committee released the *Federal Response to AIDS,* a report that condemned the lack of sufficient funds for AIDS surveillance and research. President Ronald Reagan didn't mention AIDS in a public form until September 17, 1985, and this was viewed as a lack of interest in the topic. But lack of government support was not the sole issue in funding at the time. In order for the scientific community to propose increases, there had to be adequate amounts of researchers on the receiving end. For the fiscal year of 1986, the NIH made a preliminary request for $66.1 million, but due to a lack of grant applications, that number would drop to $60.3 million [63]. To the government's credit, federal funding did increase substantially after 1984 and by 1987 had reached $411 million. This was also the first year in which AIDS funds were allocated to disease prevention and control as opposed to solely being dedicated to research.

Although the USA was successful in dramatically reducing the risk of transfusion-transmitted HIV, the epidemic would continue in other populations. Although there were differences in timing of introduction of HIV and modes of spread in Western Europe compared to the USA, current prevalence rates and deaths due to AIDS are significantly higher in the USA. As of 2008 there were 1.2 million people in the USA with HIV [64]. Even when correcting for differences in population size, this is three times higher than the prevalence in the UK [65]. Particular groups in the USA, such as intravenous drug users, would continue to acquire HIV after 1984 without needle exchange programs and drug rehabilitation programs offering opioid substitution (Fig. 6.2), while such harm reduction programs have been available in the UK since the late 1980s. The USA was dealing with a national drug problem that paralleled the emergence of HIV, and needle exchange programs were seen as solving one epidemic while fueling the other. The ban on federal funding for needle exchange programs would not be lifted until 2009, only to be put back in place in 2011 [66]. The drug crisis was centered in areas of poor socioeconomics with a large African American population, the results of which are still apparent in the prevalence of AIDS today (Fig. 6.3).

The initial stage of the HIV epidemic in the USA was marked with a paucity of conclusive scientific information, and this "uncertainty," in the face of politics, contributed to the delay and ineffective implementation of potentially helpful preventative

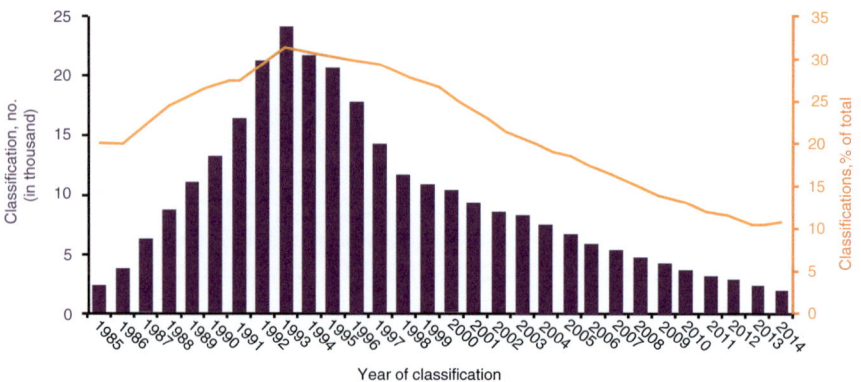

Fig. 6.2 Diagnosed HIV Infections Classified as Stage 3 (AIDS) among Persons Who Inject Drugs, 1985–2015—United States and 6 Dependent Areas. (CDC HIV Surveillance Data)

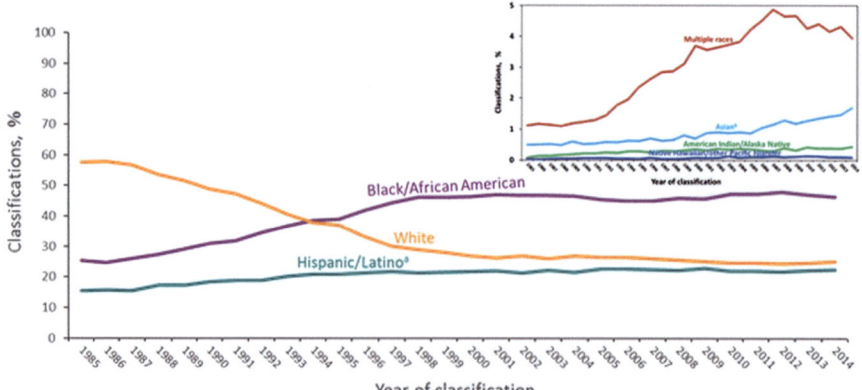

Fig. 6.3 Percentages of Stage 3 (AIDS) Classifications among Adults and Adolescents with Diagnosed HIV Infection, by Race/Ethnicity and Year of Classification, 1985–2015—United States and 6 Dependent Areas. (CDC HIV Surveillance Data)

measures. At the first public meeting held by the CDC in 1984, and many subsequent meetings, homosexual activist groups had strong representation whereas drug reform groups and minorities did not. This led to immense political pressure from the homosexual community when making decisions about public policies, blood donor screening, and health history questions. It wasn't until October of 1984 that "bathhouses" in San Francisco were ordered to be shut down by city officials. These bathhouses were known to be high-risk social clubs for homosexual males and contributed to the rapid spread of HIV in that community. It would take almost a year until bathhouses in other major cities across the nation would follow suit and close as well. An FDA recommendation to ban homosexual males from donating blood wasn't issued until September of 1985, but bans on Haitian individuals had already been in place since 1983 [67]. Of course the conversation surrounding this topic has changed in recent years due to increased sensitivity of screening tests and lower prevalence rates, but in the early 1980s, the blood bank community became susceptible to lobbying when the ban would have been most effective.

Conclusion

The HIV epidemic brought national attention to the issue of blood safety and shaped how government and medical establishments confront potential threats to blood safety from emerging pathogens. The decision-making process during the earlier stage of the HIV epidemic illustrated the complexity and challenges of making decisions with limited medical information and balancing the need to protect patient safety with considerations for blood availability and cost-effectiveness. It was also during this process that the procedures and mechanisms were developed and tested for how government agencies (CDC and FDA) work together with blood establishments to safeguard national blood supply. Prior to HIV, decision on blood safety had always rested on a balance between the strength of available evidence for the perceived threat, the potential effect on blood availability, and considerations for cost-effectiveness. The HIV epidemic was responsible for shifting this balance. The new approach for dealing with a potential new threat to blood safety would feature preemptive response based on a "zero-tolerance" principle. Much of this shift is justified. An important lesson from the HIV epidemic is that during the initial stage of the epidemic, it was very difficult for regulatory authorities and the blood establishments to have a grasp of the true risk associated with transfusion. The once quoted figure of "one in a million" HIV transfusion risk from the second joint statement from the blood bank community turned out to be a gross underrepresentation of the true risk for the time. Retrospective analysis demonstrated that the actual risk in the early 1980s was closer to 1/2500 in nonmetropolitan areas and up to one in a hundred in highest risk regions such as San Francisco in the 1980s [68–70] (Fig. 6.4). Early intervention measures such as education and self-deferral of individuals with high-risk and confidential unit exclusion proved to be very effective in reducing risk even before test-based screening technology became available [70]. Government

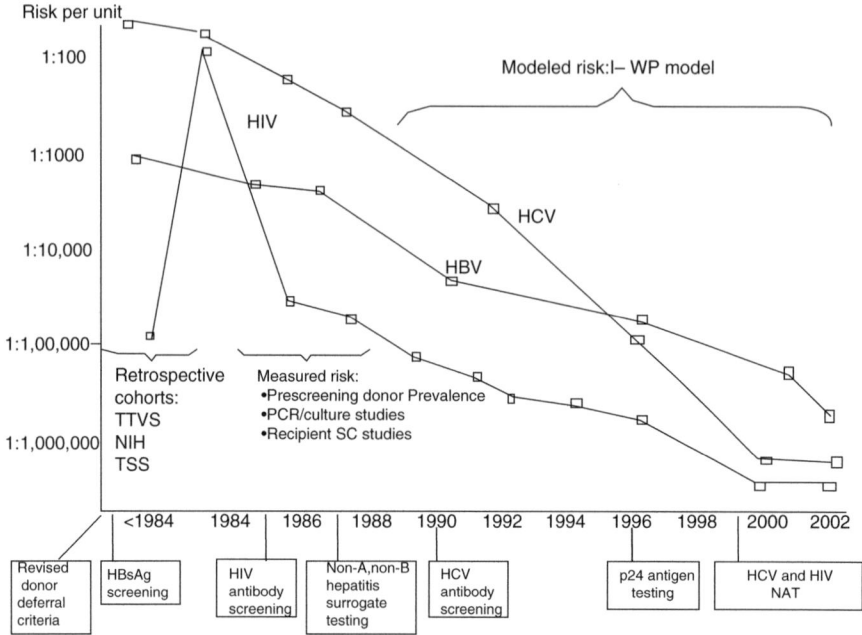

Fig. 6.4 Evolution of approaches to estimating the risks of transmission by blood transfusion for HIV, HBV, and HCV. Major interventions to reduce risks are indicated below the timeline on the X-axis. Used with permission from Busch MP. Transfusion-transmitted viral infections: building bridges to transfusion medicine to reduce risks and understand epidemiology and pathogenesis. (Reproduced with permission from John Wiley and Sons. Ref. [69])

funding and coordination of research efforts to obtain key epidemiological knowledge about the new pathogen and test development have proven to be essential for minimizing the risk to transfusion recipients. Compared to the almost 2-year lapse from the identification of HIV and the availability of a donor screening test, during the Zika epidemic of 2016, a donor screening test was developed and implemented within 5 months after the identification of Zika as a transfusion-transmitted pathogen [71, 72].

A key epidemiological metric about a pathogen is an accurate estimate of its transmission risk through transfusion. Methods for accurate risk estimation have been developed using HIV as a model for different stages of an epidemic [68–70]. More accurate risk estimation will continue to help the government and blood establishments develop evidence-based intervention policies.

The story of HIV is the story about global travel of pathogens. Although early case reports were from outside of Africa, the origin of the epidemic was eventually traced to Africa. But this did not occur until it was well into a global epidemic. Haiti's role as a HIV global stepping stone was also a retrospective realization. Moving forward, establishing infrastructures for international collaborations on developing active global pathogen surveillance programs should help the global community to more effectively identify and track potential new threats to public health as well as blood safety.

The HIV experience provided a real focus on global issues in the context of national response. In this age of globalization, one country's response to an emerging pathogen can influence how other countries react. Early response to HIV by US government agencies and blood establishments likely prompted similar response from other countries. At the same time, the USA's relatively rapid response might have also set the bar for other countries to measure their responses against, at least in the court of public opinions. This influence has continued beyond the HIV epidemic as evidenced by how the international community responded to Zika.

There is much that was learned during the HIV epidemic. It has helped to shape government policies in medical research, approaches to epidemiology and scientific research, and the social and political frames of society. We and the international community will continue to learn from it and apply the lessons to future encounters with emerging transfusion-transmitted infections.

References

1. CDC. *Pneumocystis* Pneumonia – Los Angeles. MMWR. 1981;30:1–3.
2. Van Heuverswyn F, Li Y, Neel C, Bailes E, Keele BF, Liu W, Loul S, Butel C, Liegeois F, Bienvenue Y, Ngolle EM, Sharp PM, Shaw GM, Delaporte E, Hahn BH, Peeters M. Human immunodeficiency viruses: SIV infection in wild gorillas. Nature. 2006;444(7116):164.
3. Gilbert MTP, Rambaut A, Wlasiuk G, Spira TJ, Pitchenik AE, Worobey M. The emergence of HIV/AIDS in the Americas and beyond. PNAS. 2007;104(47):18566–70.
4. Altman L. Clue found on homosexuals' precancer syndrome. The New York Times. 1982. Retrieved from http://www.nytimes.com.
5. Moskowitz LB, Kory P, Chan JC, Haverkos HW, Conley FK, Hensley GT. Unusual causes of death in Haitians residing in Miami: high prevalence of opportunistic infections. JAMA. 1983;250(9):1187–91.
6. Jaffe HW, Bregman DJ, Selik RM. Acquired immune deficiency syndrome in the United States: the first 1,000 cases. J Infect Dis. 1983;148(2):339–45.
7. Pitchenik AE, Fischl MA, Dickinson GM, et al. Opportunistic infections and Kaposi's sarcoma among Haitians: evidence of a new acquired immunodeficiency state. Ann Intern Med. 1983;98(3):277–84.
8. CDC. Follow-up on Kaposi's sarcoma and pneumocystis pneumonia. MMWR. 1981;30:409–10.
9. CDC. Update on Kaposi's sarcoma and opportunistic infections in previously healthy persons--United States. MMWR. 1982;31:294, 300–1.
10. Masur H, Michelis MA, Greene JB, et al. An outbreak of community-acquired Pneumocystis carinii pneumonia: initial manifestation of cellular immune dysfunction. N Engl J Med. 1981;305:1431–8.
11. Gottlieb MS, Schroff R, Schanker HM, et al. Pneumocystis carinii pneumonia and mucosal candidiasis in previously healthy homosexual men: evidence of a new acquired cellular immunodeficiency. N Engl J Med. 1981;305:1425–31.
12. CDC. Opportunistic Infections and Kaposi's Sarcoma among Haitians in the United States. MMWR. 1982;31:353–4, 360–1.
13. Pape JW, Liautaud B, Thomas F, et al. Characteristics of the acquired immunodeficiency syndrome (AIDS) in Haiti. N Engl J Med. 1983;309(16):945–50.

14. Pape JW, Johnson WD. Bailleire's clinical tropical medicine and communicable diseases, AIDS and HIV infection in the tropics. London, UK: Harcourt Brace; 1988. Epidemiology of AIDS in the Caribbean
15. Cayemittes M, Placide MF, Mariko S, et al. Enqûete mortalité, morbidité et utilisation des services EMMUS–e Haïti 2005–2006. Pétionville and Calverton: Institut Haïtien de l'Enfance, ORC Macro; 2006.
16. CDC. Epidemiologic notes and reports pneumocystis carninii pneumonia among persons with hemophilia a. MMWR. 1982;31:365–7.
17. CDC. Epidemiologic notes and reports possible transfusion-associated acquired immune deficiency syndrome (AIDS) – California. MMWR. 1982;31:652–4.
18. Stiehm ER, Fulginiti VA, editors. Immunologic disorders in infants and children. 2nd ed. Philadelphia: WB Saunders Company; 1980.
19. Neustadt R, Fineberg H. The swine flu affair: decisionmaking on a slippery disease. U.S. Department of Health, Education, and Welfare; 1978.
20. Foege WH. Summary report on workgroup to identify opportunities for prevention of acquired immune deficiency syndrome; 1983.
21. Abolghasemi H, Hosseini-Divkalayi NS, Seighali F. Blood donor incentives: a step forward or backward. Asian J Transfus Sci. 2010;4(1):9–13. PMC. Web. 18 Nov. 2017
22. American Association of Blood Banks; American Red Cross, and Council of Community Blood Centers. Joint Statement on Acquired Immune Deficiency Syndrome (AIDS) Related to Transfusion; 1983.
23. American Red Cross National Headquarters. Memorandum to Mr. deBeaufort from Dr. Cumming; 1983.
24. National Hemophilia Foundation; Medical and Scientific Advisory Council. Recommendations to Prevent AIDS in Patients With Hemophilia; 1983.
25. CDC. Current trends prevention of acquired immune deficiency syndrome (AIDS): report of inter-agency recommendations. MMWR. 1983;32:101–3.
26. Petricciani J. Director, food and drug administration, office of biologics. Letter to all establishments collecting human blood for transfusion; 1983.
27. Petricciani J. Director, food and drug administration, office of biologics. Letter to all establishments collecting source plasma; 1983.
28. Petricciani J. Director, food and drug administration, office of biologics. Letter to All licensed manufacturers of plasma derivatives; 1983.
29. American Association of Blood Banks; American Red Cross, and Council of Community Blood Centers. Joint Statement on Directed Donations and AIDS; 1983.
30. Stoto, et al. Federal Funding for AIDS research: decision process and results in fiscal year 1986. Rev Infect Dis. 1988;10
31. Institute of Medicine (US) Committee to Study HIV Transmission Through Blood and Blood Products. In: Leveton LB, Sox Jr HC, Stoto MA, editors. HIV and the blood supply: an analysis of crisis decisionmaking. Washington, DC: National Academies Press (US); 1995.
32. Ammann AJ, Ahrams D, Conant M, et al. Acquired immune dysfunction in homosexual men: immunologic profiles. Clin lmmunol lmmunopathol. 1983;27:3 15–25.
33. Schroff RW, Gottlieb MS, Prince HE, Chai L, Fahey JI. Immunological studies of homosexual men with immunode- ficiency and Kaposi's sarcoma. Clin lmmunol Immunopathol. 1983;27:300–14.
34. Kornfeld H, Vande Stouwe RA, Lange M, Reddy MM, Grieeo MH. -1.-lymphocyte subpopulations in homosexual men. N Engl J Med. I982;307:729–3I.
35. Galel, et al. Prevention of AIDS transmission through screening of the blood supply. Ann Rev Immunol. 1995;13
36. Simon TL, Bankhurst AD. A pilot study of surrogate tests to prevent transmission of acquired immune deficiency syndrome by transfusion. Transfusion. 1984 Sep-Oct;24(5):373–8.
37. Barré-Sinoussi F, Chermann JC, Rey F, Nugeyre MT, Chamaret S, Gruest J, Dauguet C, Axler-Blin C, Vézinet-Brun F, Rouzioux C, Rozenbaum W, Montagnier L. Isolation of a

T-lymphotropic retrovirus from a patient at risk for acquired immune deficiency syndrome (AIDS). Science. 1983;220(4599):868–71.
38. Poiesz BJ, Ruscetti FW, Gazdar AF, Bunn PA, Minna JD, Gallo RC. Detection and isolation of type C retrovirus particles from fresh and cultured lymphocytes of a patient with cutaneous T-cell lymphoma. Proc Natl Acad Sci U S A. 1980 Dec;77(12):7415–9.
39. Morgan DA, Ruscetti FW, Gallo R. Selective in vitro growth of T lymphocytes from normal human bone marrows. Science. September 1976;193(4257):1007–8.
40. Popovic M, Sarngadharan MG, Read E, Gallo RC. Detection, isolation, and continuous production of cytopathic retroviruses (HTLV-III) from patients with AIDS and pre-AIDS. Science. 1984;224(4648):497–500.
41. Gallo RC, Salahuddin SZ, Popovic M, Shearer GM, Kaplan M, Haynes BF, Palker TJ, Redfield R, Oleske J, Safai B, White G, Foster P, Markham PD. Frequent detection and isolation of Cytopathic retroviruses (HTLV-III) from patients with AIDS and at risk for AIDS. Science. 1984;224(4648):500–3.
42. Levy JA, et al. Isolation of lymphocytopathic retroviruses from San Francisco patients with AIDS. Science. 1984;225:840–2.
43. Marx JL. A virus by any other name. Science. 1985;227(4693):1449–51.
44. Helhngs JA, Theunissen H, Keur W, Siebelink-Liauw A. New developments in ELISA verification of anti-HIV screening of blood donors. J Virol Methods. 1987;17:1 1–17.
45. Jaffe HW, Darrow WW, Echenburg DF, et al. The acquired immunodeficiency syndrome in a cohort of homosexual men: a six-year follow-up study. Ann Intern Med. 1985;103(2):210–4.
46. Kalbfleisch JD, Lawless JF. Estimating the incubation time distribution and expected number of cases of transfusion-associated acquired immune deficiency syndrome. Transfusion. 1989;29:672.
47. Donegan E, Lee H, Operskalski EA, et al. Transfusion transmission of retroviruses: human T-lymphotropic virus types I and II compared with human immunodeficiency virus type 1. Transfusion. 1994;34:478–83.
48. Donegan E, Stuart M, Niland JC, et al. Infection with human immunodeficiency virus type 1 (HIV-1) among recipients of antibody-positive blood donations. Ann Intern Med. 1990;113:733–9.
49. Schreiber GB, Busch MP, Kleinman SH, Korelitz JJ. The risk of transfusion-transmitted viral infections. The retrovirus epidemiology donor study. N Engl J Med. 1996;334:1685.
50. Lackritz EM, Satten GA, Aberle-Grasse J, et al. Estimated risk of transmission of the human immunodeficiency virus by screened blood in the United States. N Engl J Med. 1995;333:1721.
51. Ward JW, Holmberg SD, Allen JR, et al. Transmission of human immunodeficiency virus (HIV) by blood transfusions screened as negative for HIV antibody. N Engl J Med. 1988;318:473.
52. Nelson KE, Donahue JG, Muñoz A, et al. Transmission of retroviruses from seronegative donors by transfusion during cardiac surgery. A multicenter study of HIV-1 and HTLV-I/II infections. Ann Intern Med. 1992;117:554.
53. Cumming PD, Wallace EL, Schorr JB, Dodd RY. Exposure of patients to human immunodeficiency virus through the transfusion of blood components that test antibody-negative. N Engl J Med. 1989;321:941.
54. Selik RM, Ward JW, Buehler JW. Trends in transfusion-associated acquired immune deficiency syndrome in the United States, 1982 through 1991. Transfusion. 1993;33:890.
55. Zou S, Dorsey KA, Notari EP, et al. Prevalence, incidence, and residual risk of human immunodeficiency virus and hepatitis C virus infections among United States blood donors since the introduction of nucleic acid testing. Transfusion. 2010;50:1495.
56. Dodd RY, Notari EP 4th, Stramer SL. Current prevalence and incidence of infectious disease markers and estimated window-period risk in the American red Cross blood donor population. Transfusion. 2002;42:975.
57. Busch MP, Glynn SA, Stramer SL, et al. A new strategy for estimating risks of transfusion-transmitted viral infections based on rates of detection of recently infected donors. Transfusion. 2005;45:254.

58. Morgenthaler JJ. Securing viral safety for plasma derivatives. Transfus Med Rev. 2001;15(3):224–33.
59. Ragni MV, Winkelstein A, Kingsley L, et al. 1986 update of HIV seroprevalence, seroconversion, AIDS incidence, and immunologic correlates of HIV infection in patients with hemophilia a and B. Blood. 1987;70:786–90.
60. Immunologic and virologic status of multitransfused patients: Role of type and origin of blood products. By the AIDS-hemophilia French study group. Blood. 1985;66:896–901.
61. Soucie JM, Evatt B, Jackson D. Occurrence of hemophilia in the United States. The hemophilia surveillance system project investigators. Am J Hematol. 1998;59(4):288–94.
62. Retrieved from https://www.census.gov/prod/www/decennial.html.
63. Stoto MA, Blumenthal D, Durch JS, Feldman PH. Federal Funding for AIDS research: decision process and results in fiscal year 1986. Rev Infect Dis. 1988;10(2):406–19.
64. Centers for Disease Control and Prevention, (CDC). HIV surveillance—United States, 1981–2008. MMWR Morb Mortal Wkly Rep. 2011;60(21):689–93.
65. Health Protection Agency. HIV in the United Kingdom: 2010 Report; 2010.
66. Weinmeyer R. Needle exchange Programs' status in US politics. AMA J Ethics. 2016 Mar 1;18(3):252–7.
67. FDA. Revised recommendations for reducing the risk of human immunodeficiency virus transmission by blood and blood products; 2015.
68. Kleinman SH, Niland JC, Azen SP, Operskalski EA, Barbosa LH, Chernoff AI, Edwards VM, Lenes BA, Marshall GJ, Nemo GJ, Norman GL, Perkins H, Pindyck J, Pitlick F, Rasheed S, Shriver K, Toy P, Tomasulo PA, Waldman A, Mosley JW, Transfusion Safety Study Group. Prevalence of antibodies to human immunodeficiency virus type 1 among blood donors prior to screening, the transfusion safety study/NHLBI donor repository. Transfusion. 1989;29:572–80.
69. Busch MP. Transfusion-transmitted viral infections: building bridges to transfusion medicine to reduce risks and understand epidemiology and pathogenesis. Transfusion. 2006;46:1624–40.
70. Busch MP, Young MJ, Samson SM, et al. Risk of human immunodeficiency virus (HIV) transmission by blood transfusions before the implementation of HIV-1 antibody screening. Transfusion. 1991;31:4–11.
71. Kuehnert MJ, Basavaraju SV, Moseley RR, Pate LL, Galel SA, Williamson PC, Busch MP, Alsina JO, Climent-Peris C, Marks PW, Epstein JS, Nakhasi HL, Hobson JP, Leiby DA, Akolkar PN, Petersen LR, Rivera-Garcia B. Screening of blood donations for Zika virus infection - Puerto Rico, April 3-June 11, 2016. MMWR Morb Mortal Wkly Rep. 2016;65(24):627–8.
72. FDA. Revised recommendations for reducing the risk of Zika Virus transmission by blood and blood components. 2016. Retrieved from www.fda.gov.

Chapter 7
vCJD Case Studies

Patricia Hewitt and Robert Will

During the 1980s questions had been raised about whether the epidemic of bovine spongiform encephalopathy (BSE) in the United Kingdom (UK) might have implications for human health. In May 1990 UK national surveillance of CJD was initiated, carried out by the National CJD Research & Surveillance Unit (NCJDRSU), in response to a recommendation made in the Southwood Committee Report of the Working Party on bovine spongiform encephalopathy (BSE), to identify any changes in the pattern of CJD that might be attributable to human infection with the agent responsible for the emergence of BSE in cattle. Such a change was recognized in 1996 when the NCJDRSU described the first ten cases of a new variant of CJD with a clinical and pathological picture distinct from that usually seen in sporadic CJD [1]. This soon became known as variant CJD (vCJD). It also soon became clear that vCJD was indeed the result of transmission of BSE from cattle to humans, through the diet, and was thus an example of a prion disease crossing the species barrier.

Very early on there was concern that vCJD might have implications for the safety of the blood supply. After the report of the first cases of vCJD, and before any link between blood transfusion and vCJD had been established, a number of blood safety measures were introduced in the UK. The precautionary principle was applied, based on the worst-case scenario that vCJD could be transmitted by blood transfusion.

The first UK blood safety response was to introduce universal leucodepletion of blood components. Although a definite scientific basis for this intervention was lacking, some preliminary work had indicated that B lymphocytes played some role

---

P. Hewitt (✉)
Department of Microbiology Services, NHS Blood and Transplant, London, UK
e-mail: patricia.hewitt@nhsbt.nhs.uk

R. Will
National CJD Research and Surveillance Unit, Western General Hospital, Edinburgh, UK

in disseminating the infectious prion. Leucodepletion was phased in by the UK blood services, starting in 1998 and fully implemented by October 1999. A further blood safety measure, introduced over the same time period, was to replace the use of UK plasma for fractionation with plasma obtained from areas with a low prevalence of BSE. This decision was in part precipitated by the complexity of the requirement to withdraw batches of product containing plasma from donors who later developed vCJD and the concern that repeated recalls would be required as new cases of vCJD in previous blood donors were confirmed. In many countries outside the UK, geographic donor deferral was introduced, so that individuals who had lived in the UK, or France, in the relevant years of the BSE epidemic were deferred from blood donation.

During 1996, a study between the four UK blood services and NCJDRSU was designed to investigate whether there was any link between CJD and blood transfusion. The study, known as the Transfusion Medicine Epidemiology Review (TMER), has been described in detail elsewhere [2]. Although it covers all types of CJD, only the part covering vCJD will be discussed.

All individuals who have a diagnosis of probable or definite vCJD and are old enough to have been blood donors are notified to the UK blood services. A search is made of national donor databases to establish whether the case was a blood donor. If there is a record of the individual, a lookback is carried out to establish the fate of all blood donations and associated issued blood components. Recipient hospitals are notified of components issued to them, and they establish the ultimate fate of the components from their laboratory records. If the blood component was transfused, the recipient is identified to the blood service and the details then shared with the NCJDRSU. Health service records are then flagged so that a copy of the death certificate will be forwarded to the NCJDRSU when the individual dies, and cause of death and associated illnesses can be determined.

For all individuals diagnosed with probable or definite vCJD, a history of transfusion is sought by enquiry from family members and from medical records. If the hospital of transfusion can be identified, then the details are forwarded to the relevant blood service which asks the hospital blood transfusion laboratory to specify what blood components have been transfused. These can then be linked with the respective donors, whose details (name and date of birth) are forwarded to the NCJDRSU for checking against its database.

The flow of information backwards and forwards between the NCJDRSU, the blood service database, blood centres, and hospitals is shown in Fig. 7.1.

When the study began in 1997 it was a research study which received ethical approval on the basis that, because there was no known link between any type of CJD and blood transfusion, the identified recipients and blood donors should not be notified.

A total of 230 cases of vCJD have now been reported worldwide, with 178 in the UK and 27 in France. Three of the UK cases have been classed as secondary, acquired through blood transfusion.

Fig. 7.1 Information flow in the TMER study

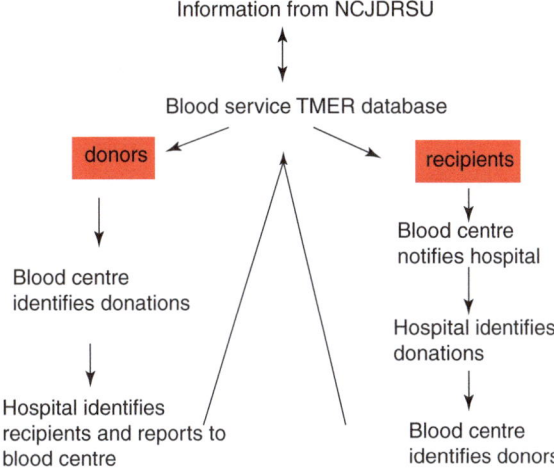

Case Study Donor 1: Donor Developed vCJD after Blood Donation

This patient in the 20–30-year age group developed anxiety and panic attacks in 1999 and was treated with antidepressants. He became apathetic and withdrawn and was referred to a psychiatrist. After some months he developed forgetfulness and confusion and was admitted to a neurology unit for investigation. On examination he was disorientated and confused with cerebellar ataxia. An MRI brain scan showed the pulvinar sign, an EEG showed slow activity and the CSF protein was elevated. The diagnosis was thought to be variant CJD, although the criteria for a probable diagnosis were not fulfilled. The patient deteriorated over a period of months and died 13 months after illness onset. Postmortem examination of the brain was carried out and showed appearance characteristic of vCJD. The patient was homozygous for methionine at codon 129 of *PRNP*, and no mutations were found on sequencing.

The patient had been reported by his family to have donated blood on 3–4 occasions. Through the TMER study, it was revealed that two blood donations had been made. A donation taken nearly 3½ years before the onset of illness had been processed into a red cell component, issued for clinical use. A second donation had been made 3 months later and issued as a red cell component. Platelets from this later donation had been incorporated into a platelet pool which was also issued for clinical use. Both the donations predated the introduction of leucodepletion.

Routine searches for the fate of the red cell component from the first donation revealed that it had been transfused into a patient in the 60–70-year age group who had undergone surgery and was still alive. The red cells from the second donation were transfused to a patient who died from the underlying disease 3 months after transfusion. The platelet pool could not be traced to an identified recipient by the hospital concerned, due to lack of records.

Case Study: Recipients Received Red Cells from Donor 1

The first patient, in the 60–70-year age group, underwent surgery in 1996 and was transfused with 5 units of non-leucodepleted red cells, including those from Donor 1. In 2002, some 6.5 years after the surgery, the patient became withdrawn and irritable. Treatment with antidepressants was started within 3 months, but the depression deteriorated, and there was a new development of a shuffling gait and repeated falls. Over the subsequent months, the patient developed blurred vision, shooting pains in the face and abdomen, fidgety movements and difficulty with motor tasks such as dressing. Six months after onset of symptoms, the patient was admitted for investigation and was noted to have dyspraxia, cognitive impairment, a shuffling unsteady gait and extensor plantar responses. Lumbar puncture was performed and revealed acellular cerebrospinal fluid (CSF) with normal constituents except for a slightly raised protein content of 0.67 g/l. An MRI brain scan was reported as normal. The patient's condition deteriorated rapidly, with onset of myoclonic jerking of the limbs; death occurred 13 months after illness onset. The cause of death was recorded as dementia, but a postmortem examination was performed and showed changes suggestive of CJD. Tissues were therefore referred to the UK NCJDRSU for review. Here, the neuropathological changes were found to be typical of those seen in vCJD, with florid plaque deposition. Prion-protein typing confirmed deposition in the brain of type 2B prion protein, pathognomic of vCJD. The patient was methionine homozygous at codon 129 of the prion protein gene (*PRNP*), with no mutations found on sequencing.

As this patient had separately been identified in the TMER study as the recipient of Donor 1, this case established the first possible link between vCJD and blood transfusion [3]. Up to this point, in the lack of any evidence of transfusion-transmission, no information had been provided to identified recipients of donors who developed vCJD at some point after blood donation, although concerns had been expressed about their "risk status". An expert multidisciplinary body, the CJD Incidents Panel, had been set up to give advice to health providers regarding incidents which might have exposed patients to a risk of transmission of vCJD. The Panel had previously considered the problem of patients who had been identified as recipients of blood components donated by individuals who had later developed vCJD and had considered in 2002/2003 that such individuals should be notified and made aware of the issue. It was acknowledged that there were difficult issues involved, with the lack of any screening or diagnostic blood test to determine whether infection was present, and the huge uncertainties that such information would bring. It was also perceived that such individuals would need extensive psychological support, and their general practitioners would require access to specialist advice and resources. Discussions were progressing slowly when the first link between a donor and a recipient, both with vCJD, was made in late 2003. At this point the Department of Health and Social Care in England decided that the risk was now at a level such that all identified recipients should be made aware with minimal delay. A notification exercise was devised and carried out shortly before Christmas 2003. As part of this exercise, the identified recipients and their clinicians were advised that they were considered "at risk of vCJD" for public health purposes by virtue of their transfusion history. Public health measures which were advised included not donating blood, organs or tissues and informing their clinicians before undergoing medical and surgical procedures so that measures such as special handling of instruments could be taken. Due to the immense effort put in by public health officials, who coordinated the notification nationally (across all four countries), and local general practitioners and infection control specialists, all but one recipient was informed in the very short time frame before the Christmas holiday period.

Separately, it was also deemed important to make further efforts to try and identify the fate of the platelet component from the donor's subsequent donation, since that recipient would be included in the "at risk of vCJD" group. The hospital was contacted once again and provided with the new information which necessitated a more intense search for the fate of the platelet pool which had been issued some 6 years earlier. The hospital had already established that at this time the record of platelet issues was not computerised and no paper records could be located. A search was then made in the laboratory system for the identity of all patients recorded to have low platelet counts on blood samples tested in the 3 days either side the date of receipt of the platelet pool. The identified patients' case notes were then examined for evidence of platelet transfusion and for confirmation of the batch number (unique identifier) of the platelets transfused. As a result of this exercise, four patients were identified who had been receiving platelet transfusions at the time in question but where batch numbers were missing from the case notes. Any of these four could therefore have been the recipient of the platelet pool under investigation. Advice was sought from the CJD Incidents Panel, which decided that in the lack of any evidence about which, if any, of the four recipients had received the platelet pool, no further action should be taken.

Some years later the old manual log books from the transfusion laboratory were found in a basement, and the fate of the platelet pool was finally established. It had been transfused to a male patient as treatment for aspirin-induced bleeding during cardiac surgery. This patient did not have a low platelet count, and was therefore not included in the notes review which had been carried out years earlier. The patient had recovered from the surgery and died 5 years later without any evidence of neurological disease and before the link to the donor who developed vCJD had been established. No postmortem had been carried out.

The first case therefore resulted in one recipient who died of vCJD, and two recipients who died of other causes within the time now recognised to reflect the incubation period for transfusion-associated vCJD.

As a result of Case 1 and the general notification exercise of identified recipients, all future cases of vCJD arising in blood donors after the time of blood donation led to notification of any identified recipients, using a standard agreed format and coordinated by the national Health Protection CJD team.

Case Study Donor 2: Developed vCJD After Blood Donation

This patient in the 20–30-year age group developed left-sided sensory disturbance in 2000, associated with apathy, withdrawal and nocturnal confusion. She then developed dysarthria and unsteadiness of gait and on examination had mild cerebellar signs. An EEG showed slow activity, and an MRI brain scan showed high signal in the pulvinar region of the thalamus. The diagnosis was thought to be probable vCJD. She deteriorated over subsequent months, developing myoclonic movements of the limbs and died 9 months after symptom onset. The diagnosis of vCJD was confirmed at postmortem and Western blot showed type 2B prion protein.

The family reported that the patient had been a regular blood donor since 1997. Through the TMER study, it was revealed that two donations had been issued: the first was made around 18 months before the onset of illness and issued as non-leucodepleted red cells and the second was 1 year later and issued as leucodepleted red cells.

Case Study: Recipients Received Red Cells from Donor 2

The non-leucodepleted red cells from Donor 2 had been transfused to an elderly patient who died from a vascular condition 5 years after transfusion. There had been no evidence of a neurological disorder. The diagnosis in the red cell donor was known at the time of death. Medico legal instruction for an autopsy was made. Protease-resistant prion protein (PrP^{res}) was detected in the spleen but not in the brain or other tissues. This was the first recorded case in the UK of autopsy detection of presumed pre- or subclinical vCJD infection [4]. This case indicated for the first time that individuals who are heterozygous at codon 129 of the *PRNP* could be infected with vCJD and raised the question whether such infection would become clinically apparent with the same length of incubation period and/or with the same clinical features as cases who are MM homozygous. As this recipient died 5 years after the blood transfusion, with no clinical or autopsy evidence of neurological disease, these questions remained unanswered.

The subsequent donation, which was issued as leucodepleted red cells, was transfused to a recipient who died of cardiac disease almost 5 years after transfusion. There had been no evidence of neurological disease before death and autopsy was not carried out.

Case Study Donor 3: Developed vCJD After Blood Donation

This patient in the 30–40-year age group developed a disturbed sleep pattern associated with vivid delusions in 2000. He became confused and described pains in the knees and tingling in the hand. His walking became ataxic with slurred speech, and his family described tremors of the limbs and twitching while asleep. All the symptoms were progressive. On examination he was confused and tearful with a rest tremor, choreiform limb movements and cerebellar signs. An EEG showed slow activity, the CSF protein was elevated and an MRI scan was degraded by movement artefact but showed high signal in the posterior thalamus and basal ganglia. The diagnosis was thought to be probable vCJD. The patient died 11 months after symptom onset and postmortem confirmed the diagnosis of vCJD. Western blot analysis showed type 2B prion protein and the patient was homozygous for methionine at codon 129 of *PRNP* and there were no mutations.

The family reported that the patient had been a regular blood donor from 1993 onwards. The TMER study identified five blood donations from which components were issued for clinical use. All of these donations occurred before the introduction of leucodepletion: five red cell and three fresh frozen plasma (FFP) components were transfused. All three FFP recipients and one red cell recipient died within 4 years of the transfusion, but the other four red cell recipients all survived more than 5 years. All these living recipients were informed that they were considered "at risk of vCJD" when the recipient notification exercise took place in late 2003. One red cell recipient, who received red cells donated 1 year and 2 months before disease onset in the donor, died of a stroke some 6 years after transfusion. No autopsy was performed. The three other red cell recipients all survived at least 7 years: two (Recipients 3 and 4) went on to develop vCJD 7 years 10 months and 8 years 4 months after the transfusion, respectively, and one survives. The two recipients who developed vCJD were both homozygous for methionine at codon 129 of *PRNP;* the surviving recipient, who was transfused with red cells donated within 1 year of the donor's development of vCJD, is known to be heterozygous.

Case Study: Recipient 3 Received Red Cells from Donor 3

This patient in the 30–40-year age group had a history of ulcerative colitis. A severe relapse some 9 years prior to presentation required a colectomy and ileostomy formation. The following year, in 1997, further surgery was performed to convert the ileostomy into an ileoanal J-pouch, but complications after surgery included pelvic bleeding, requiring further surgery and a period in intensive care. Management of the bleeding led to transfusion of 22 units of non-leucodepleted red cells, 15 units of fresh frozen plasma and 3 platelet doses. He recovered and was discharged. Six years later he presented with a short history of fluctuating exertional fatigue and impaired concentration. It was thought that these symptoms were attributable to a viral respiratory tract infection, but the symptoms continued to fluctuate. Around this time the patient and his family doctor were informed that one of the donors of the red cells transfused in 1997 had developed vCJD 20 months after donating the blood and had died after an 11-month illness. The patient was therefore considered to be at risk of vCJD. The patient was referred for neurological assessment, which was normal, including clinical cognitive assessment, routine electroencephalogram and magnetic resonance neuroimaging.

The patient improved somewhat and returned to work. Neurological review 12 months later revealed persistent symptoms of fatigue and impaired concentration, but there were no abnormal findings on clinical examination. The patient next presented 6 months later, and 7.5 years after the blood transfusion, to a specialist clinic with a complaint of progressive balance difficulties and impaired concentration. The patient reported memory problems, difficulty with recent recall and a sense of tremor in the hands with reduced manual dexterity. Over the next few weeks, he developed severe incapacitating leg pain, most prominent in the anterior thigh but affecting the whole of both legs and worsened by activity. There were hypersensitivity and paraesthesia of the feet. At this stage, examination revealed a normal mini-mental state examination (MMSE), scoring 30/30, with no evidence of dyspraxia or visuospatial dysfunction. Neurological examination was normal apart from minimal nystagmus.

Neurological decline continued over the following weeks. Six weeks later the MMSE score was 22/30; there were increasing unsteadiness and several falls, but the leg pain had lessened. Routine haematological and biochemical blood test results were normal, as was an infection screen. MR neuroimaging showed a pulvinar sign, classical of vCJD, and electroencephalogram showed nonspecific changes. The patient continued to decline, with progressive cognitive impairment, dysarthria and ataxia and became bed-bound. Death occurred 8 years and 8 months posttransfusion.

Postmortem examination of the brain confirmed the presence of disease-related PrP by immunoblotting and immunohistochemistry. The abnormal PrP was deposited in all cortical areas and in the cerebellum with abundant florid PrP plaques. Immunostaining analysis of the tonsil showed multiple lymphatic follicles containing abnormal PrP, typical to the pattern seen in vCJD. Examination of the spleen showed similar findings. The patient was homozygous for methionine at *PRNP* codon 129, as was the blood donor who had developed vCJD [5].

Case Study: Recipient 4 Received Red Cells from Donor 3

This patient was in the 70–80-year age group and had surgery requiring blood transfusion following a road traffic accident at the end of 1997. One of the non-leucodepleted red cells transfused at that time originated from Donor 3, who developed vCJD in the first half of 1999; this was the same donor as described in Case Study Recipient 3 (above). Recipient 4 was asymptomatic at the time of the recipient notification exercise in December 2003 but was offered investigation at a specialist clinic. Neurological examination just over 8 years after the transfusion was unremarkable, and an MRI brain scan showed no signal change suggestive of prion disease. Four months later the patient had developed progressive symptoms of imbalance and deteriorating cognition. Examination 2 months later demonstrated marked cognitive impairment, with cerebellar signs including impaired manual dexterity and ataxic gait. Haematological and biochemical blood tests were normal but neuropsychometry confirmed frontal and temporal deficits. A repeat MRI brain scan again showed no signal change suggestive of prion disease. *PRNP* genotyping revealed methionine homozygosity at codon 129 with no mutations.

Although the patient did not fulfil the WHO diagnostic criteria for vCJD, a tonsillar biopsy was performed: abnormal prion protein was confirmed by immunocytochemistry and Western blot examination. The patient rapidly deteriorated, became mute and bed-bound and developed dysphagia and myoclonus. Death occurred some 8 months after symptom onset, and postmortem examination demonstrated abnormal PrP in the brain and peripheral lymphoreticular tissue by immunocytochemistry [6].

Case Study Recipient 5: Received a Blood Transfusion Without an Identified Infected Donor, All Identified Donors Considered to Be "at Risk"

This patient in the 40–50-year age group had longstanding alcoholic liver disease and had suffered episodes of hepatic encephalopathy. He had a bleeding episode secondary to varices followed by a liver transplant in 1993, with significant red cell exposure during the two episodes. Sometime later he began drinking alcohol again and became confused, with a diagnosis of possible Wernicke's encephalopathy. In 1997 he developed delusions and forgetfulness. He complained his vision was not right, his speech became slurred and he began to stagger when walking. He became frightened of other people and developed twitching movements and clear memory impairment. After 6 months he was admitted for investigation and had to write on a pad to communicate because of severe dysarthria; he required one person's support to walk. He was childlike and occasionally aggressive. He had an EEG which showed no evidence of CJD and was referred for further investigation of prion disease, but then deteriorated rapidly and died before further tests could be done, 7 months after symptom onset.

Postmortem examination confirmed the diagnosis of vCJD and Western blot showed type 2B prion protein. Studies of the original liver biopsy, the transplanted liver and renal tissue from the same organ donor all showed negative results on immunocytochemistry for prion protein. The liver donor died of causes unrelated to vCJD. Through the TMER study, it was established that Recipient 5 had been exposed to blood components from 103 donors, none of whom were registered as a case of vCJD. On the balance of probabilities, it was concluded that this was most likely a primary case of vCJD, but in view of the heavy blood component exposure, transfusion-transmission could not be excluded.

Because blood transfusion remained a possible source of the patient's vCJD, all 103 blood donors were considered to be "at risk". To avoid the possible recycling of infection, it was advised that the blood donors should all be notified that they were considered the possible source of the recipient's infection and should take public health measures which included not being a donor of blood, organs or tissues. The notification exercise for these donors took place in 2005 and has been reported elsewhere [7]. Twelve years later the donors remain under passive surveillance: many person-years have now passed without any of the cohort developing vCJD [8]. A small number of the donors have died, but the cause of death is known for all of these, and there is no suggestion that any of the deaths were related to CJD. Until there are further developments, there is no method currently available to further define the risk for each of these donors, and all remain "at risk". A further risk assessment was carried out to determine whether other recipients of the 103 notified "at risk" donors could also be considered to be "at risk" of vCJD for public health purposes, but their assessed risk was less than the threshold used for notification, and no action was taken for these individuals.

Case Study Recipient 6: Developed vCJD Having Received Blood Transfusion, no Transfusion Records Available to Identify the Donors

This patient in the 10–20-year age group became very moody in 2005, with periods of aggression and tearfulness, which became more marked with time. After 6 months she developed involuntary jerking movements of the legs, difficulty walking and clumsiness of the hands. All these symptoms progressed until she needed a wheelchair to mobilise and she developed myoclonic movements of the limbs. On examination she was euphoric and had dysarthria and cerebellar ataxia. CSF examination was normal, and an EEG showed slow activity. MRI brain scan showed high signal in the pulvinar region of the thalamus, and the diagnosis was thought to be probable vCJD. The patient gradually deteriorated and died 16 months from symptom onset. Postmortem examination confirmed the diagnosis of vCJD, and Western blot showed type 2B prion protein. The codon 129 genotype was methionine homozygous and there were no mutations.

The patient had been born prematurely and was reported by her family to have had a blood transfusion shortly after birth. Through the TMER study microfilmed records of this hospital admission were retrieved which confirmed that the patient had received four top-up red cell transfusions shortly after birth. The dates of the transfusions were recorded, but other records were scanty and no batch numbers for the red cells were recorded. Because this case occurred in the same part of the country as Recipient Case 5, further investigations were carried out at the blood centre, focusing on whether it was possible that the two recipients shared a common donor. Briefly, the donation records of all 103 identified donors to Recipient 5 were examined. It was established that 18 of them had also made a donation in the time period when Recipient 6 was being transfused in early 1989. The hospitals which received the red cells were identified for all 18 donations, and in one case, this matched the hospital where Recipient 6 was transfused. The red cells were issued with a shelf life which made use for a top-up transfusion to Recipient 6 on one of the recorded dates of transfusion possible. The donor in question made 26 donations in all, and the early 1989 donation was the first. Detailed statistical analysis was performed, looking at the chance of a randomly selected donor in 1993 also having attended at the relevant time in 1989. The further investigation of this case and the possibility of a common donor to the liver transplant case above have been published [9]. The work suggested that coincidence cannot be ruled out as an explanation for the possible link of a common donor with two recipients who developed vCJD. No other recipient of the donor has developed vCJD, and the donor remains well, almost 30 years now having elapsed since the first donation. Furthermore, Recipient 6 developed vCJD 17 years after the blood transfusion, which would represent a significantly longer incubation period than for the three cases linked to donors who were known to have developed vCJD.

Case Study Recipient 7: Blood Donors and their Other Recipients Notified

Recipient 7 was in the 40–50-year age group in 2008 when she became anxious and emotionally labile and resigned from her job. Three months later she developed persistent unpleasant paraesthesia in the legs and problems with balance and walking. There were problems with memory and cognition and she began to struggle with normal day-to-day tasks. Her walking deteriorated and she needed a wheelchair and began to develop myoclonic movements of the limbs. All these symptoms deteriorated, and on admission to hospital she was disorientated and dysarthric and had cerebellar signs in the limbs. Gait was ataxic. MRI scan showed high signal in the pulvinar region of the thalamus and caudate nuclei. She was thought to have probable vCJD and tonsil biopsy was positive, in keeping with this diagnosis. The codon 129 genotype was methionine homozygous and there were no mutations. The patient gradually deteriorated and died 45 months from clinical onset.

The patient was reported to have received a previous blood transfusion, and through the TMER study it was confirmed that two units of leucodepleted red cells were transfused in 2002. The two blood donors had each given a number of blood donations both before and after 2002. The blood donors were informed that they were now considered "at risk of vCJD" and asked to stop donating. Further risk assessment was carried out, and it was established that the assessed risk to other recipients who had received blood components donated by these two "at risk" donors exceeded the threshold which has been used in the UK for considering an individual an additional risk of vCJD. A number of these recipients were already deceased by the time the index recipient was diagnosed with vCJD, but as a result of this exercise, nine surviving recipients of the two donors were notified that they were in turn considered to be at risk of vCJD. Many of these recipients were over 75 years of age when notified, and it is not surprising that some have since died, but none had developed any evidence of vCJD before death, and most survivors have now lived more than 10 years since the transfusion in question.

Summary

The TMER study was set up as a piece of research to establish whether there was any link between vCJD and blood transfusion. Animal studies of transfusion-transmission of prion diseases were also set up, using sheep which had been infected with BSE through their feed as donors to nonexposed sheep. These animal studies demonstrated transmission of BSE to recipient sheep, and such transmission occurred during the incubation period, before clinical disease appeared in the donor sheep. These results were published in 2002 [10]. By the time the first link in humans was established in late 2003, between a donor and a recipient who both developed vCJD, the TMER study had been in place for almost 6 years. What started as a research study has now passed into routine public health surveillance. The cases described in this chapter could all be investigated in such detail because there is one overarching National CJD Research & Surveillance Unit in the UK, and National Blood Services for each of the four countries, which allows close working and collaboration. The detailed surveillance which was put in place in early 1997 allowed rapid identification of the first link and facilitated the necessary public health actions.

Cases of vCJD in the UK have declined since their peak in 2000; there have been only two cases since 2011 (these two cases died in 2013 and 2016), and there has been no new case in a blood donor for many years. All four transfusion-transmission events occurred before the introduction of leucodepletion. Nevertheless, the surveillance work continues, and must continue for years to come, to ensure that a responsive system is in place to detect any second wave, or any atypical presentation of disease, which might require new public health actions.

References

1. Will RG, Ironside JW, Zeidler M, et al. A new variant of Creutzfeldt-Jakob disease in the UK. Lancet. 1996;347:921–5.
2. Urwin PJ, Mackenzie JM, Llewelyn CA, et al. Creutzfeldt-Jakob disease and blood transfusion: updated results of the UK transfusion medicine epidemiology review study. Vox Sang. 2016;110:310–6.
3. Llewelyn CA, Hewitt PE, Knight RS, et al. Possible transmission of variant Creutzfeldt-Jakob disease by blood transfusion. Lancet. 2004;363:417–21.

4. Peden AH, Head MW, Ritchie DL, et al. Preclinical vCJD after blood transfusion in a PRNP codon 129 heterozygous patient. Lancet. 2004;364:527–9.
5. Wroe SJ, Pal S, Siddique D, et al. Clinical presentation and pre-mortem diagnosis of variant Creutzfeldt-Jakob disease associated with blood transfusion: a case report. Lancet. 2006;368:2061–7.
6. Pal S, Webb T, Alner K, et al. Atypical presentation of variant Creutzfeld-Jakob disease in a 73 year old blood transfusion recipient. J Neurol Neurosurg Psychiatr. 2007;78:1014–38.
7. Hewitt PE, Moore C, Soldan K. vCJD donor notification exercise: 2005. J Clin Ethics. 2006;1:172–8.
8. Checchi M, Hewitt PE, Bennett P, et al. Ten-year follow-up of two cohorts with an increased risk of variant CJD: donors to individuals who later developed variant CJD and other recipients of these at-risk donors. Vox Sang. 2016;111:325–32.
9. Davidson LRR, Llewelyn CA, MacKenzie JM, et al. Variant CJD and blood transfusion: are there additional cases? Vox Sang. 2014;107:220–5.
10. Hunter N, Foster J, Chong A, et al. Transfusion of prion diseases by blood transfusion. J Gen Virol. 2002;83:2897–905.

Chapter 8
Case Study: West Nile Virus

Roger Y. Dodd

Introduction

The emergence of AIDS/HIV in the 1980s prompted concern that there would be additional transfusion-transmitted infections and that they would be likely to follow the same epidemiologic pattern. The emergence of West Nile virus in 1999 did fulfill the expectation that there would be new infections to manage, but unexpectedly, this was an acute infection, transmitted by mosquitoes. Nevertheless, once its threat to blood safety was recognized, preventive measures were rapidly developed and deployed.

West Nile Virus

West Nile virus (WNV) was first recognized in 1937 in the West Nile district of Uganda and was subsequently identified in birds in the Nile Delta in 1953. Currently, it is known to be present in Africa, parts of Europe, the Middle East, West Asia, and since 1999, the Americas. The virus is in the *Flavivirus* genus and belongs to the Japanese encephalitis antigenic complex of the family *Flaviviridae*. The virus is transmitted by culicine mosquitoes and can infect many vertebrates, but the amplifying hosts are birds. Humans are accidental, end-stage hosts, and there is no human-mosquito-human cycle [1, 2].

The incubation period for WNV is 2–6 days, occasionally extending to 14 days. Some 80% of infections are asymptomatic; most of those who have symptoms have

---

R. Y. Dodd
American Red Cross, Medical Office, Rockville, MD, USA

Department of Pathology, Johns Hopkins University, Baltimore, MD, USA
e-mail: Roger.Dodd@redcross.org

an acute, systemic febrile illness, commonly with headache, weakness, and myalgia or arthralgia. In some cases, there may be gastrointestinal symptoms and a transient maculopapular rash. About 1 in 150 infected individuals will have severe neuroinvasive disease, including meningoencephalitis, or acute flaccid paralysis, in some cases leading to death. There is no specific treatment, nor is there currently a human vaccine [2].

West Nile Virus and Transfusion Safety

Prior to 1999, WNV was relatively widely distributed globally, with the exception of the Americas. In general, human outbreaks were scattered and relatively small, affecting no more than a few hundred individuals. These outbreaks were self-limiting and were not seen as a threat to blood safety. However, in August 1999, a very different situation emerged in the United States. The first few cases occurred in Queens, New York City, as a cluster of six elderly patients with encephalitis and a febrile illness affecting a small number of older subjects. These cases were first thought to be St. Louis encephalitis, but the responsible agent was eventually identified as West Nile virus, appearing for the first time in the Western hemisphere. By the end of September, 17 confirmed and 20 probable cases were recognized, including 4 deaths [3]. The actual source of the virus was never definitively identified; one theory involves birds imported for the local zoo. Extensive surveillance was undertaken, and it was found that the virus spread rapidly up and down the East Coast and then West [4]. Within a few years, the virus was present in birds, mosquitoes, and humans across the entire continental United States, with outbreaks of human disease starting in early summer and continuing into the autumn months [5]. In peak years, it was estimated that there were several hundred thousand human infections and up to almost 1500 cases of human West Nile neurologic disease, some of which were fatal.

Initially, this large and unexpected outbreak of WNV was not considered to be a significant risk to blood safety, largely because of the acute nature of the infection and its rather short period of viremia in humans. However, Biggerstaff and colleagues at CDC developed and published an estimate of the risk of transmission of WNV via transfusion, and shortly after its publication in 2002 [6], the first such transmission was recognized. Eventually, 23 such transmissions were described in that same year [7], and nucleic acid tests for viral RNA were developed and implemented by the beginning of the 2003 outbreak. The FDA permitted the implementation under investigational new drug (IND) mechanisms to ensure rapid initiation prior to licensure [8, 9].

Accumulated data from the Red Cross (collecting about 40% of the US blood supply) 2003–2014 indicated that around 27 million donations had been tested and that 1576 RNA-positive donations had been identified. During this period, only one transmission to a blood recipient had been identified, and this was in a recipient of granulocytes that had been transfused before the (positive) test result had been available [10, 11].

In the United States, nucleic acid testing of blood donors has generally been achieved through testing minipools of 6 or 16 samples, depending on the technology in use. (The US regulatory agency initially required single-donation testing for Zika virus.) It soon became apparent that some donations had low levels of WNV that could not be detected in minipools, but that were nevertheless infectious, and there were a small number of resulting transfusion transmissions. This finding led to the development and refining of mechanisms to convert screening to individual donation testing in locations and times with a significant incidence of infection [10]. The process includes criteria for triggering and for ceasing individual donation testing and processes for rapid communication between blood collection sites, so that neighboring blood centers can be alerted to the need for triggering. This has resulted in a situation where the risk of transmission is minimized, and there are only very rare breakthrough infections among recipients. A nationwide total of 13 such cases were reported between 2003 and 2014 [10], and there have been 2 or 3 in the following years. The triggering approach will likely establish a model for donor testing for Zika virus as the outbreak wanes.

Extended Information

As a result of donor testing programs, a great deal of information about the pathology and epidemiology of WNV has been developed. In particular, the dynamics of infection and marker expression are well known, and it has become clear that transfusion transmission is a risk only in the early days of infection, prior to the development of detectable antibodies. As might be expected of a virus that has a non-human amplifying host, the maximum levels of viremia in humans are quite low, essentially negating the possibility of an urban, human-mosquito-human cycle [10].

An early response to risk reduction was to ask blood donors if they had any symptoms of West Nile fever before (or just after) donation, but a number of studies showed that this approach was not effective in identifying potentially infectious donations, and the approach was abandoned with the exception of routine, passive post-donation information procedures, which did not specifically target WNV [12].

It is reasonable to assume that the infection is sustained year-to-year in overwintering mosquitoes and that, given that there are new generations of birds every year, herd immunity in the amplifying host will not occur. Thus, WNV has become endemic in North America, but the size of the resulting annual outbreak is not readily predicted. Overall, however, the basis for the extent of the outbreak in North America is not well understood and seems to be very different from the rest of the world.

International Reaction to WNV

As noted above, the broad, continental epidemic and endemicity appears to be unique to North America, and reactions to this virus in other parts of the world are quite different from the widespread testing in the United States. Relatively small, self-contained outbreaks occur, particularly in Europe and are managed locally, most often by cessation of blood collection in the affected area. At the same time, there is concern about imported infection, and in many countries, individuals with recent travel from the United States are temporarily deferred from donation.

Lessons Learned

The outbreak of West Nile virus in the United States was the first example of a significant blood safety threat from an acute infection. For many years, transfusion transmission of hepatitis A virus had been recognized, but it was a rare event. West Nile refocused existing expectations that any future transfusion-transmitted infection would be chronic and parenterally transmitted, as was the case for HIV and hepatitis B and C viruses. Subsequently, outbreaks of other tropical arboviruses (such as chikungunya, dengue, and Zika) have potentially or actually threatened blood safety. However, as these viruses are predominantly spread by *Aedes* spp. mosquitoes, the risk of nationwide outbreaks in North America is absent.

A very important aspect of the emergence of WNV was the recognition of the need to establish wide-scale testing in a short period. Fortunately, this was aided by the fact that NAT was a suitable test protocol and that NAT platforms were already in widespread use. Overall, tests were developed and implemented within about 8–9 months of the decision to undertake this effort [13]. A similarly rapid response to Zika virus has been mounted in the United States, although the size of this threat seems to be much smaller and at the time or writing (2018), the epidemic in the Americas seems to be waning.

Although WNV is seasonal, the FDA required year-round testing. However it was accepted that, in times and areas with low or absent numbers of active infections, minipool testing was considered to provide an adequate assurance of safety. However it did become apparent that such an approach was not fully effective in the face of active outbreaks, and the novel concept of initiating individual donation testing was developed [10]. In essence, the minipool testing served as part of the surveillance program to identify outbreaks. Effective management of this program did include the development of a rapid communication network among blood collection sites, so that there would be awareness of outbreaks in neighboring areas and appropriate triggering of individual donation testing. There is little doubt that the various measures to identify potentially infectious donations had a substantial impact, almost eliminating the risk of transfusion-transmitted WNV. However, it is possible that such measures might not be necessary in the face of universal pathogen reduction.

References

1. Campbell GL, Marfin AA, Lanciotti RS, Gubler DJ. West Nile virus. Lancet Infect Dis. 2002;2:519–29.
2. Petersen LR, Brault AC, Nasci RS. West Nile virus: review of the literature. JAMA. 2013;310:308–15.
3. Centers for Disease Control. Outbreak of West Nile-like viral encephalitis – New York, 1999. MMWR. 1999;48:845–9.
4. Petersen LR, Hayes EB. Westward Ho? The spread of West Nile virus. N Engl J Med. 2004;351:2257–9.
5. Petersen LR, Fischer M. Unpredictable and difficult to control – the adolescence of West Nile virus. N Engl J Med. 2012;367:1281–4.
6. Biggerstaff BJ, Petersen LR. Estimated risk of West Nile virus transmission through blood transfusion in Queens, New York City. Transfusion. 2002;42:1019–26.
7. Pealer LN, Marfin AA, Petersen LR, Lanciotti RS, Page PL, Stramer SL, et al. Transmission of West Nile virus through blood transfusion in the United States in 2002. N Engl J Med. 2003;349:1236–45.
8. Stramer SL, Fang CT, Foster GA, Wagner AG, Brodsky JP, Dodd RY. West Nile virus among blood donors in the United States, 2003 and 2004. N Engl J Med. 2005;353:451–9.
9. Busch MP, Caglioti S, Robertson EF, McCauley JD, Tobler LH, Kamel H, et al. Screening the blood supply for West Nile virus RNA by nucleic acid amplification testing. N Engl J Med. 2005;353:460–7.
10. Dodd RY, Foster GA, Stramer SL. Keeping blood safe from West Nile virus: American Red Cross Experience, 2003–2012. Transfus Med Rev. 2015;29:153–61.
11. Meny GM, Santos-Zabala L, Szallasi A, Stramer SL. West Nile virus infection transmitted by granulocyte transfusion. Blood. 2011;117:5778–9.
12. Orton SL, Stramer SL, Dodd RY. Self-reported symptoms associated with West Nile virus infection in RNA-positive blood donors. Transfusion. 2006;46:272–7.
13. Dodd RY. Emerging infections, transfusion safety, and epidemiology. N Engl J Med. 2003;349:1205–6.

Chapter 9
Zika Virus

Luiz Amorim

Historical Aspects

Zika virus is an RNA virus of the *Flaviviridae* family. It was discovered in 1947 in the Zika Forest of Uganda, during monitoring of rhesus monkeys used as sentinels for the epidemiological surveillance of yellow fever [1].

The discovery occurred when the virus isolated from an infected monkey was found not to be the yellow fever virus but a distinct virus, which was named Zika in honor of the forest. The first Zika human case probably occurred in 1954, in a 10-year-old Nigerian girl. However, there remains doubt regarding the real etiology of the viral infection presented by this patient [2].

The first confirmed human cases occurred in Uganda, in 1962/1963 [3]. After this, there were several sporadic case reports on the African continent. Outside Africa, Zika's first cases were reported in Java Island, Indonesia, in 1977 [4]. There are recent retrospective seroprevalence studies, confirmed by more sophisticated molecular techniques, indicating that Zika virus was already circulating on the African and Asian continents since the 1950s, though without causing any outbreak [5].

The first outbreak of Zika in humans occurred in Yap Island, Micronesia, in 2007. The epidemic affected 5000 people, according to some estimates, which corresponded to about 75% of Yap Island's population. There were no reports of severe forms of the infection. One hundred eighty-five probable and/or confirmed cases were detected, and the overall attack rate among patients presenting to health services was estimated in 14.6 per 1000 Yap residents [6].

After this, a new epidemic would only occur in 2013, in French Polynesia; this time, the epidemic has gained large proportions, and more than 30,000 cases have been reported, with estimates that almost 100% of the population of French

L. Amorim
Hemorio Blood Center, Rio de Janeiro, Brazil
e-mail: luizamorimfilho@gmail.com

Polynesia has been reached [7], based on the estimate that only 20% of Zika's cases are symptomatic [6].

From French Polynesia, the epidemic spread to New Caledonia, Cook Islands, Easter Island, and the entire South Pacific [8]. In the French Polynesian outbreak, an association between Zika infection and Guillain-Barré syndrome (GBS) was described for the first time [7].

In 2015, the first cases of the disease were confirmed in Brazil, where the virus probably arrived in 2013 [9]. In Brazil, the epidemic took great proportions, and a fearsome neurological complication of Zika's infection—microcephaly—was quickly identified in newborns whose mothers were infected by ZIKV during pregnancy [10].

From Brazil, the virus then spread to the other countries of South America and Central America, later reaching some states in the USA, such as Florida, Texas, and California, where autochthonous cases of the disease were reported.

For this reason, and taking into account the severe consequences of Zika infection in pregnant women, the FDA stated that screening of Zika in blood donors using molecular biology techniques would be mandatory in all American states as of August 2016 (see below) [11, 12].

ZIKV is now present in more than 100 countries (Fig. 9.1) and has become one of the world's major public health concerns, especially because of its cause-effect relationship with microcephaly and other congenital and extremely serious neurological and ophthalmic lesions.

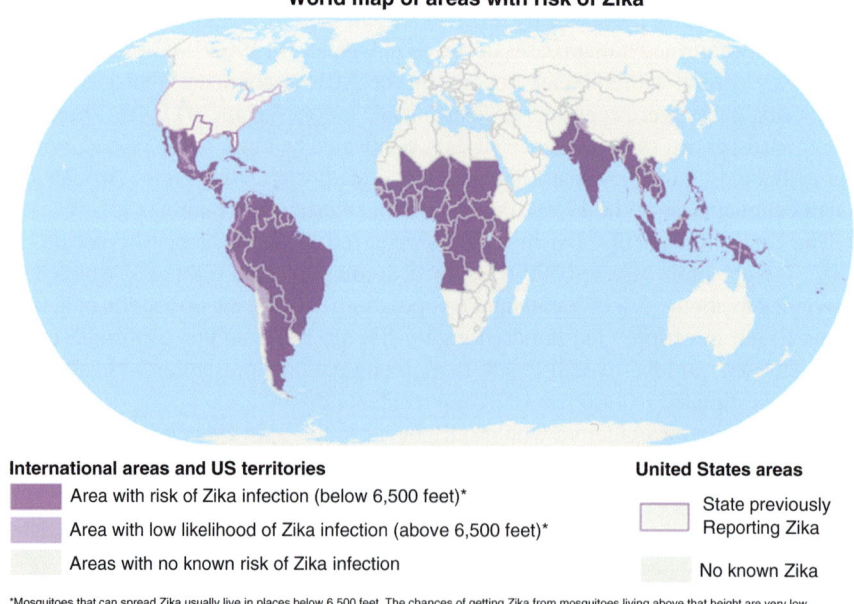

Fig. 9.1 World map of areas with Zika. (From the Centers for Disease Control, https://wwwnc.cdc.gov/travel/files/zika-areas-of-risk.pdf. Accessed 5 June 2018)

Virology

Zika virus (ZIKV) is a single-stranded, positive-sense RNA virus. It has a 10.7 kb genome, which encodes a single polyprotein that is cleaved into three structural proteins (C, prM/M, E) and seven nonstructural proteins (NS1, NS2A, NS2B, NS3, NS4A, NS4B, and NS5) [13]. ZIKV belongs to the *Flaviviridae* family, genus *Flavivirus*, and it has a great homology with the dengue virus (Fig. 9.2).

The envelope (E) glycoprotein, embedded in the membrane, allows attachment of the virus particle to the host cell receptor to initiate infection. As for other flaviviruses, antibodies against the E glycoprotein are likely to be important against protection against infection [13].

Zika virus has two lineages: Asian and African. In Africa, nonhuman primates can theoretically be involved in the maintenance of the transmission cycle, as well as the human reservoir. For the Asian lineage, humans are the main hosts [14]. ZIKV is a pathogenic and neurotropic virus, as has been shown in recent epidemics and also in animal models.

Few complete Zika virus genome sequences are available. Phylogenetic analysis of a Suriname Zika virus indicates that it belongs to the Asian genotype. It is most closely related to the strain that was circulating in French Polynesia in 2013, sharing more than 99.7% and 99.9% of nucleotide and amino acid identity, respectively [14].

The mutation in the Asian lineage may have led to the virus' adaptation to the human (as opposed to nonhuman primate) host [15]. So far, this is an unconfirmed

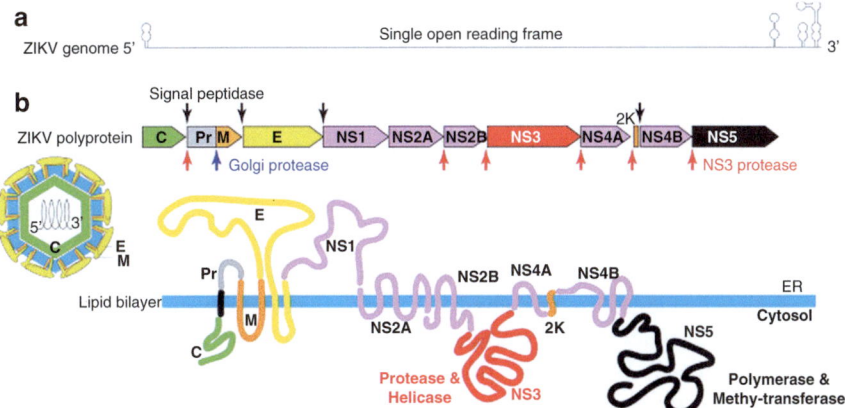

Fig. 9.2 Zika genome. (**a**) A diagram of a flavivirus genomic RNA. (**b**) Processing strategy and protein products. The polyprotein is processed at various sites by host (*red arrow heads*) and viral (*down black arrows*) proteases. NS1 is a lumenal protein that functions during replication and can also be secreted to the outside of the cell to act as a pathogenesis factor. (Reprinted from Ming et al. [76]. With permission from Elsevier)

hypothesis. There is also an unconfirmed hypothesis claiming that another mutation was responsible for severe diseases, such as congenital Zika syndrome.

Epidemiology

The vectors of ZIKV transmission are mosquitoes of the *Aedes* genus; the virus has already been isolated in *Aedes africanus*, *Aedes aegypti*—by far the most effective vector—and *Aedes albopictus hersenii*, responsible for some autochthonous cases in the USA [16]. It is now known that nonvector transmission is also possible, including by blood transfusion (see below).

A major problem in defining the precise dimensions of each epidemic is the difficulty for carrying out confirmatory tests, especially of a molecular nature, for the notified cases. This would be very important due to the clinical similarity between ZIKV infection and other arboviruses such as dengue and chikungunya, which co-circulate in many countries affected by the ZIKV. The lack of specific serological tests further complicates this task.

In the Yap Island epidemic, for example, out of 5000 presumed cases, only 49 were confirmed by viral RNA detection [6]. The estimates of 5000 cases in this island over a 3-year period are derived from seroprevalence surveys using low or moderate specificity serological tests (anti-IgG), which were (and they still are) the only ones available on a large scale for the serological diagnosis of Zika, at the time of the Yap outbreak.

The French Polynesian epidemic began in October 2013 with the reporting, including molecular proof, of three cases in the same household [5]. After these first patients, it is estimated that more than 19,000 may have been reported; as the total population of French Polynesia is approximately 270,000 people, it is possible that the infection has reached 100,000 people, almost half of the population [5].

The association between ZIKV infection and the onset of Guillain-Barré syndrome was also discovered during the epidemic in French Polynesia, where 42 cases of GBS associated with recent ZIKV infection have been described [17].

After French Polynesia, the next major epidemic—and by far the largest one—has occurred in Brazil, a country that is about 7000 miles away from French Polynesia. There is still some controversy about how the virus came to Brazil. It is very possible that it occurred in June 2013, during the Confederations Cup, a soccer tournament preparatory to the World Cup bringing together the soccer's champions from each continent. With Tahiti representing Oceania, the tournament was based in the cities of Recife and Salvador in the Northeast of Brazil, which are precisely the epicenters of the Zika epidemic in the country. This hypothesis is based on molecular epidemiology studies carried out by Rodrigues et al. [18], which showed that the age of the viral genome and the ZIKV sequencing found in Brazil corresponded to the Polynesian virus.

According to this hypothesis, it took 2 years between the introduction of the virus and the outbreak of the epidemic, since the first cases of Zika were reported as of May 2015 [9].

There are another three published hypotheses explaining how ZIKV came to be introduced into Brazil. The virus may have arrived in Brazil in June/July 2014, during the Soccer World Cup or in August 2014, during a canoe tournament—the Va'a World Sprint Championship canoe race—held in Rio de Janeiro, which included Tahitian teams [19].

Another hypothesis is that the virus introduction occurred during October 2012–May 2013, from multiple in-country sources, which is supported by the ZIVV detection in 2012 and 2013 through retrospective mosquito-based surveillance [20].

It seems more likely that the introduction of the virus occurred in the Northeast part of Brazil, from there expanding to other urban centers where the density of *Aedes aegypti* is high. In any case, the result was an epidemic of enormous proportion. The table below shows the number of Zika cases reported in Brazil from November 2015 to December 2017.

It should be noted that these numbers are probably underestimated, since the national epidemiological surveillance system for Zika, which includes compulsory reporting of cases and subsequent investigation, was only put into practice in November 2015. See Table 9.1.

At the end of 2015, Dr. de Oliveira Melo, a pediatrician working in the Northeast region, suspected that there might be some correlation between the large numbers of newborns with microcephaly and the high number of pregnant women seeking medical care with signs and symptoms of Zika infection. She started to look for scientific evidences to establish this correlation, and she rapidly succeeded (see below).

Thereafter, a number of epidemiological, virological, and even histopathological studies demonstrated that this correlation did indeed exist and was very consistent. The Brazilian Ministry of Health also started to monitor cases of microcephaly. This quickly became a huge public health problem. Table 9.2 shows the number of cases of microcephaly reported in Brazil from 2010 to 2017, as well as the number of cases in which the association with the Zika virus was confirmed.

Zika now affects more than 100 countries around the world, including US states and territories. The cumulative number of Zika cases in the USA, as of 5 April 2018, is seen in Table 9.3.

Table 9.1 Zika cases in Brazil

Year	Confirmed or probable cases	Incidence ($\times 10^5$ inhabitants)
2015 (Nov–Dec)	2401	1.2
2016	215,319	105.6
2017	4263	2.1
2018 (Jan–Feb)	705	0.3
Total	*220,287*	–

Data source: Ministry of Health Epidemiological Bulletin, 2018 [21]

Table 9.2 Notified cases of microcephaly in Brazil: 2010–2017

Year	Notified cases	Confirmed or probable Zika-associated cases	Cases under investigation	Proportion of confirmed/probable cases after investigation
2010	153	–	–	33%
2011	139	–	–	
2012	175	–	–	
2013	167	–	–	
2014	147	–	–	
2015	4120	1014	254	
2016	8599	2021	1365	
2017	2579	375	1250	
Total	16,079	3785	2869	

Data source: Ministry of Health. Epidemiological Bulletin [22]

Table 9.3 Cumulative number of Zika cases in the USA: 2016–2018

	Number of cases	Route of transmission				
		Travelers returning from affected areas	Local mosquito-borne transmission	Sexual transmission	Laboratory transmission	Unknown route
US states	5676	5392 (95%)	229 (4%)	55 (0.97%)	2 (0.035%)	1 (0.018%)
US territories	37,190	147 (0.39%)	37,043 (99.61%)	0		

Data source: Centers for Disease Control and Prevention (CDC) [11]

Clinical Manifestations of Zika Infection

The signs and symptoms of Zika infection, when they do exist, usually appear 4–7 days (on average, 6 days) after virus inoculation; the symptoms last, on average, 5 days, with reports of up to 1–2 weeks. On average, ZIKV viremia persists for 10 days after infection [23, 24].

The clinical manifestations of Zika infection are very similar to those of other arboviruses such as dengue and chikungunya. During the Zika epidemic of the Yap Islands in 2007, the main symptoms observed were macular or papular rash, which affected 90% of the patients: fever and myalgia, both present in 65% of the cases; arthritis or arthralgia of small joints, especially of the hands (65% of the cases); non-purulent conjunctivitis (55%); headache (45%); and retro-orbital pain (39%) [6].

Taking into account this seminal study, Halstead et al. [25] established a comparison between the symptoms and Zika and those of dengue and chikungunya (Table 9.4), which is very helpful for clinicians in areas where the three arboviruses co-circulate.

Table 9.4 A comparison among dengue, chikungunya, and Zika symptoms

Symptoms	Dengue	Chikungunya	Zika
Fever	++++	+++	+++
Myalgia/arthralgia	+++	++++	++
Edema of extremities	0	0	++
Maculopapular rash	++	++	+++
Retro-orbital pain	++	+	++
Conjunctivitis	0	+	+++
Lymphadenopathies	++	++	+
Hepatomegaly	0	+++	0
Leukopenia/thrombopenia	+++	+++	0
Hemorrhage	+	0	0

The Pan American Health Organization (PAHO) has created a definition for provisional Zika cases, based on patients' signs and symptoms. This definition is shown in Table 9.5

Table 9.5 PAHO: Provisional case definition of suspected acute Zika virus infection [26]

Rash or increase in body temperature (>37.2 °C), with any of the following signs/symptoms not explained by other conditions:
Arthralgia or myalgia
Non-purulent conjunctivitis
Conjunctival hyperemia
Headache
Malaise

Source: PAHO

Moreover, PAHO proposes a definition for a suspected case of Zika virus disease in geographic areas without autochthonous transmission and where there are no vectors present. In such situations, the patients should meet the above criteria and have not traveled **or** resided in a geographic area where there is known local transmission of the Zika virus **or** there is known vector presence in the 2 weeks prior to onset *or* had unprotected sex, also in the 2 weeks prior to onset, with a person who traveled, in the previous 8 weeks, to a geographic area with known local transmission of the Zika virus and/or area with known vector presence [26].

For PAHO, a probable Zika disease case affects a patient who meets the criteria of a suspected case *and* has Zika IgM antibodies, with no evidence of infection with other flaviviruses. Finally, a confirmed case, according to PAHO, would include patients meeting the criteria for a suspected case *and* having laboratory confirmation of recent Zika virus infection. This laboratory confirmation relies on RNA or Zika virus antigen in any specimen (serum, urine, saliva, tissue, or whole blood) or positive Zika IgM antibodies and plaque reduction neutralization for Zika virus titers 20 and 4 or more times greater than the titers for other flaviviruses and exclusion of other flaviviruses or, in autopsy specimens, detection of the viral genome (in fresh or paraffin tissue) by molecular techniques and/or by immunohistochemistry [26].

A very elegant review of Zika symptoms and signs was recently published based on cases seen during the Brazilian outbreak [27]. Table 9.6 summarizes the review's main findings.

Congenital Zika Syndrome (CZS)

During the outbreak of Zika in Brazil, pediatricians started to see many cases of congenital microcephaly in newborns whose mothers had Zika infection or a rash attributable to Zika during pregnancy.

At first, there was much controversy regarding the cause-effect relationship between Zika's infection and the onset of microcephaly. One of the arguments was that no microcephaly cases were reported during the epidemic in French Polynesia.

Little by little, however, evidence was emerging to dispel any doubts in this regard. Four articles in particular were determinants in the establishment of Zika as an etiologic agent of microcephaly in newborns.

The first of those four studies is published by de Oliveira Melo et al. [28]. They detected Zika virus on amniotic fluid from two pregnant women bearing a microcephalic fetus.

The second study showed Zika detection, by immunohistochemical techniques, in the tissues from four microcephalic newborns, two spontaneous miscarriages, and two newborn fatalities less than 24 h birth [29].

Then, there was a case from a Slovenian woman who lived in the Northeast part of Brazil, the epicenter of Zika infection in the country. She was pregnant and acquired Zika early in the pregnancy. Since voluntary abortion is not allowed in Brazil for this type of situation, she went back to Slovenia, where she was allowed to abort at the eighth month of pregnancy. Zika virus was found in fetal brain tissue, and the findings were confirmed by electronic microscopy [30].

Finally, ophthalmologic lesions were detected in three microcephalic newborns with cerebral calcification whose mothers had been infected with Zika during

Table 9.6 Clinical characteristics of Zika

Parameter	Zika symptoms/signs
Severity	Majority asymptomatic
Illness course	Low-grade fever with headache and arthralgia or myalgia. Followed by rash
First symptoms/phase	Low-grade fever (<38.5 °C)
Second phase/other major symptoms	Headache, mild joint pain, pruritus, conjunctivitis, fatigue
Rash details	Maculopapular rash begins on the torso or neck; spreads throughout the body; typically occurs after initial 3–4 days of fever and arthralgia/myalgia; can be pruritic
Distinguishing features	Low fever

Adapted from [27]. (Reprinted by permission from Springer Nature: He et al. [27])

pregnancy. This fourth study was the first to demonstrate that transplacental Zika transmission could also affect the fetal ocular system [31].

After that, lookback studies in French Polynesia [32] were able to trace several microcephaly cases due to pregnant infection by ZIKV; the same was seen in other countries affected by Zika outbreak, such as Colombia and Caribbean islands [33, 34].

Three years after the first reports of congenital neurological disease caused by Zika, there are more than 1000 published reports of this capital aspect of Zika virus infection. Some evidence has now arisen from all these observations.

– Infection during the first trimester of pregnancy in which the fetal brain is being formed is associated with the highest risk of microcephaly, miscarriages, and perinatal deaths. Nevertheless, the babies can also be affected even if the infection occurred in the second or third trimester of pregnancy [35].
– The cumulative prevalence of microcephalic babies in pregnant women infected by Zika, according to a meta-analysis of 8 studies (out of 930 initially reviewed), was 2.3%, if we consider only pregnancies with live birth, and 2.7% if all affected pregnancies are included [36].
– Miscarriage, stillbirth, and intrauterine growth restrictions have also been reported in association with ZIKV in pregnancy [37].
– Congenital Zika syndrome (CZS) is now much better understood. It goes far beyond microcephaly. Ocular abnormalities, hearing deficits, and several neurological problems have been described as part of this new teratogenic syndrome [38]. It is considered as a complex ensemble of neurological problems, sometimes not including microcephaly, since in many cases the babies do have neurological problems, but they present normal head circumference values. For example, in a series of 1501 cases of congenital Zika syndrome, in half of CZS confirmed cases, the babies did not show microcephaly [39].

According to the Centers for Disease Control and Prevention (CDC), the distinctive features of the CZS are microcephaly; brain abnormalities, including cerebral cortex thinning, abnormal gyral patterns, increased fluid spaces, subcortical calcifications, corpus callosum anomalies, reduced white matter, and cerebellar vermis hypoplasia; ocular findings; and congenital contracture, including unilateral or bilateral clubfoot and arthrogryposis multiplex, pronounced early hypertonia or spasticity with extrapyramidal symptoms, motor disabilities, cognitive disabilities, hypotonia, irritability or excessive crying, tremors, swallowing dysfunction, visual impairment, hearing impairment, and epilepsy [38].

– Among the neuropathologic postmortem problems already identified, there are [40]:

  - Microcephaly with ex vacuo ventriculomegaly
  - Large head circumference associated with obstructive hydrocephalus, with aqueduct distortion
  - Arthrogryposis

- Destruction of the hemispheric parenchyma
- Calcifications
- Reactive gliosis
- Cerebellar hypoplasia

The ophthalmic lesions and dysfunctions associated with ZIKV are numerous, as was shown in a series review by Paula-Freitas et al. [41]. Ophthalmologic abnormalities were present in 17 (29.3%) eyes of 10 children (34.5%); bilateral findings were seen in 7 of 10 patients presenting ocular lesions. The most common lesions were focal retinal pigment mottling and chorioretinal atrophy in 11 (64.7%) of 17 eyes with abnormalities, followed by optic nerve abnormalities. In another series, 15 (63.6%) out of 24 infants who tested positive for ZIKV infections had ophthalmic abnormalities.

Finally, there are also congenital cardiac abnormalities in babies infected by ZIKV during their intrauterine lives. A study conducted in Rio de Janeiro, Brazil [42], which included 120 children infected by ZIKV during pregnancy (confirmed by PCR), found 48 children (40%) with cardiac defects on echocardiography. Thirteen infants (10.8%) had more serious problems, such as atrial septal defect, ventricular septal defect, and patent ductus arteriosus.

Guillain-Barré Syndrome (GBS) and Other Acute Neurologic Complications

One of the most striking complications of Zika infection, besides microcephaly, is Guillain-Barré syndrome. GBS is classically associated with post-viral and post-bacterial conditions (in this case, especially after *Campylobacter jejuni* infections). It was also linked to Zika infection, for the first time, after reports from the French Polynesian outbreak [17].

There, in a period of 7 months, from October 2013 to April 2014, 42 cases of Guillain-Barré syndrome were reported [43]. In 41 cases (97.6% of the total cases observed in the period), patients had anti-Zika IgM antibodies, and 100% of the patients had neutralizing antibodies. A case-control study by Cao-Lormeau et al., in French Polynesia, demonstrated the clear association between ZIKV infection and the later appearance of Guillain-Barré syndrome [44].

In French Polynesia, the majority of patients who had GBS had previous symptoms; on average, the neurological disease manifested itself in 4–10 days (mean of 6 days) after the onset of these Zika symptoms. In this series, no patient died [43].

The incidence of GBS cases during the French Polynesian outbreak was estimated to be 0.24 per 1000 ZIKV infections, similar to the incidence of GBS after *C. jejuni* infection. A recently published meta-analysis of Zika-associated GBS cases included 165,000 cases of Zika, of which 1513 patients had GBS. Using a fixed-effect meta-analysis model, the authors estimated that 1.23% of ZIKV infection cases could progress to GBS (95% CI = 1.17–1.29%) [45].

During the great epidemic that plagued Brazil, the number of reported GBS cases has also considerably increased. Several of these cases were shown to be associated with previous and recent infection by ZIKV [46].

In Brazil, unlike the reports from French Polynesia, there were deaths caused by GBS associated with Zika infection. In addition, other post-infection neurological complications were observed, as in a series of cases that occurred in the state of Rio de Janeiro, Brazil. Besides GBS (27 cases in this series), encephalitis (5 cases), transverse myelitis (2 cases), and chronic inflammatory demyelinating polyneuropathy (1 case) were also described [47].

In this series of cases in the state of Rio de Janeiro, Brazil, there were 2 deaths (6% of the cases), and 18 patients (51%) had chronic pain 6 months after the acute illness. In a series of 50 cases in the city of Salvador, state of Bahia, mortality was exactly the same: 6% [47].

Zika-associated GBS was treated by intravenous immunoglobulin or by plasmapheresis, along with supportive care, including mechanical ventilation.

Nonvector Transmission of Zika

In addition to the probable transmission by blood transfusions (see below), the ZIKV can also be transmitted by other means, which do not involve the vector mosquito. Among these means are transmission through saliva, breast milk, sexual transmission, and laboratory contamination [48].

Transmission by Saliva

Of the four modes, transmission through saliva seems very unlikely; it is a fact that the virus has already been identified in human saliva in the acute phase of infection [49] and that there is a case report describing a possible transmission after a monkey bite, but this case was never confirmed, since it was not possible to exclude much more probable vector transmission [50].

Sexual Transmission

There is no doubt that sexual transmission of Zika does occur; the first known case occurred in 2008 in an American scientist who, returning from Senegal, transmitted the virus to his wife in the USA [51].

A review of Zika's sexual transmission, published in May 2017 [52], analyzed 18 studies reporting a total of 27 cases of sexual transmission of ZIKV. Sexual transmission occurred more frequently from man to woman (92.5% of reported cases) than from woman to man (3.7% of reported cases—just one case described); in 3.7% of the reports, the transmission occurred from man to man (again, just one case described).

The most frequent types of sexual relationship in which the virus was transmitted were unprotected vaginal intercourse (96.2%) and oral (18.5%) and anal (7.4%) sexual intercourse. The mean time between onset of symptoms in the index partner and presumed sexual transmission was 13 days (range 4–44 days) [52].

Musso and co-workers [53] longitudinally tested semen samples collected from asymptomatic blood donors. They found 45 blood donors who tested positive for ZIKV RNA in plasma during ZIKV outbreaks in Puerto Rico and Florida in 2016.

Five of the 14 (35.7%) asymptomatic blood donors provided semen samples that tested positive for ZIKV RNA. ZIKV loads range from 8.03×10^3 to 2.55×10^6 copies/mL. Plasma collected at the same time as the semen tested negative for ZIKV RNA for most ZIKV RNA-positive semen collections [53].

Transmission by Breast Milk

Transmission through breast milk was suspected when ZIKV RNA was detected in breast milk from two mothers, during the French Polynesian epidemic [54]. However, when viruses were inoculated in Vero cells, in vitro, there was no viral replication, which made the transmission via this route very unlikely. Both infants had ZIKV in their plasma, even though the viremia had started 24 h before breastfeeding begins.

Recently, Colt et al. [55] have systematically reviewed the published suspected cases of Zika transmission by breastfeeding. Of the 472 studies evaluated, only 2 were amenable to analysis. These two studies included three mother-child pairs. The first analyzed report was the one from French Polynesia, abovementioned. The second study was published by Dupont-Rouzeyrol et al. [56], in New Caledonia, a French territory in the South Pacific. Dupont-Rouzeyrol demonstrated the presence of ZIKV viral particles in the breast milk of a febrile mother on the fourth day after delivery; these viruses were successfully cultured in breast milk. However, the child did not show any symptoms or complications attributable to Zika virus infection.

More recently, there was a case report from a Venezuelan patient, who was exclusively breastfeeding her 5-month-old child [57]. She had acquired Zika infection; the virus was isolated in breast milk as well as in the child's urine. The virus was successfully cultured in milk. There was a 99% homology between the mother's and child's virus. The mother had symptoms of mild disease, whereas the child remained asymptomatic.

So far, there is no conclusive evidence that the virus is transmitted through breast milk, but it is also not possible to rule out this hypothesis. Therefore, many doubts remain about the recommendation to be made to lactating women who acquire Zika, whether or not to interrupt breastfeeding. The official recommendation from World Health Organization (WHO) [58] is that breastfeeding should not be interrupted.

Laboratory Contamination

Regarding transmission by accidental contamination in the laboratory, there is a case report from the early 1960s, corresponding to a possible laboratory contamination [3].

Zika Persistence in Body Fluids

ZIKV persistence in body fluids can be very different according to the type of fluid. In semen, for example, the virus can persist for more than 60 days in 18.2% of the studied cases. In serum, the virus persists for 8–15 days in 35% of the cases, and in 3.2% of the cases, it can persist for more than 60 days. In urine, the persistence can last to 8–15 days in 41.4% of the cases and 16–30 days in 11.2% of the cases [59].

ZIKV Transfusion-Transmission

Transmission of the Zika virus by blood transfusions turned out to be considered a concrete possibility since the studies of Musso et al. in the French Polynesian outbreak [60]. Musso and his team performed blood donor NAT tests, starting in January 2014, on minipools of three samples. In total, 1505 donors were tested. Of the total number of donors tested, 42 (2.8%) presented viremia for Zika, even though they were asymptomatic at the moment of donation. 11 (26.2%) out of the 42 positive donors developed Zika signs and/or symptoms within 3–10 days after donation.

Although there were viremic and asymptomatic donors, no cases of Zika transfusion transmission were demonstrated in the French Polynesian epidemic—but it was clear that the virus could be transmitted through blood.

The first case of transmission of Zika by blood transfusions would be reported in Brazil in 2015 and published in 2016 [61]. The case occurred in the city of Campinas, state of São Paulo, in a patient undergoing liver transplantation. The donor, asymptomatic at the time of donation, called back the blood bank 2 days later, stating that he had a fever, which he attributed to dengue. This occurred in June 2015, when it was still unknown that the Zika epidemic had arrived in Brazil. Dengue and chikungunya were investigated and excluded in the blood donor blood sample.

A few months later, in December 2015, after numerous cases of Zika were reported in Brazil, the same sample previously tested for dengue and Chik was tested for Zika, and this virus was identified by viral culture; the pre-transfusional sample of the patient was negative for Zika and the posttransfusion sample was positive.

Another probable case of Zika, also in the city of Campinas, was reported at the same time, although it was not published in a scientific journal (Addas-Carvalho, personal communication).

In March 2016, two more cases of Zika transmitted by transfusion were reported in Brazil at the National Cancer Institute in Rio de Janeiro [62]. The two cases originated from the same donation of double platelets of apheresis; one of the patients had received an allogeneic bone marrow transplant and the other had lymphoma.

In those four cases, all occurred in immunosuppressed patients, there were no signs or symptoms of posttransfusion Zika nor worsening or deterioration of the patient's clinical condition.

Table 9.7 summarizes the findings of these four probable cases of Zika transmission by blood transfusions.

A group in Ribeirao Preto City, in São Paulo state, has evaluated Zika incidence in asymptomatic blood donors, from October 2015 through May 2016, using NAT and serologic assays (IgM). The results are shown in Table 9.8, and the positive rate was surprisingly high [63].

A preliminary result from a multicentric study, in four Brazilian blood centers—Rio de Janeiro, Belo Horizonte, Recife, and São Paulo—was conducted by the Retrovirus Epidemiology Donor Study (REDS) investigators group. They screened samples coming from asymptomatic blood donors in these four centers, testing minipools of six samples by Grifols transcription-mediated amplification (TMA) multiplex assay, for dengue, Zika, and chikungunya [64]. The minipools were prepared from donations made from April 2016 through February 2017.

Table 9.7 Summary of four transfusion-transmitted Zika cases in Brazil

Case	Sex	Age	Medical condition	Involved blood component	How the case was suspected	Patient outcome
1 [61]	M	55	Liver transplantation	PC	Donor callback (post-donation)	No Zika-related symptoms
2[a]	M	38	Trauma	RBC	Patient unexplained thrombocytopenia	
3 [62]	F	54	Myelofibrosis	Double-apheresis PC	Donor callback (post-donation)	
4 [62]	F	14	Bone marrow transplantation (AML)			

[a]*Unpublished case*

Table 9.8 Zika detection in asymptomatic blood donors in Brazil

Number of tested donors	Period	Zika RNA + samples	RNA + and IgM + samples
1393 (ID-NAT)	Oct 2015–may 2016	37 (2.7%)	6/37 (13.5%)
RNA-positive samples – Viral load			
Median		7714 copies/mL	
Range		135–124,220 copies/mL	
Most frequent		10^3 copies/mL (70.3% of the positive samples)	

Adapted from Slavov et al. [63]. (Used with permission)

In this study Zika RNA was detected in 85 out of 11,284 tested minipools; since each minipool contained samples from six donors, the global incidence of viremic donors were 85:67,700 (0.12%), assuming that there was only one positive sample per pool. There was no detected case in São Paulo and Recife; if we take into account only samples from Rio de Janeiro and Belo Horizonte, then the positive rate for these two cities was 0.64%.

In Brazil, usually each whole blood donation is used to create 2.2 blood components (1 red blood cell, 1 plasma, and 1/5 of a whole blood-derived pooled platelet unit). Therefore, around 263 Zika-contaminated blood products might be transfused, although there are only four reports for transfusion-transmitted cases.

Another very important study regarding Zika detection in blood donors was the one performed in Puerto Rico, from April 2016 to September 2016 [65]. During this period, in Puerto Rico, 22,028 were tested by individual NAT test. 190 out of these 22,028 donors presented a positive NAT for Zika, and they were considered as presumptive viremic donors, which correspond to a 0.86% rate of positive cases in Puerto Rico.

Martinique, a French Caribbean territory, faced a Zika outbreak in the year 2016, alongside many other Caribbean countries. In Martinique, between January and June 10, 2016, 4129 consecutive blood donations were tested for Zika RNA. Positive NAT detection occurred in 76 blood donations (1.84%) [66].

In the USA, where the Zika individual NAT tests for blood donors have been mandatory since August 2016, the first published report describes 23 initially positive cases, after 358,786 donations from all US states were screened. Fourteen of these blood donors represented probable ZIKV infection based on reactivity on additional nucleic acid testing or anti-Zika immunoglobulin M [67].

Ten of the 14 donors reported travel to an identified ZIKV-active area within 90 days before donation (median time from end of travel to donation, 25 days; range, 6–71 days).

Three donors with travel history also had potential sexual exposure. Only seven of the 14 donations with probable ZIKV infection were detectable upon 1:6 dilution to simulate minipool testing; therefore, minipool screening would have detected only 50% of the RNA-positive donations [67]. However, it is probable that those viremic donors escaping Zika detection in minipool would not be able to transmit Zika, given their low viral load.

There is another report for Zika tests in US blood donors; a total of 1,776,190 donations were tested between February 2016 and February 2017 [68]. Altogether, 22 donations were considered true positive, corresponding to a 0.001% rate.

A risk assessment concerning Zika transfusion-transmission risk in Brazil using a Monte Carlo simulation was conducted by a collaborative group from Brazil and from Quebec, Canada [69]. The simulation took into account Brazilian official figures about Zika incidence in Brazil and in the state of Rio de Janeiro. It also considered that for each notified and confirmed (or probable) case, there should be four asymptomatic and non-notified cases.

The Zika reported incidence in Brazil and in Rio de Janeiro state was 102.9/105 person-years and 403.7/105 person-years, respectively. The formula for risk assessment

Table 9.9 Risk assessment of Zika transfusion-transmission in Brazil

Theoretical risk (Monte Carlo simulation)		
	Brazil	Rio de Janeiro state
With reported incidence	1:86,666	1:22,044
True incidence (considering 4 asymptomatic patients for 1 reported case)	1:21,666	4409

Table 9.10 Worldwide Zika positive rates in blood donors

Country	Number of donors tested	Type of test	Rate	Reference
Brazil (Rio de Janeiro and Belo Horizonte)	67,700	MP-NAT	0.64%	Custer [64]
Brazil (Ribeirão Preto city)	1393	ID-NAT	2.7%	Slavov [63]
USA	1,776,190	ID-NAT	0.01%	Pate [68]
Martinique	4129	ID-NAT	1.84%	Gallian [66]
Puerto Rico	22,028	ID-NAT	0.86%	Chevalier [65]

was as follows: [(incidence X infectious period X average donation number per donor per year) X (1-proportion of refused donors) X (1-proportion of discarded donations due to post donation information)]. Table 9.9 shows the result of this study.

The number of blood donations per year in Rio de Janeiro state is 173,000, for whole blood; considering 2.2 transfused components per donated blood, then the theoretical risk could reach 105 blood components per year, not very far from estimates by Custer et al., who estimated an annual number of 160 ZIKV-contaminated blood components in Rio de Janeiro state [64, 69].

All these publications show that Zika transmission by blood transfusion is a very concrete possibility, Zika being a considerable threat to blood safety around the world. Table 9.10 shows a summary of all the published studies related to Zika viremia in asymptomatic blood donors.

Approaches to Minimize Zika Risk and Impacts on Transfusion Medicine

Theoretically, ZIKV can affect blood safety and the blood transfusion activities in many ways. The first and most obvious way is the risk of ZIKV transfusion-transmission. So far, there are very few reported cases—four in total—without any consequences to recipients.

However, nothing is known about the risk if a Zika-contaminated blood component is transfused during pregnancy or directly to a newborn. This can be a crucial issue in areas with local transmission, even though transfusion is seldom performed during pregnancy, except in countries with many sickle cell patients, as those patients often require chronic transfusion during pregnancy.

In some countries, measures to minimize this risk are being implemented. During the French Polynesian epidemic, the local health authorities decided to transfuse only pathogen-reduced platelets and plasma, and to test blood donation for ZIKV RNA, using an in-house kit, in a minipool of three samples.

In some centers in Brazil, ZIKV RNA test is being selectively applied to a small proportion of the blood inventory, in order to avoid transfusing non-ZIKV-tested blood to pregnant women (Mendrone, personal communication).

Another important concern regards prospective donors' travel deferral. In non-endemic areas, this is a very important measure to protect blood inventory. The Food and Drug Administration (FDA) recommends a 4-week deferral period for donor candidates coming from an endemic country [70]. A risk analysis performed in Canada, using the Monte Carlo simulation, concluded that a 21-day travel deferral period would be safe enough, offering an extremely wide margin of safety [71]. The model estimated that 32 donors (range, 20–46 donors) would be able to donate while still being at risk of transmitting Zika, corresponding to a rate of 1:312,500 (range, 1:217000 to 1:500,000). None of these donors would bear ZIKV beyond 21 days; the overall risk would be less than 1:200,000,000.

Those precautionary actions are easily applicable to non-endemic countries, or in countries with few autochthonous cases, but it is hard to implement them in endemic countries. Even in non-endemic countries, where they can be easily adopted, they can contribute to decrease the eligible donor pool.

The same assumption is valid to blood component quarantine during Zika outbreak. It is a useful measure during a local epidemic, but it is very unpractical because the blood centers should put in place a structure to call blood donors in order to ask them if they have presented symptoms of arbovirus. Many donors do not answer the phone call, and very often the service has to decide if the donated blood may be used despite lack of contact with blood donors.

Interrupt the collection during the outbreak is also a valid strategy, but it requires shipping of blood from a neighbor country or from a close region free of Zika. This type of arrangement is very difficult to put in place in the developing world, especially when the majority of the country is affected by Zika.

In the USA, the FDA states that it is mandatory to defer "for 4 weeks after the resolution of symptoms a donor who reports symptoms suggestive of ZIKV that arose within 2 weeks of departure from an area with active transmission of ZIKV and/or after the resolution of symptoms a donor who reports symptoms suggestive of ZIKV that arose within 2 weeks of departure from an area with active transmission of ZIKV" [70].

This recommendation is adopted almost worldwide, but its efficacy is limited, given the high proportion of Zika asymptomatic cases (80%) [72]. Another recommendation adopted almost everywhere is to defer donors with a recent clinical history compatible with Zika for 4 weeks or 1 month after the complete resolution of symptoms and the temporary exclusion of donors for whom laboratory test results show they may recently have been infected [72].

Another safety guard band recommended by FDA is to defer donor candidates for 4 weeks after the last sexual contact with a person "who has been diagnosed with ZIKV or who traveled to or resided in an area with active transmission of ZIKV in the 3 months prior to that instance of sexual contact" [70].

Finally, many endemic countries established a formal callback policy for donors who might experiment arbovirus signs or symptoms up to 30 days after donation. The first three published ZIKV transfusion-transmitted cases in Brazil were identified in such a way.

In an unpublished study (Addas de Carvalho, personal communication) from the city of Campinas, Brazil, 2 (0.067%) out of 2954 tested donors (after callback for reporting arbovirus symptoms) were confirmed as ZIKV RNA positive (Table 9.11).

During the Zika outbreak, some blood centers in Brazil included a brief physical examination—eyes, trunk, and limb inspection—of prospective blood donors in order to look for unnoticed cutaneous rash or conjunctivitis. Very few Zika cases were identified with this step, and it has since been abandoned after the decline of the epidemic.

In the USA, as of August 2016, molecular screening for Zika became mandatory in 100% of the blood donated all over the country. The centers were allowed to use an investigational new drug (IND) test to screen the donations [70]. In October 2017, the FDA approved the first NAT test for Zika [75]. The test is still mandatory, even though the number of cases has decreased significantly. So far, as of March 2018, the only country where ZIKV screening in blood donors is mandatory is the USA [73].

The only option for ZIKV donor testing is through virus RNA detection. Anti-Zika IgM detects the virus by the fifth day after contamination, so that this test would fail to identify the vast majority of contaminated blood donors (Fig. 9.3).

IgG anti-ZIKV would not be helpful to screen blood donors, due to its late appearance during disease clinical course, after virus clearance. Moreover, virtually all the available IgG anti-ZIKV cross-react with antibodies directed to dengue virus.

Table 9.11 Results of Zika testing in donors who call back the blood center in Brazil

Year	Number of donors tested	Zika-positive results
2015	1268	1 (0.078%)
2016	1686	1 (0.059%)
Total	2954	0.067%

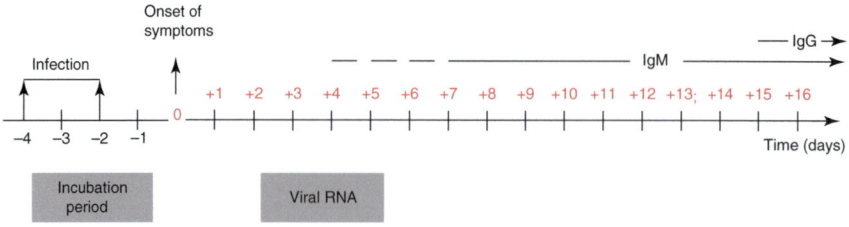

Fig. 9.3 Laboratory tests for Zika

9 Zika Virus

Pathogen Inactivation

Pathogen inactivation seems very effective against Zika virus: a log reduction of 7.5 $\log_{10}$ genome equivalents per milliliter for amotosalen + ultraviolet A (UVA)-treated platelet concentrates [74] and a 5.68 $\log_{10}$ reduction for platelet concentrates treated by ultraviolet C (UVC) [75]. The UVC method is not licensed in the USA.

The only FDA-approved method for platelet and plasma—amotosalen + UVA irradiation—offers effective protection against Zika transfusion transmission; nevertheless, it is only available, at this point, for platelets and plasma and not for red blood cell concentrates.

Table 9.12 summarizes the main approaches to reduce Zika transfusion risks as well as their pros and cons.

Table 9.12 Approaches to reduce Zika threat to blood safety

Approach		Pros	Cons	Effectivity
Donor interview	Travel deferral	Easy to be implemented; low cost	Loss of donors can affect the inventory; not applicable to endemic areas	Moderate to high (in non-endemic areas)
	Sexual deferral		Considerable loss of donors, especially in endemic areas	Low to moderate
	Donor brief physical examination	Can trace some unnoticed Zika signs	Difficult to be implemented (change of paradigm)	Low to very low
Donor callback		Can avoid transfusion of Zika (and other arbovirus)-contaminated blood	Need to have a toll-free number	Low to moderate
Donor quarantine		A way to enhance donor safety	Almost impossible in areas with important local transmission (logistic issues)	Moderate
Cease local collection and import blood		Avoid risk of Zika transfusion-transmission	Very high costs; logistic issues; can impact donors' loyalty	Very high in terms of inventory protection but very difficult to put in practice
Donor test	IgM	Relatively easy to implement; (probably) not very expensive	No test available for blood banks	Low to very low (it will miss the majority of viremic donors)
	Nat	Can adequately protect blood inventory	Very expensive; affordability issues for developing countries	Very high; cost-effective only in endemic areas
Pathogen reduction techniques		Can be implemented by the blood centers	Cost and logistic issues	High (for platelet and plasma)

Summary

Zika is definitely a new and very important threat to blood safety, since it is associated with severe clinical consequences: Zika congenital syndrome (ZCS) in neonates and Guillain-Barré syndrome (GBS) in adults.

ZCS has a high mortality and a very high morbidity; GBS mortality, at least in Brazilian cases, is also elevated (around 6%). These facts explain why the blood community is so concerned by the emergence of this virus.

Therefore, measures to protect blood inventory and to increase transfusion safety are mandatory. Whenever possible, NAT testing would contribute to significantly reduce ZIKV-contaminated blood components, but at very high cost. NAT would probably eliminate the vast majority, or even the totality, of ZIKV transfusion-transmission, since the cases missed by the test would not be infectious, due to the low viral load.

The question about NAT is whether it is worth introducing a very expensive test for a disease that will decline very quickly after the first epidemic. Experience from Yap Island and in French Polynesia shows that there was no second wave of infection after the initial outbreak.

The Brazilian experience seems to confirm this evolution of the Zika epidemic. In Brazil, after a period of 1 year (2015–2016) with a large number of cases, only sparse and sporadic reports have been observed, from July 2016 until the beginning of 2018.

It is also a matter of affordability; therefore, selective NAT, applied only to blood to be transfused in pregnant women and neonates, might be an interesting approach, despite the bioethical issues that are embedded in this type of strategy.

The second question regarding NAT testing is whether it would be possible to remove it and, in what case, if the number of disease cases in the population drops dramatically. These are two issues that are being debated by health agencies in many countries. Clearer answers will probably emerge in the next 2 years.

Many doubts persist about the transmission of ZIKV by blood: why so few cases, if many studies have shown a proportion of blood donors contaminated up to 2.8%? The transfusion-transmitted reported cases, all in Brazil, were found in immunosuppressed patients—but, nevertheless, no clinical consequences were observed.

So far, we do not have the answers for these questions, and the same is true for the question about the risk of congenital ZCS and GBS in transfusion-transmitted Zika cases.

In summary, considering the severity of ZCS and GBS associated with Zika, the blood community should make every effort to meet the challenges of Zika by taking all reasonable steps to increase blood safety with regard to the transmission of Zika by blood components.

References

1. Schwartz DA. The origins and emergence of Zika virus, the newest TORCH infection: what's old is new again. Arch Pathol Lab Med. 2017;141:18–25.
2. Macnamara FN. Zika virus: a report on three cases of human infection during an epidemic of jaundice in Nigeria. Trans R Soc Trop Med Hyg. 1954;48:139–45.

3. Simpson DI. Zika virus infection in man. Trans R Soc Trop Med Hyg. 1964;58:335–8.
4. Olson JG, Ksiazek TG, Suhandiman T. Zika virus, a cause of fever in Central Java, Indonesia. Trans R Soc Trop Med Hyg. 1981;75:389–93.
5. Musso D, Gubler DJ. Zika virus. Clin Microbiol Rev. 2016;29:487–524.
6. Duffy MR, Chen TH, Hancock WT, et al. Zika virus outbreak on Yap Island, Federated States of Micronesia. N Engl J Med. 2009;360(24):2536–43.
7. European Centre for Disease Prevention and Control. Rapid risk assessment: Zika virus infection outbreak. French Polynesia: ECDC; 2014.
8. Gubler DJ, Vasilakis N, Musso D. History and Emergence of Zika Virus. JID. 2017;216(S10):S860–7.
9. Brasil. Ministério da Saúde. Boletim epidemiológico: Monitoramento dos casos de dengue, febre de Chikungunya e febre pelo vírus Zika até a Semana Epidemiológica. 45, 2015;46(36).
10. Brasil. Ministério da Saúde. Boletim epidemiológico: Monitoramento dos casos de microcefalias no Brasil, até a semana epidemiológica. 46, 2015;46(37).
11. Hall V, Walker WL, Lindsat NP, et al. Update: noncongenital Zika virus disease cases—50 U.S. States and the District of Columbia, 2016. MMWR. 2018;67(9):265–9.
12. U.S. Department of Health and Human Services, Food and Drug Administration. Revised recommendations for reducing the risk of Zika Virus transmission by blood and blood components. https://www.fda.gov/downloads/BiologicsBloodVaccines/GuidanceComplianceRegulatoryInformation/Guidances/Blood/UCM518213.pdf. Accessed 6 June 2018.
13. Enfissi A, Codrington J, Roosblad J, Kazanji M, Rousset D. Zika virus genome from the Americas. Lancet. 2016;387:227–8.
14. Campos GS, Bandeira AC, Sardi SI. Zika virus outbreak, Bahia, Brazil. Emerg Infect Dis. 2015;21:1885–6.
15. Calvet G, Aguiar RS, Melo ASO, et al. Detection and sequencing of Zika virus from amniotic fluid of fetuses with microcephaly in Brazil: a case study. Lancet Infect Dis. 2016;16(6):553–60.
16. Katz LM, Rossmann S. Zika and the blood supply. A work in progress. Arch Pathol Lab Med. 2017;141(1):85–92.
17. Oehler E, Watrin L, Larre P, et al. Zika virus infection complicated by Guillain-Barre syndrome--case report, French Polynesia, December 2013. Euro Surveill. 2014;19(9):pii:20720.
18. Rodrigues Faria N, Azevedo RSS, MUG K. Zika virus in the Americas: early epidemiological and genetic findings. Science. 2016;352(6283):345–9.
19. Musso D. Zika virus transmission from French Polynesia to Brazil. Emerg Infect Dis. 2015;21(10):1887.
20. Ayllón T, Campos RM, Brasil P, et al. Early evidence for Zika virus circulation among Aedes aegypti mosquitoes, Rio de Janeiro, Brazil. Emerg Infect Dis. 2017;23(8):1411–2.
21. Brasil. Ministério da Saúde. Boletim epidemiológico: Monitoramento dos casos de dengue, febre de Chikungunya e febre pelo vírus Zika até a Semana Epidemiológica 9, 2018;49(13).
22. Brasil. Ministério da Saúde. Boletim epidemiológico: Monitoramento integrado de alterações no crescimento e desenvolvimento relacionadas à infecção pelo vírus Zika e outras etiologias infecciosas, até a Semana Epidemiológica 52 de 2017, 2018;49(6).
23. Lessler JT. Times to key events in the course of Zika infection and their implications: a systematic review and pooled analysis. Bull World Health Organ. 2016;1694:841–9.
24. Krow-Lucal ER, Biggerstaff BJ, Staples JE. Estimated incubation period for Zika virus disease. Emerg Infect Dis. 2017;23(5):841–5.
25. Halstead SB. Yap State Department of health Services, Plaquette Zika Virus, 9 août 2007.
26. PAHO: Provisional case definition of suspected acute Zika virus infection. http://www.paho.org/hq/index.php?option=com_content&view=article&id=11117&Itemid=41532&lang=pt. Accessed 28 Feb 2018.
27. He A, Brasil P, Siqueira AM, et al. The emerging Zika virus threat: a guide for dermatologists. Am J Clin Dermatol. 2017;18(2):231–6.
28. De Oliveira Melo AS, Malinger GR, Ximenes R. Zika virus intrauterine infection causes fetal brain abnormality and microcephaly: Tip of the iceberg? Ultrasound Obstet Gynecol. et al., 2016;47:6–7.

29. Brazil Ministry of Health. The public health Emergency Operations Center report on microcephaly. Epidemiological Week 1 of 2016. Brazil; 2016. http://portalsaude.saude.gov.br/images/pdf/2016/janeiro/13/COES-Microcefalias. Access 7 Sept 2017.
30. Mlakar J, Korva M, Tul N, et al. Zika virus associated with microcephaly. N Engl J Med. 2016;374(10):951–8.
31. Ventura CV, Maia M, Dias N, et al. Zika virus in Brazil and macular atrophy in a child with microcephaly. Lancet. 2016;387(10037):2502.
32. Besnard M, Eyrolle-Guignot D, Guillemette-Artur P, et al. Congenital cerebral malformations and dysfunction in fetuses and newborns following the 2013 to 2014 Zika virus epidemic in French Polynesia. Euro Surveill. 2016;21(13)
33. Adamski A, Bertolli J, Castañeda-Orjuela C, et al. Estimating the numbers of pregnant women infected with Zika virus and infants with congenital microcephaly in Colombia, 2015–2017. J Infect. 2018;S0163–4453(18):30082–3.
34. Ellington SR, Devine O, Bertolli J, et al. Estimating the number of pregnant women infected with Zika virus and expected infants with microcephaly following the Zika virus outbreak in Puerto Rico, 2016. JAMA Pediatr. 2016;170(10):940–5.
35. De Oliveira Melo AS, Aguiar RS, MMR A, et al. Congenital Zika virus infection: beyond neonatal microcephaly. JAMA Neurol. 2016;73:1407–16.
36. Campos Coelho AV, Crovella S. Microcephaly prevalence in infants born to Zika virus-infected women: a systematic review and meta-analysis. Int J Mol Sci. 2017;18:1714.
37. Brasil P, Pereira JP, Gabaglia CR, et al. Zika virus infection in pregnant women in Rio de Janeiro–preliminary report. N Engl J Med. 2016;375(24):2321–34.
38. Pan American Health Organization. Epidemiological alert: neurological syndrome, congenital malformations, and Zika virus infection. Implications for public health in the Americas 1 December 2015. www.paho.org/hq/index.php?option=com_docman&task=doc_view&Itemid=270&gid=32405&lang=em. Accessed 21 Dec 2017.
39. França GVA, Schuler-Faccini L, Oliveira WK, et al. Congenital Zika virus syndrome in Brazil: a case series of the first 1501 live births with complete investigation. Lancet. 2016;388:891–7.
40. Chimelli L, Avvad-Portari E. Congenital Zika virus infection: a neuropathological review. Childs Nerv Syst. 2018;34(1):95–9.
41. de Paula Freitas B, Ventura CV, Maia M, Belfort R Jr. Zika virus and the eye. Curr Opin Ophthalmol. 2017;28:595–9.
42. Orofino DHG, Passos SRL, de Oliveira RVC, et al. Cardiac findings in infants with in utero exposure to Zika virus—a cross sectional study. PLoS Negl Trop Dis. 2018;12(3):e0006362.
43. Watrin L, Ghawché F, Larre P, et al. Guillain-Barré syndrome (42 cases) occurring during a Zika virus outbreak in French Polynesia. Medicine. 2016;95(14):e3257.
44. Cao-Lormeau VM, Blake A, Mons S. Guillain-Barré syndrome outbreak caused by ZIKA virus infection in French Polynesia. Lancet. 2016;387(10027):1531–9.
45. Barbi L, Coelho AVC, Alencar LCA, Crovella S. Prevalence of Guillain-Barré syndrome among Zikavirus infected cases: a systematic review and meta-analysis. Braz J Infect Dis. 2018;22(2):137–41.
46. Styczynski AR, Malta JMA, Krow-Lucal ER, Percio J, Nóbrega ME, Vargas A. Increased rates of Guillain-Barre syndrome associated with Zika virus outbreak in the Salvador metropolitan area, Brazil. PLoS Negl Trop Dis. 2017;11(8):e0005869.
47. da Silva IRF, Frontera JA, Bispo de Filippis AM, et al. Neurologic complications associated with the Zika virus in Brazilian adults. JAMA Neurol. 2017;74(10):1190–8.
48. Chen LH, Wilson ME. Update on non-vector transmission of dengue: relevant studies with Zika and other flaviviruses. Trop Dis Travel Med Vaccines. 2016;2:15.
49. Barzon L, Pacenti M, Berto A, et al. Isolation of infectious Zika virus from saliva and prolonged viral RNA shedding in a traveller returning from the Dominican Republic to Italy, January 2016. Euro Surveill. 2016;21(10)
50. Leung GH, Baird RW, Druce J, et al. Zika virus infection in Australia following a monkey bite in Indonesia. Southeast Asian J Trop Med Public Health. 2015;46(3):460–4.

51. Foy BD, Kobylinski KC, Chilson Foy JL, et al. Probable non-vector-borne transmission of Zika virus, Colorado, USA. Emerg Infect Dis. 2011;17(5):880–2.
52. Kim CR, Counotte M, Bernstein K, et al. Investigating the sexual transmission of Zika virus. Lancet Glob Health. 2018;6(1):e24–5.
53. Musso D, Richard V, Teissier A. Detection of ZIKV RNA in semen of asymptomatic blood donors. Clin Microbiol Infect. 2017;23(12):1001.e1–3.
54. Besnard M, Lastère S, Teisier A, et al. Evidence of perinatal transmission of Zika virus, French Polynesia, December 2013 and February 2014. Eur Secur. 2014;19(13)
55. Colt S, Garcia-Casal MN, Peña-Rosas JP, et al. Transmission of Zika virus through breast milk and other breastfeeding-related bodily-fluids: a systematic review. Lancet. 2016;387(10027):1531–9.
56. Dupont-Rouzeyrol M, Biron A, O'Connor O, et al. Infectious Zika viral particles in breast-milk. Lancet. 2016;387(10023):1051.
57. Blohm GM, Lednicky JA, Márquez M, et al. Evidence for mother-to-child transmission of Zika virus through breast milk. Clin Infect Dis. 2018;66(7):1120–1.
58. WHO. Infant feeding in areas of Zika virus transmission. Summary of rapid advice guideline 29 June 2016. WHO/ZIKV/MOC/16.6.
59. Paz-Bailey G, Rosenberg ES, Doyle K, et al. Persistence of Zika virus in body fluids—preliminary report. N Engl J Med. 2017; https://doi.org/10.1056/NEJMoa1613108.
60. Musso D, Nhan T, Robin E, et al. Potential for Zika virus transmission through blood transfusion demonstrated during an outbreak in French Polynesia, November 2013 to February 2014. Euro Surveill. 2014;19
61. Barjas-Castro ML, Angerami RN, Cunha MS, et al. Probable transfusion-transmitted Zika virus in Brazil. Transfusion. 2016;56(7):1684–8.
62. Motta IJ, Spencer BR, Cordeiro da Silva SG, et al. Evidence for transmission of Zika virus by platelet transfusion. N Engl J Med. 2016;375(11):1101–3.
63. Slavov SN, Hespanhol MR, Rodrigues ES, et al. Zika virus RNA detection in asymptomatic blood donors during an outbreak in the northeast region of São Paulo State, Brazil, 2016. Transfusion. 2017;57(12):2897–901.
64. Custer B, Gonçalez T, Gao K, et al. Zika, chikungunya and dengue virus incident infections in blood donors in Brazil: implications for blood safety and public health surveillance. Transfusion. 2017;57(3S):27A.
65. Chevalier MS, Biggerstaff BJ, Basavaraju SV, et al. Use of blood donor screening data to estimate Zika virus incidence, Puerto Rico, April–August 2016. Emerg Infect Dis. 2017;23(5):790–5.
66. Gallian P, Cabi A, Richard P, et al. Zika virus in asymptomatic blood donors in Martinique. Blood. 2017;129(2):263–6.
67. Galel SA, Williamson PC, Busch MP, et al. Zika-positive donations in the continental United States. MP Transfusion. 2017;57(3pt2):770–8.
68. Pate LL, Williamson PC, Busch MP. Detection of Zika in United States blood donations using cobas® Zika on the cobas 6800/8800 systems. Transfusion. 2017;57(3S):26A.
69. Amorim L, Germain M, Delage G, et al. Risk assessment for Zika virus transfusion transmission in Brazil using Monte Carlo simulation. Transfusion. 2017;57(3S):26A.
70. FDA. Revised recommendations for reducing the risk of Zika Virus transmission by blood and blood components. https://www.fda.gov/downloads/biologicsbloodvaccines/guidancecomplianceregulatoryinformation/guidances/blood/ucm518213.pdf. Accessed 15 Dec 2017.
71. Germain M, Delage G, O'Brien SF, et al. Mitigation of the threat posed to transfusion by donors traveling to Zika-affected areas: a Canadian risk-based approach. Transfusion. 2017;57(10):2463–8.
72. WHO: Zika virus and safe blood supply: questions and answers. http://www.who.int/features/qa/zika-safe-blood/en/. Accessed 12 Jan 2018.
73. Food and Drug Administration. FDA approves first test for screening Zika virus in blood donations. https://www.fda.gov/NewsEvents/Newsroom/PressAnnouncements/ucm579313.htm. Accessed 2 Nov 2017.

74. Santa Maria F, Laughhunn A, Lanteri MC, et al. Inactivation of Zika virus in platelet components using amotosalen and ultraviolet A illumination. Transfusion. 2017;57(8):2016–25.
75. Fryk JJ, Marks DC, Hobson-Peters J, et al. Reduction of Zika virus infectivity in platelet concentrates after treatment with ultraviolet C light and in plasma after treatment with methylene blue and visible light. Transfusion. 2017;57(11):2677–82.
76. Ming G-l, Tang H, Song H. Advances in Zika virus research: stem cell models, challenges, and opportunities. Cell Stem Cell. 2016;19(6):690–702.

Part III
Current Concerns

Chapter 10
The Emergence of Zoonotic Pathogens as Agents of Concern in Transfusion Medicine

Louis M. Katz

Our Historic Challenges: The Reactive Paradigm

Among the "classic" transfusion-transmitted infections (TTIs), person-to-person transmission was the important route of donor infection, and we *reacted* to incontrovertible evidence of a clinical burden in transfusion recipients. These included syphilis, malaria, hepatitis B, hepatitis C, and HIV (originally a nonhuman primate zoonosis). Over time, epidemiologic and other scientific data about risk were examined with the aim of developing (roughly sequentially) overlapping mitigation strategies that included (1) the virtual elimination of paid blood donors in the United States, (2) donor risk education to promote self-deferral, (3) explicit deferral criteria to be applied at the time of the donor interview, and (4) laboratory testing to reduce donation of infectious blood by donors who might have limited understanding of and/or were reluctant to recognize or admit their "behavioral" risks. The morbid impacts of these historical agents on many thousands of recipients make the disadvantages of reactive approaches obvious—one need not look further than the thousands of transmissions of HIV and non-A and non-B hepatitis (i.e., before the description of HCV) [1]. In part resulting from shortcomings enumerated in the Institute of Medicine report, the US blood community has explored more precautionary and proactive applications of these approaches to the assessment and mitigation of infectious risks in recent decades.

Surrogate testing using donor testing for alanine aminotransferase and antibody to the hepatitis B core antigen was an early initiative in this direction before the identification of hepatitis C virus and the availability of specific assays [2–4]. Testing for human T-lymphotropic retrovirus types I/II (HTLVs) in the United States was another early effort at a more proactive approach to donor screening [5, 6]. Infection with HTLV-I was known to cause acute T-cell leukemia and

L. M. Katz
America's Blood Centers, Washington, DC, USA
e-mail: lkatz@americasblood.org

myelopathy, albeit with low disease penetrance, and infection was present in healthy individuals who would otherwise qualify as donors. Transfusion transmission was documented, but the attendant disease burden was poorly characterized. In the wake of events caused by another retrovirus (HIV), antibody testing was required in the United States in 1988. Controversy about its impact and cost-effectiveness persists [7].

During the last 30 years, additional nonspecific measures have been deployed in furtherance of transfusion safety. These include stringent process controls: in the United States, "current good manufacturing practices" (cGMP) from the Code of Federal Regulations [8] prevent distribution for transfusion of blood from unacceptable donors and donations that manages to enter the supply chain. Development and deployment of ever more complex information systems cleared by the Food and Drug Administration as medical devices (blood establishment computer systems) have been required to support these kinds of quality systems. Finally, with a litany of real and purported adverse outcomes attendant on transfusion (infectious but also serious non-infectious hazards), the clinical cascades that ultimately expose a patient to transfusion are under scrutiny under the rubric of "patient blood management."

All these approaches contribute to the impressive safety of transfusion from *recognized* infections in the developed world [9]. Pathogen reduction processes for labile blood components are proactive solutions but remain aspirational, as they are not yet available for all components, and will not be potent against all agents. Further, consensus on the health economic justification for pathogen reduction is absent when viewed from a societal perspective.

Emerging Zoonotic Agents: Toward a more Proactive Approach

Overlaying our history with these classic pathogens is "new" pathogen emergence and discovery. Identification of new agents is accelerating. The number of viral species recognized to infect human is predicted to rise from less than 10 in 1900 to more than 200 by 2020, with the large majority of the increase since 1960 (Fig. 10.1) [10]. The reasons are diverse and beyond the scope of this chapter, but a shrinking globe puts pathogens from the sub-Saharan rain forest within 24 h of a blood center in the Northern Plains. Urbanization, especially when combined with poverty and overcrowding, and human changes of and encroachment into diverse ecologic niches change host, pathogen, and vector relationships. Alterations of climate and animal husbandry also affect reservoir, pathogen, and vector distributions. New discovery systems like next-generation sequencing and metagenomics identify *potential* pathogens in the environment, wildlife reservoirs, and humans (our microbiome), well before disease associations are even considered. Social media via the Internet brings us nearly instantaneous news and speculation about new diseases and

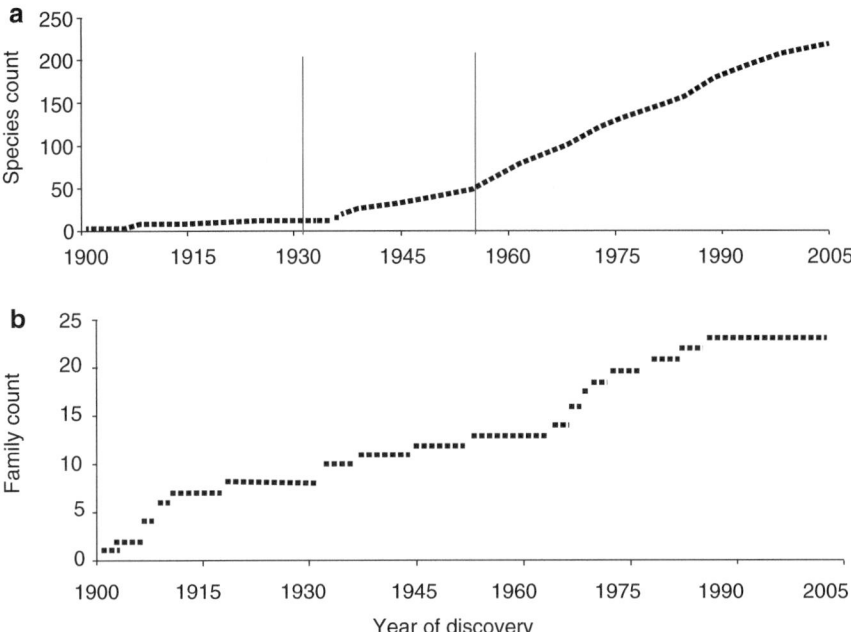

Fig. 10.1 New viruses infecting humans. Discovery curves for human viruses. (**a**) Virus discovery curve by species. Cumulative number of species reported to infect humans. Statistically significant upward breakpoints are shown (vertical lines). (**b**) Virus discovery curve by family. Cumulative number of families containing species reported to infect humans [10]. (Data source: Woolhouse et al. [89])

outbreaks from anywhere in the world. How do we integrate, or decide not to, the potential threats into our blood safety regime? Our difficult task in the transfusion medicine community is choosing a proactive framework within which to approach emerging infections despite initially incomplete information about their impacts on transfusion safety.

WNV, the severe acute respiratory syndrome coronavirus (SARS-CoV), *Trypanosoma cruzi*, Zika, and *Babesia microti* are recent demonstrations that zoonotic infections, as they emerge (or emerge in our consciousness), become targets for intervention. There are many other zoonotic and/or arthropod-borne agents for which we have not implemented mitigation measures (beyond the requirement that donors are well when they give) but about which we need to think. They include, but are by no means restricted to, dengue, chikungunya, MERS-CoV, Nipah, Hendra, the severe fever with thrombocytopenia syndrome virus (SFTSV), Bourbon and Powassan viruses, Mayoro virus, the tick-borne agents (*Erlichia sp.*, *Anaplasma phagocytophilum*) and *Leishmania*. These agents persist in arthropods and/or nonhuman vertebrate reservoirs with spillover into human populations either by contact or vector transmission. Tick-borne infections are not further considered herein.

Zoonotic infections, excluding HIV, have certainly had less clinical impact in transfusion medicine than the classic sexually and parenterally transmitted agents, but, especially under epidemic scenarios, several are presently prominent in conversations about if and when to intervene for blood safety. In this context, we have taken to speculating on the need for interventions for pathogens for which transfusion transmission, when the asymptomatic presence of an agent is biologically plausible, is theoretical. This is indeed proactive, in contrast to our historical approach, but risks a response (and consumption of scarce resources) where none is appropriate. In the best light, this is "precautionism."

In a perfect world, we will answer four questions about a putative transfusion-transmitted agent before recipients are infected to prospectively inform consideration, development, and deployment of mitigation strategies [11].

1. Is the agent present in the blood of otherwise qualified donors?
2. Is the agent parenterally transmissible (by blood, organ/tissue transplantation), or is such transmission biologically plausible?
3. Will the agent survive in contemporary blood components to be transmitted?
4. Does the agent, if transmitted, pose a material clinical risk after transfusion— Does it cause significant illness among susceptible transfusion recipients?

Unfortunately, with current surveillance and pathogen discovery techniques in an increasingly interconnected world, the answers to these questions are not available or are incomplete when decision-making must be started—that is, initial responses are necessarily considered in a precautionary context. The question of a "correct" process by which we ought to select agents to examine for risk before reports of transfusion transmission come to light is unanswered [12]. Several historical examples are provided that describe how we have actually approached some of these pathogens.

Historical Zoonoses (Excluding HIV)

Variant Creutzfeldt-Jakob Disease (vCJD)

vCJD is a zoonotic transmissible spongiform encephalopathy (TSE) that spreads from bovines to humans, mainly in the United Kingdom. Precautionary deferrals were required before the recognition of transfusion transmission based largely on the occurrence of TSEs (sporadic CJD, Kuru et al.) in humans, the presence of the vCJD prion in the reticuloendothelial system of apparently food-borne human cases, and a precedent of parenteral transmission of the prion that causes classic or sporadic CJD [13]. These deferrals aim to prevent an adverse outcome that has proven to be very rare, even in the United Kingdom epicenter of the bovine spongiform encephalopathy epidemic [14]. The cost has been the ongoing loss of many thousands of donors for residence in and travel to (and transfusion in some) the countries with risk. In addition to difficult donor counseling sessions, the estimates of donor loss ranged as high as 5% in the United States [15, 16]. We will likely maintain them until concerns about theoretical subsequent waves of the vCJD epidemic, largely related to incubation periods associated with polymorphisms in the human prion protein gene, are adjudicated [17, 18].

West Nile Virus (WNV)

Mitigation strategies for the mosquito-borne avian pathogen WNV were implemented after the recognition of a single transmission of the virus from a blood donor to an organ donor and forward to the organ recipients [19]. An emergency response ramped up over several weeks in 2002, using an incomplete understanding of the level of risk being addressed based on clinical information from the cases and modeling data that had been produced before observation of those transmissions [20, 21]. Twenty-three blood recipient infections were documented (retrospectively) during that first season [22]. These were in the context of 4156 WNV cases reported to CDC [23]. Within less than 1 year after the first case report, minipool nucleic acid tests were developed and implemented across the US blood supply. In subsequent seasons, strategies to trigger individual donation testing with increased sensitivity evolved and, despite persistent endemic activity in the United States, transfusion transmission WNV has been essentially eliminated [24].

Severe Acute Respiratory Syndrome Coronavirus (SARS-CoV)

SARS-CoV is an enveloped RNA viral respiratory pathogen of zoonotic origin causing significant mortality. First identified in Asia during 2003, it spread from Asia to North America with sporadic travel-associated cases and subsequent extensive localized healthcare-associated (nosocomial) transmission. SARS was met with an FDA guidance for immediate implementation requiring the interrogation of US blood donors about a history of SARS, potential exposure to cases, and travel to or residence in areas during the 14 days before presentation to donate. Temporary deferral was required if "risk" was present. This was based on the theoretical possibility of asymptomatic viremia and isolation of the virus from tissues outside the respiratory tract, presumably as a result of blood-borne spread. These interventions occurred absent any clinical evidence of parenteral or transfusion risk [25]. SARS-CoV RNA was subsequently found in patient plasma as early as day 2 after onset of symptoms [26, 27], but there are still no data on infectious viremia in the incubation period or among asymptomatic contacts of cases on which to judge the plausibility of parenteral transmission. The requirement for donor screening was allowed to lapse 90 days after CDC lifted the last travel alerts and SARS has not reemerged.

Ebola Virus

Ebola, recognized in 1976, spreads from an animal reservoir to humans unpredictably. The massive West African Ebola outbreak in 2014–2016 resulted in promulgation of FDA guidance to prevent transfusion transmission of a pathogen not recognized to be transmitted by this route. That response was predicated on the observation that the virus is present in blood and body fluids, direct contact with which is associated with a highly morbid infection [28].

Zika Virus

Zika virus, a nonhuman primate virus that has spilled over into human populations causing a pandemic, is covered elsewhere, but its example bears repetition here. Its nucleic acid is present in the blood of asymptomatic individuals (including donors), US donors have frequent travel to affected areas outside the mainland United States, the major vector is present in areas of the mainland United States, and sexual transmission is a documented, if poorly quantitated, route of infection [29, 30]. Driven by the recognition of severe clinical outcomes among infants infected in utero (and neurologic morbidity in a proportion of infected adults), investigational individual-donation nucleic acid screening for Zika virus was implemented emergently in the United States in 2016. This was absent evidence of clinically significant morbidity associated with receipt of blood from viremic donors. At this writing, there have been three apparent transfusion transmissions of the virus published, all in Brazil, with none causing recognizable morbidity [31, 32]. CDC investigators have estimated the cost for the emergency implementation of Zika screening in US collection facilities at $137,000,000 annually [33].

"Newer" Zoonoses

As interesting as the examples above, where interventions have been required or widely implemented voluntarily, is a list (by no means exhaustive) of potential pathogens for which we have not acted. The examples chosen are epidemic pathogens (somewhere) and exemplify the difficulties faced when trying to assess the risks of transfusion-transmitted infection, with particular reference to the four questions.

Dengue and Chikungunya Viruses

Aedes mosquitos transmit both dengue, a *Flavivirus*, and chikungunya, an *Alphavirus*. They cause explosive epidemics, primarily in tropical and subtropical regions of the developing world, and manifest asymptomatic viremia; vector-borne infections are associated with morbidity and, in the case of dengue, mortality. The large global areas affected by dengue and chikungunya overlap those with endemic malaria, and temporary malaria deferral for travel to these areas surely provides partial protection of the blood supply in unaffected areas. However, the use of malaria deferral is clearly an incomplete approach [34], failing to address risks associated with malaria-free areas and from autochthonous transmission in the United States or other non-endemic countries where competent vectors are established (e.g., as has been seen sporadically with dengue in the United States [35]).

Dengue, while not strictly zoonotic, has a sylvan nonhuman primate-mosquito cycle in addition to the urban human-mosquito cycle responsible for human epidemics. Our response to dengue risk, or lack thereof, is informative of considerations used to address emerging pathogens. It is the most common human arboviral infection in the world (recent estimates suggest that more than 390,000,000 million infections occur annually) [36]. Human infections can range from asymptomatic to a lethal hemorrhagic fever. It is increasing in incidence worldwide, and transfusion transmission has been documented (albeit infrequently) [37–39]. Accordingly, dengue was labeled a priority agent in an AABB Transfusion-Transmitted Disease Committee exercise [11]. However, to date, no interventions are being seriously considered in the United States, beyond the requirement that donors be well when they are bled and what is contributed by malaria deferrals. For donors with risk for dengue from travel or outbreaks, who can be identified prior to donation, management strategies that temporarily restrict their donations or use (currently investigational) donor screening tests have been considered or used with variable costs and impacts on the availability of donors [40–43]. Recent data, using nucleic acid amplification tests, suggest that the clinical burden after transfusion transmission may be quite modest and not require action [44]. In this study from Brazil, 16 susceptible transfusion recipients of blood from dengue RNA-positive donors were clinically indistinguishable from susceptible controls who did not. Five exposed recipients experienced probable dengue transmissions, and one was a possible infection. Surveillance for the clinical sequelae of transfusion transmission is clearly a priority as the blood community considers the relevance of this virus.

Chikungunya originated in Africa where, historically, it circulated in a sylvan cycle among forest-dwelling *Aedes* mosquitos and nonhuman primates, with occasional human spillover. Human infection is generally symptomatic but was thought to be benign. However, during the recent pandemic, the occurrence of severe joint pain persisting for many weeks and months was recognized [45]. A mutation in the viral envelope protein allowed its adaptation to and high-level replication in the cosmopolitan vector *Aedes albopictus* [46]. Subsequently, the virus emerged from Africa as a pandemic that spread across the Indian Ocean, Asia, and the Pacific starting in 2005, reaching the Americas (St. Martin in the Caribbean) in late 2013 [38, 47]. The explosive (attack rate >30%) 2005–2006 epidemic on Reunion Island in the Indian Ocean was met with suspension of the collection of red blood cells and plasma on the island, their importation from Metropolitan France, and the emergent introduction of pathogen reduction for platelets collected from local at-risk donors [48]. The virus can be transmitted by IV inoculation of monkeys [49]. Modeling exercises suggest a substantial risk of transmission by blood [50, 51]. Donor testing in the Caribbean using nucleic acid tests during 2014–2015 identified 0.19–0.54% of tested donors to be "RNA-emic" [52, 53]. The positive units were discarded if prospectively tested or de-linked, so recipient outcomes are not available.

Internationally, and during its spread in the Americas where more than 2,000,000 cases have been reported to the Pan American Health Organization from 2014 to mid-September 2017 [54], transfusion transmission has been neither recognized nor alleged. No transfusion medicine interventions are planned in the United States beyond continued surveillance. Limited local transmission in South Florida provoked a scaled response depending on the case load, monitoring in conjunction with local public health, addition of travel deferrals for potential exposures in epidemics ex-US, proactive donation quarantine in zip codes with autochthonous cases and callback to assure the donor remained well before components could be distributed for transfusion, and zip code-based staged cessation of collections for local cases beyond a predetermined threshold number [55].

The absence of recognized or alleged transfusion-associated morbidity from these two viruses may be a result of several things. It may be nearly impossible to recognize such events against a background of epidemic vector-borne transmission, especially when transfused cohorts might have risk from both sources. In non-epidemic locations, the diagnosis may never be considered by clinicians unfamiliar with a potential for parenteral transmission. The infections can be clinically nonspecific, patients ill enough to require transfusion may have multiple sources of fever, and (in the experience of this infectious diseases clinician) febrile patients are generally not asked for a recent transfusion history, i.e., clinical surveillance is passive and limited. Finally, there are important pathogenic differences between mosquito transmission and parenteral transmission that relate to the effects of arthropod mediators injected with virus and the innate immune or inflammatory responses associated with vector transmission [56].

The pathogen reduction techniques being developed for labile components are likely effective against both viruses [57]. Likewise, multiple steps in the manufacture of plasma derivatives should make their risk de minimis. These include wet heat, dry heat, lyophilization, solvent-detergent treatment, and nanofiltration. The purification steps used to manufacture plasma-derived medicinal products including cold ethanol or chemical precipitation and chromatographic steps should further mitigate risk.

The Middle East Respiratory Syndrome Coronavirus (MERS-CoV)

In contrast to SARS-CoV, no interventions have been required in response to MERS-CoV. This enveloped RNA betacoronavirus emerged as a human pathogen in 2012 [58] and has been reported subsequently from 27 countries. The infection is endemic on the Arabian Peninsula where the large majority of cases have occurred or originated. Cases are occasionally exported elsewhere [59]. MERS-CoV causes respiratory infection including pneumonia and respiratory failure with an incubation period of days but up to 2 weeks. Gastrointestinal signs and symptoms may also occur. Treatment is supportive, and effective prophylactic measures have not been described.

Symptomatic MERS-CoV infection is associated with a high-mortality (≈35%) respiratory illness in humans, but asymptomatic infections (relevant to concerns about transfusion) have been recognized during aggressive laboratory investigation of contacts of cases, and infection is certainly considerably less lethal than the mortality reported for recognized disease [60]. From emergence to September 2017, 2081 laboratory-confirmed cases have been reported (82% from the Kingdom of Saudi Arabia). 21.5% have had no or mild symptoms. 46.8% had severe disease or died [61]. Two imported infections have been recognized in the United States, both in 2014, affecting healthcare workers exposed in Saudi Arabia. The potential for more extensive transmission outside the endemic area is exemplified by the large 2015 outbreak of healthcare-associated infection in South Korea (185 linked cases) where the index patient was a traveler to the Middle East [62]. The ultimate reservoir is not established, but the agent is likely to have evolved in bats and then was transmitted to camels [63, 64]. Direct contact with dromedary camels and consumption of raw camel milk have been suspected epidemiologically to be routes of primary infection and MERS-CoV transmission to humans [65]. Secondary cases are predominantly in healthcare settings in the absence of or with nonadherence to standard infection prevention and control strategies.

Transfusion transmission of MERS-CoV is neither reported nor suspected to date, and there is no such precedent with other coronaviruses. The occurrence of asymptomatic infection is obviously problematic, however [58]. Evidence for viremia is rarely sought but, where evaluated to date, has been confined to severely ill patients. The index patient in a family cluster in Tunisia in 2013 had viral sequences amplified by PCR from serum after more than a week of illness [66]. Another patient, with fatal infection, had sequences detected 4 weeks after onset of the illness, but was not apparently tested earlier [67]. In neither case was infectious virus sought. One hundred ten Saudi blood donors were seronegative for neutralizing antibodies [68], but there are no systematic studies looking for asymptomatic RNAemia or viremia in higher-risk cohorts such as contacts of cases. The most recent formal WHO MERS-CoV risk assessment includes no mention of a risk from transfusion-transmitted infection [69], nor does the European CDC rapid risk assessment of communicable diseases risk associated with the 2017 Hajj [70]. Given the low number of cases outside of the Middle East, and the apparent requirement for close contact with ill patients for person-to-person transmission to occur (esp. to healthcare workers), it does not appear that specific travel or risk deferrals are appropriate. Continuous monitoring (i.e., systematic "horizon scanning") for changes in the epidemiology and clinical pathology of MERS to be alert to changes that would suggest some risk of parenteral spread and transfusion risk seems an appropriate response.

In 2013, the AABB TTD emerging infections working group rejected the use of specific screening questions and referenced the FDA guidance on SARS for donors who spontaneously provide a history of exposure or illness [71]. Were a donor to provide such information during screening, the deferral criteria used for SARS (14 days from the last exposure and 28 days from completion of treatment and resolution of illness) seem rational, if wholly empirical.

Riboflavin and ultraviolet light and amotosalen with ultraviolet light have been reported to inactivate >4 and >5 logs of MERS-CoV in plasma [72, 73]. Data on platelets, RBC, and whole blood are not available. The manufacturing steps used for plasma derivatives should render such medicines safe.

Nipah and Hendra Viruses

Nipah, Hendra (and the apparently nonpathogenic Cedar virus), are *Henipaviruses* are from the *Paramyxovirinae* family. They are currently confined to South Asia and Australia (Fig. 10.2) [74]. Nipah is an emerging bat zoonosis, which spills over into humans to cause human infections ranging from inapparent to lethal encephalitis. It is an enveloped RNA virus sharing 70–90% amino acid homology across regions of the genome with Hendra virus. Nipah emerged in Malaysia in 1998–1999 where bats infected swine and the swine infected humans. During that outbreak of encephalitis and respiratory illness, there were approximately 300 human cases and more

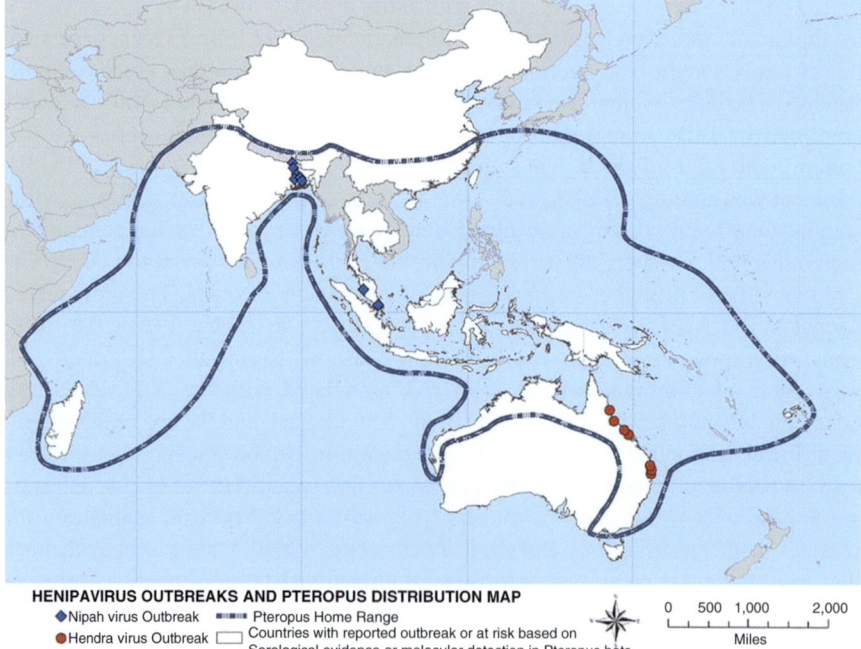

Fig. 10.2 Geographic distributions of Nipah (blue diamonds) and Hendra infections (red circles), with home range of *Pteropus* bats (blue line). (Source: Centers for Disease Control and Prevention, National Center for Emerging and Zoonotic Infectious Diseases (NCEZID), Division of High-Consequence Pathogens and Pathology (DHCPP), Viral Special Pathogens Branch (VSPB). https://www.cdc.gov/vhf/nipah/outbreaks/distribution-map.html. Accessed 4 Oct 2017)

than 100 deaths [75, 76]. The clinical spectrum seems variable across geographically separate outbreaks. Treatment is supportive, but the antiviral ribavirin has been used in uncontrolled circumstances with some success. No effective prophylaxis (medication, immunoglobulin, or vaccine) has been reported. The human incubation period has ranged from 4 days to 2 months (90% ≤14 days), and there is, again, some variation according to the location of the outbreak. Direct contact with the respiratory secretions of infected swine that generally have a mild illness (apparently infected by consumption of mangoes contaminated with bat urine) was the source of the index outbreak. Bats of the genus *Pteropus* ("flying foxes") appear to be the natural reservoir and can infect a variety of mammalian secondary hosts (i.e., felines, canines, swine, and equines). An outbreak in Bangladesh was associated with the consumption of date palm sap, again contaminated by infected bats. Direct contact with infected bats may also result in transmission. Human-to-human transmissions, including family and healthcare associated, are documented. There is indirect evidence (i.e., lacking virus isolation or nucleic acid tests) of reactivation of latent, chronic infection resulting in recurrent CNS disease and death [77–79]. Despite recurrent outbreaks, especially in Bangladesh and India, there have been no allegations of transfusion transmission, and little attention has been paid to implications for blood safety.

Hendra virus is closely related to Nipah at the sequence level. Recognized human Hendra virus infection is much rarer than Nipah, with seven cases and four deaths recognized since the first equine outbreak in Australia in 1994 [80]. Horses are infected after contact with infected urine from *Pteropus* bats. A total of 53 outbreaks of equine respiratory illness involving more than 70 horses have all been confined to the northeast coast of Australia [81]. There is no evidence of the infection before its 1994 emergence after serological studies on a number of vertebrate and invertebrate repository samples. It causes a spectrum of human illness from nonspecific fever to flu-like syndromes to fatal encephalitis, generally as a consequence of spillover from equine infections. Treatment is supportive. No effective prophylaxis is available. The incubation period is from 5 to 21 days from exposure. Transmission to humans occurs mainly after direct contact during the care of sick horses or at the time of their autopsies. In early studies, recipient horses were infected intravenously using homogenates of the spleen and lung from two of the index horses. Postmortem lung, liver, kidney, and spleen from a human decedent were infectious in tissue culture [70]. In one case of CNS infection, the patient recovered but had recurrent neurological illness over a year later and died. There are no reports alleging transfusion transmission.

There is a small amount of evidence for an acute, low-level viremia for Nipah virus, and one might expect the same for Hendra. Pathologic studies demonstrate that respiratory and vascular endothelial cells are important targets for both Nipah and Hendra. How they spread from the portal of entry, likely the respiratory epithelium, is not fully characterized. In later stages of clinical infection, pulmonary endothelium is infected, and small vessel vasculitis ensues. They are believed to enter the bloodstream at that point and disseminate as free and cell-associated virus [82, 83] and gain entry to the central nervous system. At least one mouse model has discounted the requirement for viremia for development of encephalitis with Hendra [84]. Direct evidence of human viremia has not been provided for either virus. Whether an asymptomatic infected individual sustains a potentially infectious viremia has not been addressed. Blood donor studies have not been published.

Donor screening, whether by health history or in vitro assays, has not been proposed for either of these viruses. Donor questions to understand exposure risk can be developed and implemented at need, in the event of outbreaks that might affect blood donors. High-throughput assays are not available, although diagnostic assays might be repurposed for this indication if the need arose.

Donor deferral strategies for a history of exposure or infection will, necessarily, be empiric. For a history of exposure, they would be some multiple of the maximum credible incubation period (e.g., perhaps 6 weeks for Hendra and 6 months for Nipah). Since some proportion of infections are asymptomatic, donor reentry with a negative diagnostic serology might be considered. A history of infection is more problematic, given the apparent persistence of some Nipah infections and a single case report of relapsing Hendra in the CNS. A lifetime deferral is defensible for both viruses after clinical infection.

In an outbreak context (potentially including travel to areas experience significant activity) or when a donor is diagnosed with one of these viral infections, it seems reasonable for a blood collection organization to have (generic) procedures to guide a recall of co-components of donations from exposed or ill donors from within some reasonable interval before donation. These would reflect their incubation periods and the best data on the presence and duration of putative viremia. It would be prudent to perform a lookback to recipients of blood transfused before such a recall was undertaken, for the purposes of assessing their likelihood of having been infected. Likewise, an allegation of transfusion transmission should be carefully evaluated and the need to evaluate donors assessed.

Appropriate studies of pathogen reduction for labile blood products have not been published for either Nipah or Hendra, but similar viruses (i.e., enveloped RNA viruses) are effectively inactivated by the processes being advanced for approval in the United States. Likewise, one would expect that one or more of the specific viral inactivation, removal and purification steps in commercial plasma fractionation processes, would eliminate risk from derivatives.

Looking Forward

The foregoing depict a very *ad hoc* process for recognizing and responding to emerging infectious threats to transfusion safety, whether zoonotic, arthropod-borne, or others. Given the unpredictability attending the emergence of a specific pathogen, this is perhaps inevitable. That said, that new pathogens will emerge is axiomatic. The task for infectious diseases and epidemiology experts in the blood community is to be sensitive to this inevitability and to spend real effort anticipating which agents of many candidates pose material threats that bear forethought and planning. To that end, the emerging infections subgroup at AABB has engaged in developing a toolkit to guide that process (Fig. 10.3). The most critical activity is "horizon scanning" that daily surveils a spectrum of online and print resources to identify new and emerging human pathogens. These include media reports, professional meetings, organizational and peer-reviewed publications, open source and subscription websites (e.g., ProMED [85], CDC.gov, WHO.int, PAHO.org, and many others), and personal networks. Perhaps difficult element for horizon scanning is effective hemovigilance. This requires of clinicians the routine elicitation of a transfusion history as they establish a differential diagnosis in patients with apparent infections, so that they can ask themselves the four questions we have proposed as critical for imputing blood as a "vector."

Criteria for more detailed review include the *de novo* identification or expansion of the range of a pathogen, especially its involvement in an outbreak; reports of transmission by organ and tissue transplantation; infection following parenteral inoculation via needle stick and laboratory accidents; an association with injection drug use or sexual activity; a close relationship to a recognized TTI; and actual allegations of transfusion transmission.

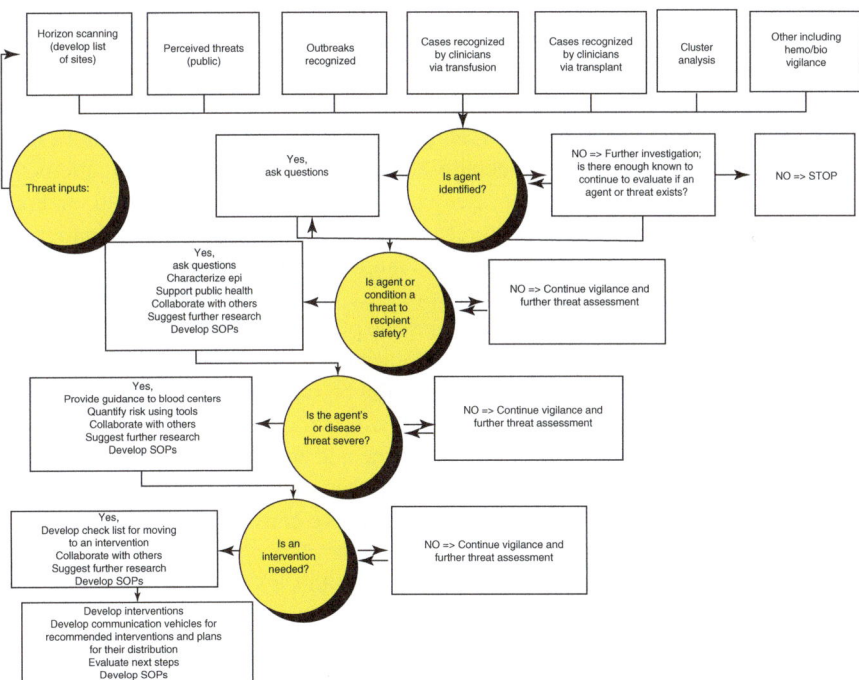

Fig. 10.3 Outline of AABB emerging infectious diseases subgroup's toolkit including the framework for recognition, assessment, and management of EID agents for risk of transfusion-associated transmission and disease. SOP standard operating procedure [24]. (Used with permission from: Stramer SL and Dodd RY for the AABB Transfusion-Transmitted Diseases Subgroup [90])

The role and effectiveness of advanced molecular techniques (e.g., pathogen discover via metagenomics or next-generation sequencing and other non-culture-based techniques) to study clinically infected patients for diagnostic indications and populations (including blood donors) to elucidate the human microbiome and explore new disease associations are not yet clear. False alarms will occur when members of the "normal human flora" are discovered. TT virus (an anellovirus) was discovered using representational difference analysis for the amplification of nucleic acids in patients with posttransfusion non-A, B, and C hepatitis [86], causing its brief consideration as a target for interventions in transfusion medicine, but any association of the ubiquitous virus with either transfusion pathology or other illness was eventually refuted. More recently, next-generation sequencing was applied to sera from 204 US patients with acute liver failure of unknown etiology and failed to identify unexpected pathogens [87].

With the suspicion that a new infection threatens blood transfusion recipients, a risk must be quantified, initially using provisional clinical and epidemiological descriptions that will be refined over time. Online risk modeling tools to accomplish these analyses are being developed for transfusion medicine [88], with the critical, if obvious, caveat that the precision of their output is wholly dependent on input parameters. These are necessarily least precise in the earliest stages of emergence when initial preparedness decisions must be made generally and specifically with regard to transfusion safety. There are critical data needed to inform any quantitative assessment of the importance of a potential pathogen. A "routine" search for and reports of the presence of the infectious agent (or the imperfect surrogates, nucleic acids, and antigens) in the blood of asymptomatic individuals at risk would be a valuable standard operating procedure during epidemiologic investigations of emerging infections; this does not often occur early and before the blood community must respond to a potential threat. Likewise, prospective determination of pathogen survival through contemporary component production, processing, and storage should be a research priority.

When we conclude that material risk may be present, interventions must be considered and prioritized. They will range from information and education to donor queries and deferrals. For example, would it not be rational in the temperate world to consider a blanket travel deferral of several weeks for donors visiting tropical and subtropical venues where acute arthropod-borne and zoonotic agents are common? Donor testing and determining the role of pathogen reduction techniques are more aggressive responses to greater perceived risk. These considerations are all, necessarily, cyclic, iterative processes. The pivotal role of risk-based decision-making from a societal perspective is covered elsewhere in this book.

References

1. Institute of Medicine. Committee to study HIV transmission through blood and blood products. In: Leveton LB, Sox Jr HC, Stoto MA, editors. HIV and the blood supply: an analysis of crisis decision-making: consensus study report. Washington, DC: National Academy Press; 1995.

2. Alter HJ, Purcell RH, Holland PV, et al. The relationship of donor transaminase (ALT) to recipient hepatitis: impact on blood transfusion services. JAMA. 1981;246:630–4.
3. Koziol DE, et al. Antibody to hepatitis B core antigen as a paradoxical marker for non-A, non-B hepatitis agents in donated blood. Ann Intern Med. 1986;04:488–95.
4. Stevens CE, et al. Hepatitis B virus antibody in blood donors and the occurrence of non-A, non-B hepatitis in transfusion recipients: an analysis of the transfusion-transmitted viruses study. Ann Intern Med. 1984;104:488–95.
5. US Food and Drug Administration. HTLV-1 antibody testing (11/29/88). At https://www.fda.gov/downloads/biologicsbloodvaccines/guidancecomplianceregulatoryinformation/other-recommendationsformanufacturers/memorandumtobloodestablishments/ucm063001.pdf. Accessed 27 Oct 2017.
6. Centers for Disease control and Prevention and the US Public Health Service working group. Guidelines for counseling persons infected with Human T-Lymphotropic type 1 (HTLV-1) and type 2 (HTLV-2). Ann Intern Med. 1993;118:448.
7. Marano G, Vaglio S, Pupella S, et al. Human T-lymphotropic virus and transfusion safety: does one size fit all? Transfusion. 2016;56:249–60.
8. Current good manufacturing practice regulations relevant to blood establishments can be found in 21 CFR parts 210, 211, 600, 606, 610, and 640. At https://www.accessdata.fda.gov/scripts/cdrh/cfdocs/cfcfr/CFRSearch.cfm?
9. Zou S, Stramer SL, Dodd RY. Donor testing and risk: current prevalence, incidence, and residual risk of transfusion-transmissible agents in US allogeneic donations. Trans Med Rev. 2012;26:119–28.
10. Woolhouse MEJ, Scott F, Hudson ZR, et al. Human viruses: discovery and emergence. Philos Trans R Soc Lond B. 2012;367:2864–71.
11. Stramer SL, Hollinger FB, Katz LM, et al. Emerging infectious disease agents and their potential threat to transfusion safety. Transfusion. 2009;49:1S–29S.
12. Stramer S. State of the art: Current perspectives in transfusion-transmitted infectious diseases: emerging and re-emerging infections. ISBT Science Series. 2014;9:30–6.
13. US Food and Drug Administration. Guidance for industry: revised precautionary measures to reduce the possible risk of transmission of Creutzfeldt-Jakob disease (CJD) and new variant Creutzfeldt-Jakob Disease (nvCJD) by blood and blood products; 1999.
14. Bennett P, Daraktchiev M. vCJD and transfusion of blood components: an updated risk assessment. 2013. At https://www.gov.uk/government/publications/vcjd-and-transfusion-of-blood-components-updated-risk-assessment. Accessed 2 Oct 2017.
15. US Food and Drug Administration. Guidance for industry. Revised preventive measures to reduce the possible risk of transmission of Creutzfeldt-Jakob disease (CJD) and variant Creutzfeldt-Jakob disease (vCJD) by blood and blood products. 2002. https://www.fda.gov/downloads/biologicsbloodvaccines/guidancecomplianceregulatoryinformation/guidances/blood/ucm307137.pdf.
16. Murphy EL, Connor D, McEvoy P, et al. Estimating blood donor loss due to the variant CJD travel deferral. Transfusion. 2004;44:645–50.
17. Mok T, Jaunmuktane Z, Joiner S, et al. Variant Creutzfeldt–Jakob Disease in a Patient with Heterozygosity at PRNP Codon 129. N Engl J Med. 2017;376:292–4.
18. Fernandez-Borges N, Espinosa JC, Marin-Moreno A, et al. Protective effect of Val_{129}-PrP against bovine spongiform encephalopathy but not variant Creutzfeldt-Jakob disease. Emerg Infect Dis. 2017;23(9):1522–30.
19. US Centers for Disease Control and Prevention. West Nile virus infection in organ donor and transplant recipients—Georgia and Florida, 2002. MMWR. 2002;51:790.
20. Petersen LR, Marfin AA, Gubler DJ. West Nile Virus. JAMA. 2003;290:524–8.
21. Biggerstaff BJ, Petersen LR. Estimated risk of West Nile virus transmission through blood transfusion during an epidemic in Queens, New York City. Transfusion. 2002;42:1019–26.
22. Pealer LN, Marfin AA, Petersen LR, et al. Transmission of West Nile Virus through blood transfusion in the United States in 2002. N Engl J Med. 2003;349:1236–45.
23. O'Leary DR, Marfin AA, Montgomery SP, et al. The epidemic of West Nile virus in the United States, 2002. Vector Borne Zoonotic Dis. 2004;4:61–70.

24. Glynn SA, Busch MP, Dodd RY, et al. Emerging infectious agents and the nation's blood supply: responding to potential threats in the 21st century. Transfusion. 2013;53:438–54.
25. Food and Drug Administration. Guidance for Industry. Recommendations for the assessment of donor suitability and blood product safety in cases of suspected severe acute respiratory syndrome (SARS) or exposure to SARS. 2003. At https://www.fda.gov/biologicsbloodvaccines/guidancecomplianceregulatoryinformation/guidances/blood/ucm075016.htm. Accessed 2 Oct 2017.
26. Ng LFP, Wong M, Koh S, et al. Detection of severe acute respiratory syndrome coronavirus in blood of infected patients. J Clin Micro. 2004;42:347–50.
27. Wang W-K, Fang C-T, Chen H-L, et al. Detection of severe acute respiratory syndrome coronavirus RNA in plasma during the course of infection. J Clin Micro. 2005;43:962–5.
28. US Food and Drug Administration. Recommendations for assessment of blood bonor eligibility, donor deferral and blood product management in response to Ebola Virus; Guidance for Industry. At https://www.fda.gov/BiologicsBloodVaccines/GuidanceComplianceRegulatoryInformation/Guidances/Blood/default.htm. Accessed 30 Oct 2017.
29. US Food and Drug Administration. Revised recommendations for reducing the risk of Zika virus transmission by blood and blood components guidance for industry. At https://www.fda.gov/downloads/BiologicsBloodVaccines/GuidanceComplianceRegulatoryInformation/Guidances/Blood/UCM518213.pdf. Accessed 30 Oct 2017.
30. Katz LM, Rossmann SN. Zika and the blood supply: a work in progress. Arch Path Lab Med. 2017;141:85–92.
31. Barjas-Castro ML, Angerami RN, Cunha MS, et al. Probable transfusion transmitted Zika virus in Brazil. Transfusion. 2016;56:1684–8.
32. Motta IJF, Spencer BR, Cordiero SG, et al. Evidence for transmission of Zika virus by platelet transfusion. N Engl J Med. 2016;375:1101–3.
33. Ellingson KD, Sapiano MRP, Haas KA, et al. Cost projections for implementation of safety interventions to prevent transfusion-transmitted Zika virus infection in the United States. Transfusion. 2017;57:1625–33.
34. Spencer BR, Katz LM. Estimating the impact of a potential dengue travel deferral. Transfusion. 2011;51(s3):3–4A.
35. Morens DM, Fauci AS. Dengue and hemorrhagic fever: a potential threat to public health in the United States. JAMA. 2008;299:214–6.
36. World Health Organization. Dengue control: epidemiology. At http://www.who.int/denguecontrol/epidemiology/en/. Accessed 2 Oct 2017.
37. Wilder-Smith A, Chen LH, Massad E, et al. Threat of dengue to blood safety in dengue-endemic countries. Emerg Infect Dis. 2009;15:8–11.
38. Teo D, Ng LC, Lam S. Is dengue a threat to the blood supply? Transfus Med. 2009;19:66–77.
39. Matos D, et al. Probable and possible transfusion transmitted dengue associated with NS1 antigen-negative but RNA confirmed-positive red blood cells. Transfusion. 2015;56:215–22.
40. Seed CR, Kiely P, Hyland CA, Keller A. The risk of dengue transmission by blood during a 2004 outbreak in Cairns, Australia. Transfusion. 2009;49:1482–7.
41. Clive R. Seed PhD, Donor and product safety policy unit. Australian Red Cross Blood Services, Melbourne AU.
42. Stramer SL, Linnen JM, Carrick JM, et al. Dengue viremia in blood donors identified by RNA and detection of dengue transfusion transmission during the 2007 dengue outbreak in Puerto Rico. Transfusion. 2012;52:1657–66.
43. Spencer BR, Stramer S, Dodd R, et al. Survey to estimate donor loss to a 14- or 28-day travel deferral for mitigation of CHIKV, DENV and other acute infections. Transfusion Plenary abstract P1-030A. 2015;55(S3):3A.
44. Sabino EC, Loureiro P, Lopes ME, et al. Transfusion-transmitted dengue and associated clinical symptoms during the 2012 epidemic in Brazil. J Infect Dis. 2016;213:694–702.
45. Weaver SC, Lecuit M. Chikungunya virus and the global spread of a mosquito-borne disease. N Engl J Med. 2015;372:1231–9.

46. Schuffenecker I, Iteman I, Michault A, et al. Genome microevolution of chikungunya viruses causing the Indian Ocean outbreak. PLoS Med. 2006;3:1058–70.
47. Staples JE, Breiman RF, Powers AM. Chikungunya fever: an epidemiological review of a re-emerging infectious disease. J Infect Dis. 2009;49:942–8.
48. Rasogles P, Angelini-Tibert MF, Simon P, et al. Transfusion of platelet components prepared with photochemical pathogen inactivation treatment during a Chikungunya virus epidemic in Ile de La Réunion. Transfusion. 2009;49:1083–91.
49. Labadie K, Larcher T, Joubert C, et al. Chikungunya disease in nonhuman primates involves long-term viral persistence in macrophages. J Clin Invest. 2010;120:894–906.
50. Brouard C, Bernillon P, Quatresous I, et al. Estimated risk of Chikungunya viremic blood donation during an epidemic on Reunion Island in the Indian Ocean, 2005 to 2007. Transfusion. 2008;48:1333–41.
51. Appassakij H, Promwong C, Rujirojindakul R, et al. The risk of blood transfusion–associated Chikungunya fever during the 2009 epidemic in Songkhla Province, Thailand. Transfusion. 2015;54:1945–52.
52. Gallian P, de Lamballerie X, Salez N, et al. Prospective detection of chikungunya virus in blood donors, Caribbean 2014. Blood. 2014;123:3679–81.
53. Chiu CY, Bres V, Yu G, et al. Genomic assays for identification of chikungunya virus in blood donors, Puerto Rico, 2014. Emerg Infect Dis. 2015;21:1409–13.
54. Pan American Health Organization. Chikungunya: Data, Maps and Statistics. http://www.paho.org/hq/index.php?option=com_topics&view=readall&cid=5927&Itemid=&lang=en. Accessed 2 Oct 2017.
55. LeParc GF, Reik RA. A strategy to manage the risk of dengue and chikungunya virus disease in the donor population. Transfusion. 2015;55(s3):17A.
56. Pingen M, Bryden SR, Pondeville E, et al. Host inflammatory response to mosquito bites enhances the severity of arbovirus infection. Immunity. 2016;44:1455–69.
57. Tan L, Lam S, Ling Low S, et al. Evaluation of pathogen reduction systems to inactivate dengue and chikungunya viruses in apheresis platelets suspended in plasma. Adv Infect Dis. 2013;3:1–9.
58. Zaki AM, van Boheemen S, Bestebroer TM, et al. Isolation of a novel coronavirus from a man with pneumonia in Saudi Arabia. N Engl J Med. 2012;367:1814–20.
59. Zumala A, Hui DS, Perlman S. Middle East Respiratory Syndrome. Lancet. 2015;386:995–1007.
60. World Health Organization. Middle East Respiratory Syndrome (MERS-CoV). At http://www.who.int/mediacentre/factsheets/mers-cov/en/. Accessed 6 Oct 2017.
61. World Health Organization. WHO MERS-CoV global summary and assessment of risk. At www.who.int/emergencies/mers-cov/risk-assessment-july-2017.pdf. Accessed 23 Oct 2017.
62. US Centers for Disease Control and Prevention. Middle East Respiratory Syndrome (MERS). At https://www.cdc.gov/coronavirus/mers/about/index.html. Accessed 5 Oct 2017.
63. Ithete NL, Stoff berg S, Corman VM, et al. Close relative of human Middle East respiratory syndrome coronavirus in bat, South Africa. Emerg Infect Dis. 2013;19:1697–9.
64. Memish ZA, Mishra N, Olival KJ, et al. Middle East respiratory syndrome coronavirus in bats, Saudi Arabia. Emerg Infect Dis. 2013;19:1819–23.
65. Hemida MG, Al-Naeem A, Perera RAPM, et al. Lack of Middle East respiratory syndrome coronavirus transmission from infected camels. Emerg Infect Dis. 2015;21:699–701.
66. Abroug F, Slim A, Ouanes-Besbes L, et al. Family cluster of Middle East Respiratory Syndrome Coronavirus infections, Tunisia, 2013. Emerg Infect Dis. 2014;20:1527–30.
67. Poissy J, Goffard A, Parmentier-Decrucq E, et al. Kinetics and pattern of viral excretion in biological specimens of two MERS-CoV cases. J Clin Virol. 2014;1:275–8.
68. Gierer S, Hofmann-Winkler H, Albuali WH, et al. Lack of MERS coronavirus neutralizing antibodies in humans, Eastern Province, Saudi Arabia. Emerg Infect Dis. 2013;19:2034–6.
69. World Health Organization. MERS-CoV global summary and assessment of risk-July 2017. At http://www.who.int/emergencies/mers-cov/en/. Accessed 6 Oct 2017.

70. European Centers for Disease Control. Rapid Risk Assessment: Public health risks related to communicable diseases during the Hajj 2017, Saudi Arabia, 30 August – 4 September 2017. At https://ecdc.europa.eu/en/publications-data/rapid-risk-assessment-public-health-risks-related-communicable-diseases-during. Accessed 7 Oct 2017.
71. AABB. Middle East Respiratory Syndrome Coronavirus. At http://www.aabb.org/tm/eid/Documents/middle-east-respiratory-syndrome-coronavirus.pdf.
72. Keil SD, Bowen R, Marschner S. Inactivation of Middle East respiratory syndrome coronavirus (MERS-CoV) in plasma products using a riboflavin-based and ultraviolet light-based photochemical treatment. Transfusion. 2016;56:2948–52.
73. Hindawi SI, Hashem AM, Damanhouri GA, et al. Efficient inactivation of MERS-CoV in human plasma with amotosalen and UVA light. Transfusion. 2017;57(s3):190A.
74. US Centers for Disease Control and Prevention. https://www.cdc.gov/vhf/nipah/outbreaks/distribution-map.html. Accessed 4 Oct 2017.
75. US Centers for Disease Control and Prevention. Outbreak of Hendra-like virus—Malaysia and Singapore, 1998-1999. MMWR. 1999;48:265–9.
76. Chua KB, Bellini WJ, Rota PA, et al. Nipah virus: a recently emergent deadly paramyxovirus. Science. 2000;288:1432–5.
77. US Centers for Disease Control and Prevention. Nipah Virus (NiV): Signs and symptoms. At https://www.cdc.gov/vhf/nipah/symptoms/index.html. Accessed 4 Oct 2017.
78. Tan CT, Goh KJ, Wong KT, et al. Relapsed and late onset Nipah encephalitis. Ann Neurol. 2002;51:703–8.
79. Chong HT, Tan CT. Relapsed and late-onset Nipah encephalitis, a report of three cases. Neurol J Southeast Asia. 2003;8:109–12.
80. Murray K, Selleck P, Hooper P, et al. A morbillivirus that caused fatal disease in horses and humans. Science. 1995;268:94–7.
81. World Health Organization. Hendra virus (HeV) infection. At http://www.who.int/csr/disease/hendra/en/. Accessed 4 Oct 2017.
82. Wong KT, Shieh WJ, Kumar S, et al. Nipah Virus Pathology Working Group () Nipah virus infection: pathology and pathogenesis of an emerging paramyxoviral zoonosis. Am J Pathol. 2002;161:2153–67.
83. Escaffre O, Borisevich V, Rockx B. Pathogenesis of Hendra and Nipah virus infection in humans. J Infect Dev Ctries. 2013;7(4):308–11.
84. Dups J, Middleton D, Yamada M, et al. A new model for Hendra virus encephalitis in the mouse. PLoS One. 2012;7(7):e40308. https://doi.org/10.1371/journal.pone.0040308.
85. International Society for Infectious Diseases. About ProMED. At http://www.promedmail.org/aboutus/. Accessed 31 Oct 2017.
86. Nishizawa T, Okamoto H, Konishi K, et al. A novel DNA virus (TTV) associated with elevated transaminase levels in posttransfusion hepatitis of unknown etiology. Biochem Biophys Res Commun. 1997;241:92–7.
87. Somasekar S, Lee D, Rule J, et al. Viral surveillance in serum samples from patients with acute liver failure by metagenomic next-generation sequencing. Clin Infect Dis. 2017;65:1477–85.
88. Kiely P, Gambhir M, Cheng AC, et al. Emerging infectious diseases and blood safety.: modeling the transfusion-transmission risk. Trans Med Rev. 2017;31:154–64.
89. Woolhouse MEJ, Howey R, Gaunt E, et al. Temporal trends in the discovery of human viruses. Proc R Soc B. 2008;275:2111–5.
90. Stramer SL and Dodd RY for the AABB Transfusion-Transmitted Diseases Subgroup. Transfusion-transmitted emerging infectious diseases: 30 years of challenges and progress. Transfusion. 2013;53(10 pt2):2375–83.

Chapter 11
Tick-Borne Infections: Beware the Tortoises Among Us

David A. Leiby

Introduction

Worldwide vector-borne agents of disease continue to emerge and play ever-increasing roles as threats to blood safety likely influenced by several factors including climate and weather, changing ecosystems, human behavior, economic development, and changes in land use [1]. Among mosquito-borne agents, the triumvirate of dengue, chikungunya, and Zika viruses has joined West Nile virus as recognized risks for transmission by blood transfusion. However, with the exception of West Nile virus, which demonstrates an established zoonotic life cycle, most outbreaks associated with mosquito-borne agents of concern are ephemeral in nature and quickly transition to naïve populations in new geographic locations. In contrast, tick-borne agents are generally zoonotic in nature, remaining entrenched where first identified, spreading slowly from the areas of initial establishment to new geographic regions. Tick-borne and mosquito-borne agents are thus analogous to Aesop's *Tortoise and the Hare*, respectively. While mosquito-borne agents have garnered most of the popular media's attention, this chapter will focus on those tick-borne agents or "tortoises," which in their steady plodding fashion pose expanding and ongoing threats to blood safety.

Tick-borne agents meet many of the prerequisites for transfusion transmission. Firstly, during active infections many tick-borne agents are present in the peripheral blood. While some agents like spirochetes of *Borrelia miyamotoi* (agent of relapsing fever) are free in peripheral blood, many tick-borne agents exploit intracellular niches enhancing the likelihood of transmission by blood transfusion: erythrocytes (*Babesia microti*), monocytes (*Ehrlichia chaffeensis*), and granulocytes (*Anaplasma phagocytophilum, Ehrlichia ewingii*). Secondly, most tick-borne agents are capable

---

D. A. Leiby
Division of Emerging and Transfusion-Transmitted Diseases OBRR/CBER,
U.S. Food and Drug Administration, Silver Spring, MD, USA
e-mail: david.leiby@fda.hhs.gov

of surviving blood processing (e.g., leukoreduction, irradiation) and storage conditions (i.e., 4 °C). As will be discussed, several cases of transfusion transmission associated with *A. phagocytophilum* have implicated leukoreduced blood products. In contrast, the relative inability of *B. burgdorferi* to survive storage at 4 °C has been suggested as a contributing factor to the absence of Lyme transmission cases. Lastly, upon introduction into a blood recipient, tick-borne agents are capable of establishing infections (e.g., *B. microti*, Colorado tick fever virus, *Rickettsia rickettsii*, etc.). The likelihood of establishing infection is enhanced by at-risk recipients including those who are immunocompromised, multiply transfused, demonstrate geographic or seasonal risk, or receive transfusions in the absence of effective interventions.

One approach in reviewing tick-borne agents that pose blood safety threats is to list all the agents which pose a potential risk or that have been implicated in transfusion cases. While this didactic approach can be effective, this chapter will take a slightly different slant by focusing on the vector, using the concept of the microbial "guild." A guild can be defined as a group of unrelated species sharing a common resource, in this case the so-called deer or black-legged tick, *Ixodes scapularis*. As such, *I. scapularis* is known to be the vector for *Borrelia burgdorferi*, *B. microti*, *A. phagocytophilum*, *B. miyamotoi*, and Powassan virus. In many instances the geographic distribution of these agents is overlapping, and coinfections in patients are not uncommon. While *I. scapularis* is limited to North America, it is interesting to note that similar *Ixodes* sp. in northern latitudes of Europe and Asia also harbor guilds of comparable tick-borne agents.

The present discussion of the *I. scapularis* guild of agents will not focus on *B. burgdorferi* or *B. microti*. In the case of Lyme disease, tens of thousands of clinical cases have been reported in the United States and worldwide since *B. burgdorferi* was first identified as the etiologic agent of disease in 1982 [2]. While *B. burgdorferi* case reports continue to increase across the United States and the geographic range of the agent continues to expand, no cases of transfusion-associated Lyme disease have been reported to date. The reasons for the absence of transfusion cases are not clear but anecdotally have been attributed to the limited period of time the agent is present in peripheral blood and its reported low tolerance of blood storage conditions. In contrast, *B. microti* is routinely present in peripheral blood, survives blood storage at 4 °C for up to 42 days [3], and was initially implicated in 159 cases of transfusion transmission [4]; however, this number now likely exceeds 200 cases. Multiple high-quality reviews and research studies focused on *B. microti* have been published that describe transfusion-transmitted babesiosis and associated mitigation efforts in detail [5–7]; thus reiteration is unnecessary. As envisioned, this review is designed to be forward thinking and horizon scanning. Therefore, it will focus on three other members of the *I. scapularis* guild: *A. phagocytophilum* which has been implicated in an increasing number of transfusion cases, the newly described *B. miyamotoi* whose survival in blood products and transmission by blood transfusion in animal models has been documented, and the lesser known Powassan virus, unusual in that it is a tick-borne flavivirus, a group of viruses (e.g., West Nile, dengue, etc.) that have been transmitted by blood transfusion.

Anaplasma phagocytophilum

Foremost among recently emergent agents transmitted by the deer tick is *Anaplasma phagocytophilum*, the etiologic agent of human granulocytic anaplasmosis (HGA) [8]. *A. phagocytophilum*, first identified in 1994 (originally named *Ehrlichia* sp.) [9, 10], is an obligate intracellular Gram-negative rickettsial bacterium that infects neutrophils and is endemic to the Northeast, Upper Midwest and portions of the Mid-Atlantic United States [11, 12]. Since becoming reportable in 1999, HGA cases have increased annually from 348 in 2000 to 2782 cases in 2013 [13, 14], but these numbers likely represent underestimates. Similarly, since the first case of transfusion-transmitted anaplasmosis (TTA) was reported in 1999 [15], case reports have become more frequent, suggesting that *A. phagocytophilum* may pose an increasing blood safety risk.

Biology and Epidemiology

A. phagocytophilum is endemic worldwide in the northern latitudes of North America, Europe, and Asia. As indicated above, in the United States, it is primarily endemic to the northeast, upper Midwest, and portions of the mid-Atlantic, but the geographic range continues to expand. In general, its distribution in the United States reflects the range of the primary vector, *I. scapularis*, but the western black legged tick (*I. pacificus*) has also been linked to cases along the Pacific coast [16]. Nymphal and adult ticks of *I. scapularis* and *I. pacificus* are capable of infecting humans and causing disease. Reservoir hosts are not well understood, but the primary reservoir hosts are thought to be the white-footed mouse (*Peromyscus leucopus*) and the eastern chipmunk (*Tamias striatus*) [17, 18]. The geographic range of *A. phagocytophilum* continues to expand in large part due to reforestation, geographic extension of tick vectors, and an increase in the white-tailed deer population [16, 19, 20]. Initial transmission to humans usually requires the tick vector to be attached for at least 24 h [21], and similar to other tick-borne agents, transmission peaks during the summer months.

Clinical Features/Diagnosis/Treatment

Following successful transmission by an infected tick bite, symptoms normally appear 5–10 days later but may take as long as 3 weeks [21]. Infections with *A. phagocytophilum* can range from asymptomatic to more severe disease demonstrating fever, headache, malaise, myalgia, low platelet and white blood cell levels, and elevated liver enzymes, potentially leading to adult respiratory distress syndrome, renal failure, neurologic disorders, and death in less than 1% of clinical cases [22].

Upon the establishment of infection, bacteria multiply as microcolonies, referred to as morulae, within cytoplasmic inclusions of neutrophils. In symptomatic cases, the acute bacteremic phase generally lasts only 1–2 weeks [23, 24] but has not been well characterized in asymptomatic patients. As for many tick-borne diseases, persons with attenuated immune responses are at greater risk for increased severity of symptoms and potential complications. Similarly, HGA cases are more frequently reported in males and persons over 40 years of age [13].

Infection with *A. phagocytophilum* can be diagnosed by direct detection, serology, and/or molecular techniques [13]. For direct detection, identification of intracellular morulae in neutrophils by microscopic examination of stained blood smears is diagnostic. Similarly, the presence of IgM or IgG antibodies by IFA or ELISA is indicative of infection with *A. phagocytophilum*. However, confirmation of infection usually relies upon a fourfold rise in IgG titers in paired serum samples or positive detection of *A. phagocytophilum* DNA in blood by PCR. Although more laborious, diagnosis can also be made through isolation of the agent in cell culture. Treatment regimens are effective, leading to rapid resolution of infection and usually rely upon doxycycline, rifampin, and/or levofloxacin [22].

Seroprevalence and Incidence

There have been limited seroprevalence studies performed to date, perhaps in part due to a lack of suitable assays. Overall cross-sectional seroprevalence in endemic areas is 3.7%, ranging from 14.9% in Northwest Wisconsin to 0.6–0.9% in Connecticut [25–27]. Perhaps a more reliable measure of HGA is incidence reports provided to the CDC. As stated previously, cases reported to the CDC have increased dramatically since HGA became notifiable in 1999. The incidence of HGA has also increased, from 1.4 cases (per million persons) in 2000 to 6.1 in 2010, but the case fatality rate has remained at <1% [13]. HGA case reports are concentrated in six states, with over 90% of reported US cases originating from New York, Connecticut, New Jersey, Rhode Island, Minnesota, and Wisconsin. However, these case numbers likely represent an underestimate as many cases go unreported or unrecognized due to generalized symptoms that are similar to other common infections.

Transfusion Transmission/Survival in Blood

The intracellular niche of *A. phagocytophilum*, coupled with survival under blood storage conditions for at least 30 days [15], enhances its potential for transmission by blood transfusion. To date there have been at least ten cases of TTA; all cases involved immunocompromised recipients >34 years of age, and all but one case was reported in the last 10 years [15, 28–34]. With the exception of one case reported from Slovenia, all cases of TTA occurred in the United States: Minnesota ($n = 3$),

Wisconsin ($n = 2$), Rhode Island ($n = 2$), Connecticut ($n = 1$), and Massachusetts ($n = 1$). Among infected recipients, six were female and four were male. Implicated blood components primarily were red blood cell units, both leukoreduced and non-leukoreduced, but two cases were reported from platelets [31, 34], one that implicated a 5-day-old leukoreduced apheresis platelet unit and the other from a whole blood-derived leukoreduced platelet pool. When specifically mentioned in the case reports, implicated red cell units ranged in age from 8 to 30 days. Patients were generally treated with doxycycline or rifampin and subsequently recovered with the exception of one patient who died of underlying trauma unrelated to anaplasmosis [31]. Of note, one TTA case involved a pregnant patient with thalassemia trait who delivered a healthy full-term girl [33]. The baby was tested for *A. phagocytophilum* by PCR and found negative.

Strategies for Mitigating Risk

Current options for mitigating risk associated with *A. phagocytophilum* are limited. As for other tick-borne diseases, recognition of infection is rarely linked with an associated tick bite. Attempts to query donors about recognition and exposure to ticks have proven to be largely ineffective [26]. While research and diagnostic assays (e.g., IFA, NAT) for HGA are currently available, there are no licensed blood screening assays for *A. phagocytophilum*. In part the absence of blood screening assays may reflect an industry view that current levels of risk associated with HGA do not suggest a need for blood screening. It has been suggested that based on their intracellular niche (i.e., intragranulocytic), cells infected with *A. phagocytophilum* may be removed by leukoreduction. However, studies examining the impact of leukoreduction filters indicate that they remove some, but not all infected cells [35]. Thus, leukoreduction likely reduces transmission risk, but does not prevent transfusion transmission. Indeed, as indicated above, several cases of TTA have implicated leukoreduced red cell products, and one case implicated a leukoreduced apheresis platelet unit. Lastly, based on studies with *Orientia tsutsugamushi* [36, 37], a related rickettsial agent that causes scrub typhus, pathogen inactivation (PI) may provide a viable option for preventing TTA, but at present PI is only licensed in the United States for use with selected plasma and platelets products, not red cell products which pose a far greater risk.

Borrelia miyamotoi

A relatively recent addition to the guild of agents residing in and transmitted by the deer or black-legged tick (*I. scapularis*) is the spirochete *Borrelia miyamotoi*, which along with several other agents causes relapsing fever. The first human infection attributed to *B. miyamotoi* was described in Russia in 2011 [38]; thereafter human cases have been described in the United States, Japan, and Europe. To date, no cases of transfusion-transmitted *B. miyamotoi* have been reported, but at least two studies using animal models suggest that transmission by blood transfusion is feasible.

Biology and Epidemiology

B. miyamotoi is a bacterium (i.e., spirochete) that causes relapsing fever and is remotely related to the *Borrelia* associated with Lyme disease. In 1994, *B. miyamotoi* was first identified in Japan from an *Ixodis persulcatus* tick, the local vector for Lyme disease [39]. In the United States, *B. miyamotoi* was initially described in *I. scapularis* ticks from Connecticut in 2001 [40]. Subsequently the agent has been detected throughout the range of *I. scapularis* in the Northeastern and upper Midwestern United States and in association with *I. pacificus* ticks on the West Coast of the United States [41]. The earliest US cases of human infection with *B. miyamotoi* were reported in 2013 [42, 43], and the first large case series was described in 2015 [44]. Transmission likely occurs primarily via infected nymphal and adult ticks; however, larval ticks theoretically may also transmit infection due to transovarial transmission from infected female ticks [40]. Studies in mice indicate that single infected *I. scapularis* nymphs are capable of transmitting infection within the first 24 h of feeding, and transmission probability increases with duration of nymphal attachment [45].

Clinical Features/Diagnosis/Treatment

Infections with *B. miyamotoi* are characterized by fever, chills, and headache (severe in most patients), often accompanied by body and joint pain with fatigue. Unlike Lyme disease, rash is rarely observed (only 8% of patients) and, when present, reportedly does not appear as an erythema migran [44, 46]. Reoccurring fever is reported in approximately 4–10% of clinical cases. More severe complications can include meningoencephalitis, leukopenia, thrombocytopenia, and elevated liver enzymes. In one large case study ($n = 97$), the mean age of infection was 55 years old (range 12–88), and 57% were males [44].

Detection of infection relies upon blood smears or laboratory-based assays for detection of antibodies by ELISA or Western blot and by PCR detection of bacterial DNA. Spirochetes can be detected by immunofluorescence using Wright- or Giemsa-stained smears of blood or CSF specimens [42, 46]. Antibody-based assays often rely upon detection of glycerophosphodiester phosphodiesterase (GlpQ) antigen, which is not detected in Lyme borreliosis patients [47]. GlpQ reportedly is insensitive for detection of acute disease but is useful for detection of resolved or convalescent infections. Similarly, most PCR assays have used primers that target the GlpQ gene [48], but others have targeted the flagellin gene [40, 42]. Treatment regimens generally include doxycycline, but amoxicillin and ceftriaxone are also reportedly effective. Doxycycline is the preferred initial therapy, since it is also effective for treatment of Lyme disease and HGA, which may present as coinfections [42–44, 46].

Seroprevalence and Incidence

Given that the first *B. miyamotoi* infections in the United States were just reported in 2013, seroprevalence and incidence reports are extremely limited. Two studies published by Krause and colleagues used an ELISA with confirmatory Western blot to detect anti-GlpQ antibodies in selected populations from *B. miyamotoi* endemic and non-endemic regions [43, 49]. In healthy populations found in the endemic regions (Block Island and Prudence Island, Rhode Island; Brimfield, Massachusetts), seroprevalence ranged from 1% (6/584) to 3.9% (25/639), while in non-endemic regions (Tempe, Arizona; Miami, Florida), none (0/300) were confirmed positive. In 299 patients evaluated for Lyme, 9 (3.2%) were confirmed positive for *B. miyamotoi* [43], while among 194 patients with acute Lyme borreliosis, 19 (9.8%) were positive for *B. miyamotoi* [49]. These results suggest increased risk due to likely vector exposure and a propensity for coinfections. Corroborating data were provided by a seroprevalence study from the Netherlands [50], where *I. ricinus* ticks are frequently infected with *B. miyamotoi* [51]. Using a GlpQ-Luminex assay, Jahfari et al. identified antibodies to *B. miyamotoi* in 3/150 (2%) blood donors, 12/120 (10%) forest workers, and 4/54 (7.4%) confirmed Lyme neuroborreliosis patients. Again, rates were higher in those populations with greater exposure to ticks (i.e., forest workers, Lyme patients), and coinfections were not uncommon.

Transfusion Transmission/Survival in Blood

As mentioned previously, no cases of transfusion-transmitted *B. miyamotoi* have been reported to date. However, cases have been reported for similar relapsing fever agents, *B. recurrentis* and *B. duttoni* [52, 53]. Unlike clinical cases of Lyme disease, infections with relapsing fever agents demonstrate prolonged and recurrent spirochetemia, thereby increasing the risk of transfusion transmission. Taken together, these observations suggest that *B. miyamotoi* may pose a blood transfusion risk. Using murine models, Krause and colleagues investigated the transmission of *B. miyamotoi* via fresh or stored red blood cells [54]. Mice were transfused with *B. miyamotoi*-infected murine blood that had been freshly collected or stored for 7 days. Immunocompromised recipient mice (i.e., SCID) demonstrated motile spirochetes for up to 28 days posttransfusion with fresh or stored infected red cells. In immunocompetent mice (i.e., DBA/2, C57BL/6), spirochetemia was transient, with clearance observed by 5 days posttransfusion. Consequently, it appears that immunocompromised mice may be at greater risk for infection, particularly after blood transfusion.

Corroborating evidence was provided by a related study examining the distribution and survival of *B. miyamotoi* in human blood components stored under standard blood bank conditions [55]. Freshly collected whole blood (tubes and whole blood units) was inoculated with culture-derived *B. miyamotoi* or *B. miyamotoi*-infected plasma and separated into representative components: red blood cells, plasma, and platelets. In vivo, immunocompromised mice (i.e., CB17 SCID) injected with representative samples obtained from all components before storage and from red blood cells stored for up to 42 days developed infection. Wild-type mice (*Peromyscus leucopus*) were similarly infected but at lower rates. Neither mouse strain became infected when inoculated with plasma that had been frozen for 30 days at −20 °C. In vitro experiments demonstrated survival of *B. miyamotoi* for 42 days in leukoreduced and non-leukoreduced red cells, for 5 days in platelet units, but spirochetes failed to remain viable in plasma frozen at −20 °C for 30 days. Based on these two studies, *B. miyamotoi* appears to survive standard blood bank storage conditions, with the exception of freezing, and may pose a transmission risk for transfusion of human blood components.

Strategies for Mitigating Risk

As already discussed for *A. phagocytophilum*, mitigation strategies for tick-borne infections are limited. Questions regarding tick exposure are ineffective and would be particularly problematic for *B. miyamotoi* since larval ticks theoretically may transmit infection. Blood screening assays are not available and given the absence of blood transfusion cases are not likely needed at this time. However, since transfusion cases have been associated with other relapsing fever agents and based on the studies describing transmission of *B. miyamotoi* in mouse blood transfusion models, along with the survival of the agent in stored blood products, the potential for transfusion transmission needs to be monitored going forward. Pathogen inactivation remains a potential option, but specific studies describing inactivation of *B. miyamotoi* have not been published, and the absence of licensed technology to inactivate red cell products currently precludes this option.

Powassan Virus

Powassan virus (POWV) is a tick-borne flavivirus found primarily in the United States and Canada, which like other members of this tick-associated guild are transmitted by *I. scapularis*. As a tick-borne flavivirus, POWV is somewhat unique since most flaviviruses are transmitted to humans by mosquito vectors. POWV was first identified as a human pathogen in 1958 following its isolation from the brain of a 5-year-old boy living in Powassan, Ontario, who died of acute encephalitis [56]. Since its initial discovery, the incidence of human infection with POWV appears to be steadily rising in Canada and the United States [57]. Between the 10-year period from 2007 to 2016, over 75 cases of Powassan encephalitis were reported in the United States [58], but during 2017 alone, 30 cases have been tentatively reported through the end of the year [59]. Disease manifestations range from a febrile illness to neurologic disease, with severe complications and death in 10% of patients [58].

Biology and Epidemiology

POWV can be broadly classified into two genotypes based on phylogenetics that are related to geographic distribution, tick vectors and reservoir hosts [60]. POWV or lineage I has been identified in Russia, Canada, and the United States. In North America, POWV has been reported primarily in the North Central (i.e., Michigan, Wisconsin, and Minnesota) and Northeastern United States (i.e., Connecticut and Massachusetts) and along the east coast. Similarly, this genotype has also been reported from the Canadian provinces of Ontario, Alberta, British Columbia, and Quebec. Throughout these areas the virus is maintained predominately by *I. cookei* and the groundhog (*Marmota monax*) or the striped skunk (*Mephitis mephitis*) [61–63]. Lineage II is commonly referred to as the deer tick virus (DTV), which was isolated from its primary vector *I. scapularis* in 1997 and is maintained in white-footed mouse (*Peromyscus leucopus*) reservoir hosts [64, 65]. DTV primarily occurs in New England but has been reported from Nova Scotia to Virginia. POWV and DTV are reported to be serologically indistinguishable, but phylogenetic distinctions are demonstrable. Nucleotide sequencing indicated a high level of genetic similarity for POWV and DTV: 84% by nucleotide sequence identity and 94% amino acid identity [66]. For the remainder of this discussion, POWV will be used to represent both lineages.

As already stated, POWV is transmitted to humans via tick vectors, primarily by *I. scapularis* and *I. cookei*. Unlike other tick-borne infections (e.g., *B. microti, A. phagocytophilum*, etc.) that require the vector to feed for 24–48 h to successfully transmit infections, POWV is transmitted within hours of tick attachment, reportedly as rapidly as 15 min [67]. Indeed, in a 2016 case from Eastern Connecticut in which a 5-month-old infant contracted infection, the estimated time for tick attachment was less than 3 hours [68]. Such rapid viral transmission complicates efforts to prevent infection that are based on physical examination and rapid removal of ticks (i.e., tick checks) after potential exposure outdoors. Coupled with the relatively small size for nymphal stages of *Ixodes* ticks, the likelihood of transmission is increased.

Clinical Features/Diagnosis/Treatment

POWV can cause severe encephalitis in humans. Following infection, the incubation period is 1–5 weeks, but as for many tick-borne infections, most patients do not recall a tick bite associated with the onset of infection and subsequent symptoms [60]. Most infections are characterized initially by fever, sore throat, drowsiness, headache, and disorientation [69]. Disease progression leading to encephalitis often demonstrates fever, vomiting, respiratory distress, loss of coordination, speech difficulties, paralysis, and seizures. Long-lasting neurologic sequelae occur in 50% of survivors including memory problems, hemiplegia, muscle wasting, and severe headaches. Approximately 10% of encephalitis cases are fatal [60]. Diagnosis of neuroinvasive POWV is dependent upon clinical disease criteria and one or more laboratory criteria [70]. Clinical criteria indicative of POWV disease are a fever of ≥ 38 °C, any signs or symptoms of peripheral or central nervous system dysfunction documented by a physician, and the absence of a more likely clinical explanation. Diagnostic laboratory criteria include POWV isolation; detection of viral nucleic acid/antigen in blood, cerebrospinal fluid, tissue, or other body fluids; $\geq$ fourfold change in POWV-specific quantitative antibody titers in paired serum; POWV-specific IgM antibodies in CSF for arboviruses endemic to the region where exposure occurred; or POWV-specific IgM antibodies in serum with confirmatory POWV-specific neutralizing antibodies in the same or a later specimen [70]. Currently there are no vaccines to prevent POWV infection, nor are there specific drug treatments available. High-dose corticosteroids have been used to treat neuroinvasive disease, but their true efficacy is not known. A few reports indicate that POWV encephalitis has been treated with intravenous immunoglobulin.

Seroprevalence and Incidence

Formal seroprevalence studies for POWV have not been performed to date. However, clinical case reports provide a partial understanding of the virus's distribution and recent increase in reported cases. Over the past 10 years, approximately 75 cases of POWV disease have been reported [58]. Cases were clustered in the Northeast and Midwest, with the highest number of cases reported from Minnesota ($n = 20$), New York ($n = 16$), and Wisconsin ($n = 16$) during the period from 2006 to 2015. Case reports appear to be increasing, particularly with six or more cases reported each year beginning with 2009. Concomitant with the rise of POWV cases in humans, the seroprevalence of POWV in the deer population, particularly in the Northeast, has trended dramatically higher [71]. Thus, these observations suggest emerging and expanding areas for exposure risk to POWV leading to clinical cases in humans.

Transfusion Transmission/Survival in Blood

Despite the apparent increase in human infections, no cases of transfusion-transmitted POWV have been reported to date. Formal investigations of POWV in peripheral blood of patients and survival in blood components are lacking. However, transmission by blood transfusion has been documented for other flaviviruses (e.g., dengue virus, Zika virus, Japanese encephalitis virus) [72–74], as well as for other agents from the *I. scapularis* guild (i.e., *B. microti*, *A. phagocytophilum*) [4, 34]. Since POWV continues to demonstrate an expanding area of risk and a concomitant rise in reported cases, ongoing surveillance for potential transmission cases is prudent going forward.

Strategies for Mitigating Risk

Similar to *A. phagocytophilum* and *B. miyamotoi*, mitigation options for POWV are limited at this time. The current absence of transmission risk does not suggest the need for blood screening (i.e., NAT), and efficacy has not been demonstrated by PI, although based on experience with analogous flaviviruses (e.g., Zika, dengue), PI would likely be effective [75, 76]. While risk factor questions for tick exposure have been shown to be ineffective for other tick-borne agents [26], they would be particularly problematic for POWV given the relatively short period (i.e., 15 min) required for transmission of the agent following tick attachment [67].

Closing Thoughts

Tick-borne agents have been described as posing a cornucopia of threats to transfusion medicine [77]. The current chapter opted to focus on three agents associated with the *I. scapularis* guild that pose emerging threats to blood safety. Among these three agents, *A. phagocytophilum* raises particular concern and deserves ongoing attention due to demonstrable transfusion transmission that appears to be increasing in frequency. However, there are also other tick-borne agents that have been transmitted by blood transfusion including *B. microti*, Colorado tick fever virus, *Ehrlichia ewingii*, and *Rickettsia rickettsii* [78–80], while *Ehrlichia chaffeensis* has been implicated in transmission via renal transplant [81]. Thus, there are a wide variety of "tortoises" or tick-borne agents that pose potential blood safety threats. Similar to Aesop's tortoise, tick-borne agents steadily plod forward, relentlessly moving into new geographic regions where they remain deep-rooted, causing public health issues for the foreseeable future that must not be ignored.

Disclaimer This work reflects the views of the author and should not be construed to represent FDA's views or policies.

References

1. Lederberg JSR, Oakes SC Jr, editors. Institute of Medicine (U.S.). Committee on Emerging Microbial Threats to Health. Emerging infections: microbial threats to health in the United States. Institute of Medicine. Washington DC: National Academy Press; 1992.
2. Burgdorfer W, Barbour AG, Hayes SF, et al. Lyme disease-a tick-borne spirochetosis? Science. 1982;216:1317–9.
3. Johnson ST, Cable RG, Leiby DA. Lookback investigations of *Babesia microti*-seropositive blood donors: seven-year experience in a *Babesia*-endemic area. Transfusion. 2012;52:1509–16.
4. Herwaldt BL, Linden JV, Bosserman E, et al. Transfusion-associated babesiosis in the United States: a description of cases. Ann Intern Med. 2011;155:509–19.
5. Leiby DA. Transfusion-transmitted *Babesia* spp. bull's-eye on *Babesia microti*. Clin Microbiol Rev. 2011;24:14–28.
6. Moritz ED, Winton CS, Tonnetti L, et al. Screening for *Babesia microti* in the U.S. Blood Supply. N Engl J Med. 2016;375:2236–45.
7. Vannier E, Krause PJ. Human babesiosis. N Engl J Med. 2012;366:2397–407.
8. Dumler JS, Barbet AF, Bekker CP, et al. Reorganization of genera in the families *Rickettsiaceae* and *Anaplasmataceae* in the order *Rickettsiales*: unification of some species of *Ehrlichia* with *Anaplasma*, *Cowdria* with *Ehrlichia* and *Ehrlichia* with *Neorickettsia*, descriptions of six new species combinations and designation of *Ehrlichia equi* and 'HGE agent' as subjective synonyms of *Ehrlichia phagocytophila*. Int J Syst Evol Microbiol. 2001;51:2145–65.
9. Chen SM, Dumler JS, Bakken JS, et al. Identification of a granulocytotropic *Ehrlichia* species as the etiologic agent of human disease. J Clin Microbiol. 1994;32:589–95.
10. Bakken JS, Dumler JS, Chen SM, et al. Human granulocytic ehrlichiosis in the upper Midwest United States. A new species emerging? JAMA. 1994;272:212–8.
11. Aguero-Rosenfeld ME, Donnarumma L, Zentmaier L, et al. Seroprevalence of antibodies that react with *Anaplasma phagocytophila*, the agent of human granulocytic ehrlichiosis, in different populations in Westchester County, New York. J Clin Microbiol. 2002;40:2612–5.
12. Dumler JS, Choi KS, Garcia-Garcia JC, et al. Human granulocytic anaplasmosis and *Anaplasma phagocytophilum*. Emerg Infect Dis. 2005;11:1828–34.
13. Centers for Disease Control and Prevention. Anaplasmosis. 2013. Available at: http://www.cdc.gov/anaplasmosis/index.html. Accessed 29 Dec 2017.
14. Centers for Disease Control and Prevention. Notice to Readers: Final 2013 Reports of Nationally Notifiable Infectious Diseases. MMWR Morb Mortal Wkly Rep. 2014;63:702–15.
15. Eastlund T, Persing D, Mathiesen D, et al. Human granulocytic ehrlichiosis after red cell transfusion [abstract]. Transfusion. 1999;39 Suppl:117S.
16. Eisen RJ, Kugeler KJ, Eisen L, et al. Tick-Borne Zoonoses in the United States: persistent and emerging threats to human health. ILAR J. 2017;58(3):319–35.
17. Walls JJ, Greig B, Neitzel DF, et al. Natural infection of small mammal species in Minnesota with the agent of human granulocytic ehrlichiosis. J Clin Microbiol. 1997;35:853–5.
18. Keesing F, McHenry DJ, Hersh M, et al. Prevalence of human-active and variant 1 strains of the tick-borne pathogen *Anaplasma phagocytophilum* in hosts and forests of eastern North America. Am J Tro Med Hyg. 2014;91:302–9.
19. Ostfeld RS, Brunner JL. Climate change and *Ixodes* tick-borne diseases of humans. Philos Trans R Soc Lond Ser B Biol Sci. 2015;370:20140051.
20. Spielman A. The emergence of Lyme disease and human babesiosis in a changing environment. Ann N Y Acad Sci. 1994;740:146–56.

21. Goodman JL. Human granulocytic anaplasmosis. In: Goodmam JL, Dennis DT, Sonenshine DE, editors. Tick-borne diseases of humans. Washington, DC: ASM Press; 2005. p. 218–38.
22. Dumler JS, Madigan JE, Pusterla N, et al. Ehrlichioses in humans: epidemiology, clinical presentation, diagnosis, and treatment. Clin Infect Dis. 2007;45(Suppl 1):S45–51.
23. Bakken JS, Dumler JS. Clinical diagnosis and treatment of human granulocytotropic anaplasmosis. Ann N Y Acad Sci. 2006;1078:236–47.
24. Schotthoefer AM, Meece JK, Ivacic LC, et al. Comparison of a real-time PCR method with serology and blood smear analysis for diagnosis of human anaplasmosis: importance of infection time course for optimal test utilization. J Clin Microbiol. 2013;51:2147–53.
25. JW IJ, Meek JI, Cartter ML, et al. The emergence of another tickborne infection in the 12-town area around Lyme, Connecticut: human granulocytic ehrlichiosis. J Infect Dis. 2000;181:1388–93.
26. Leiby DA, Chung AP, Cable RG, et al. Relationship between tick bites and the seroprevalence of *Babesia microti* and *Anaplasma phagocytophila* (previously *Ehrlichia sp.*) in blood donors. Transfusion. 2002;42:1585–91.
27. Bakken JS, Goellner P, Van Etten M, et al. Seroprevalence of human granulocytic ehrlichiosis among permanent residents of northwestern Wisconsin. Clin Infect Dis. 1998;27:1491–6.
28. Annen K, Friedman K, Eshoa C, et al. Two cases of transfusion-transmitted *Anaplasma phagocytophilum*. Am J Clin Pathol. 2012;137:562–5.
29. Jereb M, Pecaver B, Tomazic J, et al. Severe human granulocytic anaplasmosis transmitted by blood transfusion. Emerg Infect Dis. 2012;18:1354–7.
30. Alhumaidan H, Westley B, Esteva C, et al. Transfusion-transmitted anaplasmosis from leukoreduced red blood cells. Transfusion. 2013;53:181–6.
31. Townsend RL, Moritz ED, Fialkow LB, et al. Probable transfusion-transmission of *Anaplasma phagocytophilum* by leukoreduced platelets. Transfusion. 2014;54:2828–32.
32. Centers for Disease Control and Prevention. *Anaplasma phagocytophilum* transmitted through blood transfusion - Minnesota, 2007. MMWR Morb Mortal Wkly Rep. 2008;57:1145–8.
33. Shields K, Cumming M, Rios J, et al. Transfusion-associated *Anaplasma phagocytophilum* infection in a pregnant patient with thalassemia trait: a case report. Transfusion. 2015;55:719–25.
34. Fine AB, Sweeney JD, Nixon CP, et al. Transfusion-transmitted anaplasmosis from a leukoreduced platelet pool. Transfusion. 2016;56(3):699–704.
35. Proctor MC, Leiby DA. Do leukoreduction filters passively reduce the transmission risk of human granulocytic anaplasmosis? Transfusion. 2015;55:1242–8.
36. Rentas F, Harman R, Gomez C, et al. Inactivation of *Orientia tsutsugamushi* in red blood cells, plasma, and platelets with riboflavin and light, as demonstrated in an animal model. Transfusion. 2007;47:240–7.
37. Belanger KJ, Kelly DJ, Mettille FC, et al. Psoralen photochemical inactivation of *Orientia tsutsugamushi* in platelet concentrates. Transfusion. 2000;40:1503–7.
38. Platonov AE, Karan LS, Kolyasnikova NM, et al. Humans infected with relapsing fever spirochete *Borrelia miyamotoi*, Russia. Emerg Infect Dis. 2011;17:1816–23.
39. Fukunaga M, Takahashi Y, Tsuruta Y, et al. Genetic and phenotypic analysis of *Borrelia miyamotoi* sp. nov., isolated from the ixodid tick *Ixodes persulcatus*, the vector for Lyme disease in Japan. Int J Syst Bacteriol. 1995;45:804–10.
40. Scoles GA, Papero M, Beati L, et al. A relapsing fever group spirochete transmitted by *Ixodes scapularis* ticks. Vector Borne Zoonotic Dis. 2001;1:21–34.
41. Mun J, Eisen RJ, Eisen L, et al. Detection of a Borrelia miyamotoi sensu lato relapsing-fever group spirochete from *Ixodes pacificus* in California. J Med Entomol. 2006;43:120–3.
42. Gugliotta JL, Goethert HK, Berardi VP, et al. Meningoencephalitis from *Borrelia miyamotoi* in an immunocompromised patient. N Engl J Med. 2013;368:240–5.
43. Krause PJ, Narasimhan S, Wormser GP, et al. Human *Borrelia miyamotoi* infection in the United States. N Engl J Med. 2013;368:291–3.
44. Molloy PJ, Telford SR 3rd, Chowdri HR, et al. *Borrelia miyamotoi* disease in the Northeastern United States: a case series. Ann Intern Med. 2015;163:91–8.

45. Breuner NE, Dolan MC, Replogle AJ, et al. Transmission of *Borrelia miyamotoi* sensu lato relapsing fever group spirochetes in relation to duration of attachment by *Ixodes scapularis* nymphs. Ticks Tick Borne Dis. 2017;8:677–81.
46. Krause PJ, Barbour AG. *Borrelia miyamotoi*: The Newest Infection Brought to Us by Deer Ticks. Ann Intern Med. 2015;163:141–2.
47. Schwan TG, Schrumpf ME, Hinnebusch BJ, et al. GlpQ: an antigen for serological discrimination between relapsing fever and Lyme borreliosis. J Clin Microbiol. 1996;34:2483–92.
48. Ullmann AJ, Gabitzsch ES, Schulze TL, et al. Three multiplex assays for detection of *Borrelia burgdorferi* sensu lato and *Borrelia miyamotoi* sensu lato in field-collected *Ixodes* nymphs in North America. J Med Entomol. 2005;42:1057–62.
49. Krause PJ, Narasimhan S, Wormser GP, et al. *Borrelia miyamotoi* sensu lato seroreactivity and seroprevalence in the northeastern United States. Emerg Infect Dis. 2014;20:1183–90.
50. Jahfari S, Herremans T, Platonov AE, et al. High seroprevalence of *Borrelia miyamotoi* antibodies in forestry workers and individuals suspected of human granulocytic anaplasmosis in the Netherlands. New Microbes New Infect. 2014;2:144–9.
51. Fonville M, Friesema IH, Hengeveld PD, et al. Human exposure to tickborne relapsing fever spirochete *Borrelia miyamotoi*, the Netherlands. Emerg Infect Dis. 2014;20:1244–5.
52. Hira PR, Husein SF. Some transfusion-induced parasitic infections in Zambia. J Hyg Epidemiol Microbiol Immunol. 1979;23:436–44.
53. Nadelman RB, Wormser GP, Sherer C. Blood transfusion-associated relapsing fever. Transfusion. 1990;30:380–1.
54. Krause PJ, Hendrickson JE, Steeves TK, et al. Blood transfusion transmission of the tick-borne relapsing fever spirochete *Borrelia miyamotoi* in mice. Transfusion. 2015;55:593–7.
55. Thorp AM, Tonnetti L. Distribution and survival of *Borrelia miyamotoi* in human blood components. Transfusion. 2016;56:705–11.
56. Mc LD, Donohue WL. Powassan virus: isolation of virus from a fatal case of encephalitis. Can Med Assoc J. 1959;80:708–11.
57. Hermance ME, Thangamani S. Powassan virus: an emerging Arbovirus of public health concern in North America. Vector Borne Zoonotic Dis. 2017;17:453–62.
58. Centers for Disease Control and Prevention. Powassan Virus. Available at: https://www.cdc.gov/powassan/. Acceessed 14 Dec 2017.
59. Centers for Disease Control and Prevention. MMWR Morb Mortal Wkly Rep. 2018;66(52):ND–1025. https://www.cdc.gov/mmwr/volumes/66/wr/pdfs/mm6652md-H.pdf. Accessed: January 24, 2018
60. Ebel GD. Update on Powassan virus: emergence of a North American tick-borne flavivirus. Annu Rev Entomol. 2010;55:95–110.
61. McLean DM, Best JM, Mahalingam S, et al. Powassan virus: summer infection cycle, 1964. Can Med Assoc J. 1964;91:1360–2.
62. Johnson HN. Isolation of Powassan virus from a spotted skunk in California. J Wildl Dis. 1987;23:152–3.
63. Main AJ, Carey AB, Downs WG. Powassan virus in *Ixodes cookei* and Mustelidae in New England. J Wildl Dis. 1979;15:585–91.
64. Telford SR 3rd, Armstrong PM, Katavolos P, et al. A new tick-borne encephalitis-like virus infecting New England deer ticks, *Ixodes dammini*. Emerg Infect Dis. 1997;3:165–70.
65. Ebel GD, Campbell EN, Goethert HK, et al. Enzootic transmission of deer tick virus in New England and Wisconsin sites. Am J Trop Med Hyg. 2000;63:36–42.
66. Kuno G, Artsob H, Karabatsos N, et al. Genomic sequencing of deer tick virus and phylogeny of powassan-related viruses of North America. Am J Trop Med Hyg. 2001;65:671–6.
67. Ebel GD, Kramer LD. Short report: duration of tick attachment required for transmission of powassan virus by deer ticks. Am J Trop Med Hyg. 2004;71:268–71.
68. Tutolo JW, Staples JE, Sosa L, et al. Notes from the field: Powassan virus disease in an infant - Connecticut, 2016. MMWR Morb Mortal Wkly Rep. 2017;66:408–9.
69. Smith R, Woodall JP, Whitney E, et al. Powassan virus infection. A report of three human cases of encephalitis. Am J Dis Child. 1974;127:691–3.

70. Centers for Disease Control and Prevention. Arboviral diseases, neuroinvasive and non-neuroinvasive 2015 case definition. Available at: https://wwwn.cdc.gov/nndss/conditions/arboviral-diseases-neuroinvasive-and-non-neuroinvasive/case-definition/2015/. Accessed 29 Dec 2017.
71. Nofchissey RA, Deardorff ER, Blevins TM, et al. Seroprevalence of Powassan virus in New England deer, 1979–2010. Am J Trop Med Hyg. 2013;88:1159–62.
72. Sabino EC, Loureiro P, Lopes ME, et al. Transfusion-transmitted dengue and associated clinical symptoms during the 2012 epidemic in Brazil. J Infect Dis. 2016;213:694–702.
73. Barjas-Castro ML, Angerami RN, Cunha MS, et al. Probable transfusion-transmitted Zika virus in Brazil. Transfusion. 2016;56:1684–8.
74. Cheng VCC, Sridhar S, Wong SC, et al. Japanese encephalitis virus transmitted via blood transfusion, Hong Kong, China. Emerg Infect Dis. 2018;24:49.
75. Santa Maria F, Laughhunn A, Lanteri MC, et al. Inactivation of Zika virus in platelet components using amotosalen and ultraviolet A illumination. Transfusion. 2017;57:2016–25.
76. Musso D, Richard V, Broult J, et al. Inactivation of dengue virus in plasma with amotosalen and ultraviolet A illumination. Transfusion. 2014;54:2924–30.
77. Leiby DA, Gill JE. Transfusion-transmitted tick-borne infections: a cornucopia of threats. Transfus Med Rev. 2004;18:293–306.
78. Wells GM, Woodward TE, Fiset P, et al. Rocky mountain spotted fever caused by blood transfusion. JAMA. 1978;239:2763–5.
79. Regan J, Matthias J, Green-Murphy A, et al. A confirmed *Ehrlichia ewingii* infection likely acquired through platelet transfusionClin Infect Dis. 2013;56:e105–7.
80. Randall WH, Simmons J, Casper EA, Philip RN. Transmission of Colorado tick fever virus by blood transfusion. MMWR Morb Mortal Wkly Rep. 1975;24:422–7.
81. Sadikot R, Shaver MJ, Reeves WB. *Ehrlichia chaffeensis* in a renal transplant recipient. Am J Nephrol. 1999;19:674–6.

Part IV
International Collaboration

Chapter 12
International Collaboration for Improving Global Blood Safety and for Monitoring and Responding to Potential Microbial Threats

Jose Ramiro Cruz, Rene Berrios Cruz, Jorge Duque Rodríguez, and Silvina Kuperman

Introduction

The recognition in the 1970s and 1980s that highly pathogenic infectious agents could be transmitted by blood transfusions [1–4] led to the notion that the blood components used to treat patients needed to be pathogen-free. Measures to prevent contaminated blood components from being transfused include the deferral of potentially infected donors and the implementation of laboratory tests to screen blood donations for the presence of antibodies, microbial antigens, and microbial nucleic acids [5–12]. For the prevention of currently recognized transfusion-transmissible infections (TTI), the World Health Organization (WHO) recommends that all blood donations in every country of the world be screened for human immunodeficiency (HIV), hepatitis B (HBV) and hepatitis C (HCV) viruses, and *Treponema pallidum* [13]. Although the WHO recommends that testing for *Trypanosoma cruzi* (*T. cruzi*), malaria, and human T-lymphotropic viruses (HTLV) be carried out in all units of blood collected only in endemic countries, non-endemic

---

In Memoriam
Gabriel Adrian Schmunis
July 26, 1939–April 9, 2017

J. R. Cruz (✉)
International Affairs Committee, Grupo Cooperativo Iberoamericano de Medicina Transfusional, Ashburn, VA, USA
e-mail: jcruz62004@aol.com

R. Berrios Cruz
Ministry of Health, National Blood Service, Managua, Nicaragua

J. Duque Rodríguez
Facultad de Medicina, Area de Investigacion, Universidad Autonoma de Chihuahua, Chihuahua, Mexico

S. Kuperman
Centro Regional de Hemoterapia, Hospital de Pediatria Garrahan, Buenos Aires, Argentina

© Springer International Publishing AG, part of Springer Nature 2019
H. Shan, R. Y. Dodd (eds.), *Blood Safety*,
https://doi.org/10.1007/978-3-319-94436-4_12

countries have implemented ad hoc laboratory measures to prevent transmission of *T. cruzi* associated with blood donors who emigrated from endemic areas [14–16]. All nations should test for the presence of cytomegalovirus only when blood components are intended for especially susceptible groups of patients [13]. Other prion, viral, bacterial, and parasitic agents also have the potential to emerge as threats to blood safety [17–19]. The probability of these, and other emerging pathogens, to enter the blood supply depends on their prevalence in the general population, their mode of natural transmission, the duration of their asymptomatic infections, their persistence in the human bloodstream, their capacity to withstand the environmental conditions of processing and storing blood components, and the availability of laboratory tests to detect their presence in donated blood [20–22].

The application of donor deferral and laboratory testing strategies has significantly reduced but not eliminated TTI, giving rise to metrics intended to estimate the risk of TTI in different settings and conditions [23–25]. The concept of blood safety emerged from aiming at the preparation and transfusion of blood components with minimal risk of transmitting infectious agents [26]. Because transfusions were shown not to be risk-free, patient surveillance systems were put in place to monitor TTI and to identify—as well as to implement—additional interventions to prevent them [27, 28]. Hemovigilance gradually evolved into more comprehensive processes to reduce untoward and unintended effects of blood transfusion and blood donation [29]. The efforts to reduce adverse reactions among blood donors and transfused patients, to protect blood safety, and to guarantee timely access to and appropriate use of sufficient blood components represent the current concept of blood transfusion safety [30].

This chapter intends to provide insight on how international cooperation may promote global blood safety, within the context of transfusion safety, by using case studies in Ibero-American countries and with a perspective derived from the concept of "global health" proposed by the Institute of Medicine in 2009 [31]: "Global blood safety is the goal of attaining the safest possible blood for all patients in all nations by establishing universal voluntary altruistic blood donation, pertinent and precise laboratory blood testing, and appropriate preparation of blood components. It can be attained by combining surveillance, training, research, oversight, governance, and collaboration among stakeholders."

Ibero-America

Ibero-America comprises 19 Spanish- and Portuguese-speaking countries of North, Central, and South America and the Caribbean [32], with a population of 606 million inhabitants in 2015 [33] (Table 12.1).

The two Ibero-American countries with very high Human Development Index (HDI) have 60 million inhabitants, which represent 10% of the population, while the six nations with medium HDI are home to 55 million people, a 9% share of the total number of inhabitants. The obvious implication is that 91% of Ibero-Americans

Table 12.1 Human Development Index (HDI), population indicators, Human Health Index (HHI), and blood safety indicators of Ibero-American countries, 2015

Country	HDI	Population × 1000		HHI	Blood collection	Donors (%)		TTI markers (%)		
		Total	In poverty			Deferred	Voluntary	HBsAg, HCV, HIV	Anti-HBc	Anti-*T. cruzi*
Countries with very high HDI										
Chile	0.847	17,924	2581	0.922	239,549	22.3	28.5	0.06	NR	0.13
Argentina	0.827	42,155	13,571	0.866	1.025,679	14.2	45.7	1.06	0.93	1.50
Countries with high HDI										
Uruguay	0.795	3430	333	0.880	90,471	23.4	51.4	0.53	0.79	0.19
Panama	0.788	3988	917	0.885	56,294	NR	7.0	0.73	1.74	0.52
Costa Rica	0.776	5002	1085	0.922	75,732	22.5	60.4	0.45	0.90	0.13
Cuba	0.775	11,249	NR	0.912	416,923	4.6	100	1.78	NR	NA
Venezuela	0.767	31,293	6165	0.841	299,879	NR	5.8	0.98	2.56	0.31
Mexico	0.762	125,236	57,859	0.885	2.167,733	28.5	3.8	0.87	NR	0.37
Brazil	0.754	203,657	17,718	0.830	3.089,122	19.3	61.3	0.77	1.30	0.22
Peru	0.740	31,161	7073	0.843	NR	NR	NR	NR	NR	NR
Ecuador	0.739	16,226	4154	0.831	246,769	15.9	68.3	0.85	0.15	0.34
Colombia	0.727	49,529	13,770	0.831	795,688	18.0	91.1	0.70	1.56	0.38
Dominican Republic	0.722	10,652	3249	0.822	78,515	23.0	11.2	1.27	1.18	NA

(continued)

Table 12.1 (continued)

| Country | HDI | Population × 1000 | | HHI | Blood collection | Donors (%) | | TTI markers (%) | | |
		Total	In poverty			Deferred	Voluntary	HBsAg, HCV, HIV	Anti-HBc	Anti-*T. cruzi*
Countries with medium HDI										
Paraguay	0.683	7033	1561	0.804	85,997	7.7	10.2	0.93	2.75	2.37
El Salvador	0.680	6426	2243	0.809	92,819	25.0	17.0	0.35	NR	2.65
Bolivia	0.674	11,025	4256	0.727	108,072	29.4	40.9	0.85	NR	2.51
Nicaragua	0.645	6257	1859	0.844	74,955	9.0	100	0.61	NR	0.34
Guatemala	0.640	16,255	9639	0.802	126,222	25.9	5.4	1.16	3.14	0.93
Honduras	0.625	8424	2493	0.828	71,637	15.7	18.6	0.65	1.62	0.74
Total		606,992	150,526 24.3%[a]		9,142,056 159/10,000[b]					

Data from Refs. [34–37]
[a]Proportion of population living below poverty line, except Cuba
[b]Donation rate, except Peru
NR not reported, *NA* not applicable

reside in areas of very high or high HDI. There are, however, differences in the level of human development within each of the countries, with some provinces showing a significant lower HDI than the national index [38, 39]. One fourth of Ibero-Americans, 150 million, live in poverty [35]. Mexico, Brazil, Colombia, and Argentina account for 103 million (68%) poor Ibero-Americans, a fact that is associated with the size of their national populations. The available data show that the proportion of individuals living below the poverty line is higher in medium HDI countries, 40%, than in those with very high HDI and high HDI, 27% and 24%, respectively (Chi^2 = 8.55, p < 0.0139, goodness of fit test [40]). This situation has potential implications for the ability of large segments of the population to access and utilize health services, as shown by the Human Health Index (HHI). Although there is a direct correlation between national HDI and national HHI in Ibero-America (r_s = 0.7902, p = 0.00028, Spearman rank-order correlation test [41]), Argentina, Venezuela, and Brazil have HHI that are at least four ranks lower than their corresponding HDI, while Costa Rica, Mexico, Ecuador, and Nicaragua show the opposite trend. The disparities in national development, in financial resources, and in the access to basic services are factors that contribute to the individual's health status, to his travel patterns, and to his willingness to emigrate.

Transfusion-Transmissible Infections in Ibero-America

The United Nations AIDS (UNAIDS) Program estimates that there were 1.7 million people living with HIV in Ibero-America by the end of 2015, with 72% of the cases in Brazil, Colombia, Mexico, and Venezuela [42]. The estimated prevalence of HIV in the general population is 0.4%. The highest estimated prevalence rates among those aged 15–49 years old, however, are in Guatemala (1.5%), Peru (1.3%), El Salvador (1.2%), and Ecuador (1.1%). HIV infections are more common in urban settings and along commercial corridors, with transgender women, men who have sex with men, male and female sex workers, and people who inject illegal drugs being at higher risk [42, 43].

According to the Pan American Health Organization (PAHO), created in 1904 as the Pan American Sanitary Bureau to coordinate international activities to control infectious diseases in the Americas and which became the Regional Office of WHO in 1948 [44], the information available in 2015 about hepatitis B and hepatitis C in Ibero-American countries was either incomplete or unstandardized [45]. A more recent PAHO report, however, estimates 0.33% prevalence of HBV infection among the general Ibero-American population, with around two million HBV chronically infected individuals [46]. Other population-based studies showed that, in Ibero-American countries, children 5–9 years old are more likely than adults to be infected with hepatitis B [47]: in Argentina, Chile, Cuba, the Dominican Republic, Ecuador, Peru, Paraguay, and Uruguay, the prevalence of hepatitis B was 2–4% among adults; it was less than 2% in the remaining nations. The epidemiology of HBV is likely to differ within countries, as shown by the findings in Brazil, where the overall prevalence of anti-HBc antibodies was found to be 8%, with regional rates ranging from 1.2% in Fortaleza to 21% in Manaus [48].

PAHO estimates that the prevalence of chronic HCV infection in Ibero-American countries is 0.65% [46]. Estimates of the Global Burden of Disease [49] place all 19 Ibero-American countries in regions where the HCV prevalence rates fall between 1.2% and 1.6% and the proportions of viremic individuals range from 70% to 80.2% [49]. The prevalence rates of HCV infection among the general population are 1.6% for Brazil and Paraguay; 1.5% for Argentina, Chile, Uruguay, and Venezuela; 1.4% for Colombia, Costa Rica, the Dominican Republic, El Salvador, Guatemala, Honduras, Mexico, and Nicaragua; 1.2% for Bolivia, Ecuador, Panama, and Peru; and 0.8% for Cuba. Interestingly, prevalence and viremic rates are directly correlated [49]. In every country the estimated age-specific prevalence rates are highest, reaching 4%, in persons older than 55 years of age [50]. Estimates of infection for high-risk groups, such as illegal drug users, men who have sex with men, sex workers, and prison inmates, may attain 20% [51].

The WHO in 2015 estimated that there were 5.7 million people infected with *T. cruzi* in the 17 continental endemic Ibero-American countries, with Argentina, Brazil, Colombia, and Mexico accounting for 69% of all those individuals who harbor *T. cruzi* [52]. The countries with the highest prevalence rates of infection are Bolivia (6.104%), Argentina (3.640%), Paraguay (2.130%), Ecuador (1.379%), El Salvador (1.297%), Guatemala (1.230%), Venezuela (1.055%), Colombia (0.956%), and Honduras (0.917%). Countries with lower HDI are more likely than countries with higher HDI to be included in this group (Chi^2 = 3.397, p = 0.0065, goodness of fit test, [41]). Intra-country variations have been reported in the prevalence of *T. cruzi* infections either among blood donors or among pregnant women [53, 54]. An inversed relationship exists between the prevalence of infection in pregnant women (range 0.60 to 11.8%) and the HDI of the 23 Argentinian provinces where they live ([39, 53], r_s = − 0.4308, p = 0.0199765, Spearman rank order correlation test [41]).

Malaria, mainly due to *Plasmodium vivax* and *Plasmodium falciparum,* is endemic in 16 of the 19 Ibero-American countries, the exceptions being Chile, Cuba, and Uruguay [55]. The number of yearly cases fell to 426,151 in 2011 in the 16 nations and continued to decrease, reaching 358,473 confirmed cases in 2014 [56], when 20 adjoining municipalities in Brazil, Colombia, Peru, and Venezuela accounted for 48% of all new cases. Foci of high incidence occurred also in Guatemala, Honduras, Mexico, and Nicaragua, while Argentina, Costa Rica, El Salvador, and Paraguay each reported fewer than ten cases during that year [56]. In 2015, however, Colombia, the Dominican Republic, Ecuador, Guatemala, Honduras, Nicaragua, and Peru reported incremented numbers of cases, a trend that continued in Colombia, Ecuador, and Venezuela in 2016 [57]. Furthermore, autochthonous cases were reported in Costa Rica and Cuba in 2016, prompting the PAHO to issue an Epidemiological Alert on 15 February 2017 [57].

Dengue, chikungunya, and Zika viruses have become prevalent in Ibero-American countries [58], where over 2.2 million cases of dengue were detected and reported during 2016 [59]. Although Brazil accounted for 66% of all infections, Paraguay and Nicaragua showed the highest annual incidence rates, while Chile,

Cuba, and Uruguay had the lowest [59]. Eighteen Ibero-American nations, the exception being Uruguay, reported 500,202 cases of chikungunya in 2016 [60]. Bolivia, Brazil, and Honduras had the most infections per inhabitant. Chile and Cuba had no autochthonous cases and Panama had only six [60]. The national surveillance systems identified 11 cases of chikungunya infection that were acquired in other countries and imported into Bolivia, Ecuador, Panama, and Peru. The Ibero-American national surveillance systems, however, did not detect the early local circulation of Zika virus in their territories [61, 62], and it was not until Brazil reported the first cases of fetal microcephaly that public health attention was drawn into it [63]. Since 2015, and up to 28 February 2017, there have been 603,472 cases of Zika infection reported to PAHO [64], with Honduras, Colombia, and Venezuela showing the highest incidence rates. Chile and Uruguay have not had any autochthonous cases. The importation of 565 (0.09%) cases has been reported by 11 countries.

Potential Implications for Global Blood Safety

Ibero-Americans infected with HIV, HBV, HVC, *T. cruzi*, *Plasmodium*, dengue, chikungunya, or Zika viruses can, in turn, be the source of infections to other individuals who live in their own local communities or in other places they may visit or emigrate into. Natural modes of transmission include exposure to contaminated body fluids (via intimal physical contact, through fomites, or congenitally in utero) and vector-borne [42, 65–69]. The period of infectivity may precede, include, and follow the symptomatic phase of the disease, which may happen days, weeks, months, and even years after the initial infection, or not happen at all [65–69]. Asymptomatic, infected individuals who are not aware of the risk factors or behaviors for acquiring one of these infections are not likely either to be tested or to seek medical care for their condition [70, 71]. Additionally, the absence of signs and symptoms of infection allows infected persons to live normal lives, including traveling within their own countries or internationally. Human mobility and social dynamics are recognized as important factors in the spread of communicable diseases [72, 73].

Every year, there are over 60 million international departures from the 19 Ibero-American countries (Table 12.2, [74]). Because of current donor deferral criteria, blood donation in foreign countries is highly improbable during short-time trips [75, 76]. Risk behaviors for HIV, HBV, HCV, and sexual transmission of Zika, however, may occur among adult travelers [77–79]. Adequate application of donor deferral criteria related to illegal drug use and sexual practices should prevent blood donation from locals who might have become infected.

On the other hand, visitors to Ibero-America from other regions of the world may be exposed to microbes that threaten global blood safety. Each year, there are over 80 million international travelers to Ibero-American countries [80], some of whom may acquire infections prevalent locally [81]. A portion of those infections may be

Table 12.2 International travel from and to Ibero-American Countries, 2015, 2016

Country	Outbound travel × 1000		International arrivals × 1000	
	2015	2016	2015	2016
Countries with very high HDI				
Chile	3359	3553	4478	5641
Argentina	7807	10,297	5736	5559
Countries with high HDI				
Uruguay	2217	1715	2396	3037
Panama	740	770	2109	2007
Costa Rica	919	1036	2660	2925
Cuba	580	724	3491	3968
Venezuela	1539	1530	857[a]	601
Mexico	19,603	20,223	32,093	35,079
Brazil	9469	8528	6306	6578
Peru	2595	2751	3456	3744
Ecuador	1398	1551	2542	1418
Colombia	3860	3795	2978	3317
Dominican Republic	478	500	5600	5959.3
Countries with medium HDI				
Paraguay	1008	1503	1215	1308
El Salvador	1618	1804	1402	1434
Bolivia	965	1048	871[a]	959
Nicaragua	925	981	1386	1504
Guatemala	1130	1195	1464	1906
Honduras	692	NR	914	271
Total	60,902	63,504	81,954	87215.3
Annual increase (%)		5.4		6.4

Data from Refs. [74, 80]
[a]Data for 2014
HDI Human Development Index, *NR* Not reported

asymptomatic, allowing returning travelers to offer donating blood in their countries of origin [82]. Again, the application of current donor deferral criteria should prevent blood from being donated during the window periods of those infections which are routinely tested for.

Special attention should be given to persons who travel specifically to seek medical care in Ibero-America. According to *Patients Beyond Borders* [83], 14 million individuals travel each year for health reasons. Three Ibero-American countries, Brazil, Costa Rica, and Mexico, are among the world's 10 top destinations, receiving around 1.5 million patients each calendar year. Cardiovascular, orthopedic, and oncologic conditions, which are very likely to require blood transfusions, are among the most common reasons for receiving dedicated international medical care, usually provided by hospitals that are accredited by international bodies [83]. Accreditation of patient care facilities usually considers the availability of and the access to the safest possible blood. Incidental hospitalizations associated with emergencies, however, may be surrounded by different and possibly substandard conditions that hinder timely access to blood for transfusion, a factor associated with the lack of voluntary blood donors and with administrative procedures that limit donation by nonresident foreigners [84]. Emergency medical care of foreigners should be considered within the realm of local health systems.

A different situation emerges when Ibero-Americans immigrate to other countries. Table 12.3 summarizes data showing that over 21 million nationals from the 19 nations live in the United States, Canada, Spain, and Portugal alone [85–87]. Lower but still significant numbers of Ibero-Americans have immigrated to other European countries, such as Italy, France, Germany, Greece, Sweden, and Norway [88], and within Ibero-America itself [89]. Historical high incidence, long-term asymptomatic infections, lack of awareness about the disease, poor access to diagnosis, and weaknesses of the health systems in the immigrants' countries of origin contributed to the globalization of *T. cruzi* infections and its associated Chagas'

Table 12.3 Number of Ibero-Americans living in Canada, Portugal, Spain, and the United States

Country of origin	Country of foreign residence				
	Canada	Portugal	Spain	United States	Total
Countries with very high HDI					
Chile	38,140	259	20,397	95,104	153,900
Argentina	16,915	618	86,921	181,233	285,687
Countries with high HDI					
Uruguay	5500	116	26,581	43,971	76,168
Panama	3650	a	a	103,625	107,275
Costa Rica	5335	a	a	90,109	95,444
Cuba	21,440	575	39,775	1,210,674	1,272,444
Venezuela	18,165	3368	28,188	255,320	305,041
Mexico	96,055	278	10,700	11,643,298	11,750,331
Brazil	25,395	49,678	30,242	361,374	466,689
Peru	34,385	277	90,906	445,921	571,489
Ecuador	20,115	330	376,233	441,257	837,935
Colombia	76,580	574	225,504	699,399	1,002,057
Dominican Republic	16,715	71	58,126	1,063,239	1,138,151
Countries with medium HDI					
Paraguay	3425	69	8557	34,749	46,800
El Salvador	63,965	a	a	1,352,357	1,416,322
Bolivia	3780	77	52,587	78,093	134,537
Nicaragua	11,445	a	a	256,171	267,616
Guatemala	20,765	a	a	927,595	948,360
Honduras	8720	a	a	599,030	607,750
aCentral America		108	9761		9869
Total	490,490	56,398	1,064,458	19,882,519	21,493,865

Data from Refs. [85–87]
aPanama, Costa Rica, El Salvador, Nicaragua, Guatemala, Honduras listed as "Central America" by Padilla and Peixoto [86]

disease, for example [90–94]. The implications of migration are further exemplified by the occurrence of congenital Chagas' disease among children born in non-endemic countries to mothers who grew up in *T. cruzi*-endemic areas [95, 96]. It is, therefore, not surprising that transmission of *T. cruzi* has been associated with organ transplantation and blood transfusion in non-Ibero-American countries [97, 98], prompting regulatory agencies and blood collection organizations to implement preventive measures [99–101].

Blood Safety in Ibero-America

The interest in blood safety in Ibero-America dates back to the 1940s, when the first statement regarding the potential transfusion-associated transmission of *T. cruzi* was published in Brazil by Dias [cited in 102]. The report of the first cases of post-transfusion *T. cruzi* infection in 1952 [103] raised awareness among Brazilian physicians, prompting several studies on seroprevalence of anti-*T cruzi* antibodies among blood donors [cited in 102] and reports of transfusion-associated cases of *T. cruzi* infections in Brazil, Panama, Argentina, and Venezuela in the following 10 years (from Table 2, in [101]). PAHO included a table summarizing the prevalence of anti-*T cruzi* antibodies in blood donors of 13 Ibero-American countries in a 1990 report on health conditions in the Americas [104]. The same PAHO publication listed the prevalence rates of anti-HIV antibodies among blood donors from seven Ibero-American nations, which showed the highest values, 7%, in remunerated donations [105]. The report, however, did not present blood bank data on viral hepatitis markers.

The first article that discussed the risk of transfusion transmission of HIV, HBV, HCV, and *T. cruzi* in multiple Ibero-American countries was published in 1998, using data from either 1993 or 1994 [25]. Because none of the 12 countries reported universal screening for the 4 agents, and derived from the high prevalence rates of markers (medians 2.05, 8.30, 4.40, and 14%, respectively) for HIV, HBV, HCV, and *T cruzi*, the authors estimated that, during the year of the study, there were 6385 viral and 2589 *T. cruzi* infections transmitted through transfusions. Information from 13, 14, 17, and 19 Ibero-American nations published later indicated that, by 2001, only 6 of them had achieved universal screening for all required TTI and that the prevalence rates of all markers had decreased when compared to those found in 1994 [106–109]. As a consequence, the risk of TTI in Ibero-America was deemed lower, but still unacceptable, and susceptible to improvement by eliminating replacement and paid donation, reducing the number of blood banks, and implementing quality assurance measures [110]. These recommendations were supported by subsequent communications on the occurrence of high proportions of both false-negative and false-positive test results, primarily concentrated in the smaller laboratories which participated in national programs of external evaluation of performance of TTI screening [111–113]. A 9-country multicenter study carried out from 2003 to 2004 in 3499 multi-transfused patients found that 20%, 14.5%, and 2.1% of them were positive for HCV, HBV, and HIV, respectively [114–123]. The findings not only correlated well with the risk estimates presented by Schmunis and his collaborators but also showed the importance of both universal screening and voluntary blood donation for improving blood safety [25, 110, 123]. The situation in 2013 was still suboptimal, as judged by two facts. First, 4 Ibero-American countries where the prevalence of the 4 TTI markers added to 0.24%, 1.46%, 1.68%, and 3.49% failed to test 31, 191 units for HIV, 35,255 for HBV, 38,041 for HCV, and 133,671 for *T. cruzi* [124]. Second, 29 laboratories of 18 countries reported 1.6% of falsely reactive and 2.9% of falsely negative results in programs of external evaluation of performance [125]. Additionally, 55 infectious adverse reactions to transfusion were reported by individuals from 7 different countries who participated in a survey [126]. This type of survey is a common mechanism for collecting information on adverse reactions to transfusions in Ibero-America, where official public documentation indicates that countrywide hemovigilance systems are functional only in Colombia and Brazil [127, 128].

Can Blood Safety Be Improved in Ibero-America?

In the absence of structured, current countrywide information on actual numbers of infections associated with transfusions, estimations of blood safety in the 19 Ibero-American countries can be based only on indirect indicators, such as proportions of voluntary blood donation, rates of donor deferral, and prevalence of TTI markers among blood donors [25, 110]. The data in Table 12.4, with the addition of those for Peru in 2013 [124], were used to allocate the nations into three groups according to their proportion of VBD.

Group I, with VBD less than 11%, consisted of Mexico, Peru, Guatemala, Venezuela, Panama, and Paraguay; Group II, with VBD between 11% and 51.4%, included the Dominican Republic, El Salvador, Honduras, Chile, Bolivia, Argentina, and Uruguay; while Group III comprised those countries with VBD above 60%, Costa Rica, Brazil, Ecuador, Colombia, Cuba, and Nicaragua. The corresponding proportions of deferred donors of viral TTI markers and *T. cruzi* antibodies were categorized in relation to the median of each indicator and considered "deficient" when they were above that value. Chile was excluded from the statistical analysis because it reported confirmed TTI-positive donations, while the other nations defined reactive donations using screening test results. This arrangement left six countries in each Group. Out of the 29 deficient indicators, 16 were found in Group I, 9 in Group II, and 4 in Group III, demonstrating that countries with higher VBD have lower probability of deferring donors and of finding HIV, HBV, HCV, and *T. cruzi* markers among their donors (goodness of fit test, $Chi^2 = 8.78$, 2df, $p = 0.0124$, [129]). Other observations have shown that Ibero-American countries with lower proportion of VBD are more likely to have more blood banks per 100,000 inhabitants [130], a fact that justifies the proposal to centralize blood collection and processing in larger out-of-hospital blood centers. Centralizing blood collection and

Table 12.4 Blood safety indicators, according to level of voluntary, altruistic blood donation, in Ibero-American countries, 2015

Country	Proportion of voluntary donors (%)	Proportion of deferred donors (%)	Prevalence of TTI markers (%) HBsAg, HCV, HIV	Anti-HBc	Anti-*T cruzi*
Countries with very low (less than 11%) voluntary blood donation					
Mexico	3.8	**28.5**	0.87	NR	0.37
Peru (2013)	4.6	**29.7**	**1.17**	**4.19**	**0.88**
Guatemala	5.4	**25.9**	**1.16**	NR	0.34
Venezuela	5.8	NR	0.98	**2.56**	0.31
Panama	7.0	NR	0.73	**1.74**	**0.52**
Paraguay	10.2	7.7	**0.93**	**2.75**	**2.37**
Countries with low and intermediate (11–60%) voluntary blood donation					
Dominican Republic	11.2	**23.0**	**1.27**	1.18	NA
El Salvador	17.0	**25.0**	0.35	NR	**2.65**
Honduras	18.6	15.7	0.65	**1.62**	**0.74**
Chile	28.5	**22.3**	0.06[a]	NR	0.13
Bolivia	40.9	**29.4**	0.85	NR	0.34
Argentina	45.7	14.2	**1.06**	0.93	**1.50**
Uruguay	51.4	**23.4**	0.53	0.79	0.19
Countries with high and very high (more than 60%) voluntary blood donation					
Costa Rica	60.4	**22.5**	0.45	0.90	0.13
Brazil	61.3	19.3	0.77	1.30	0.22
Ecuador	68.3	15.9	0.85	0.15	0.34
Colombia	91.1	18.0	0.70	**1.56**	**0.38**
Cuba	100	4.6	**1.78**	NR	NA
Nicaragua	100	9.0	0.61	NR	0.34
Median value	*29.75*	*20.9*	*0.85*	*1.43*	*0.355*
Countries in analysis		16	18	12	16

Data taken from Table 14.1
[a]TTI testing results confirmed as positive. Chi^2 for distribution of "deficient indicators" (in bold) among the three groups of countries = 8.78, 2 df, $p = 0.0124$.

processing will also result in more efficient and precise TTI screening and easier implementation of national quality assurance programs [111–113]. In fact, taking blood collection out of all the hospitals, eliminating coerced replacement donation, and centralizing blood processing in only two centers were interventions implemented by Nicaragua, with the support of international collaborators, which improved national blood transfusion safety indicators [131, 132].

In 2002, Nicaragua started the national initiative to centralize its national blood collection and processing system, based on the Regional Plan of Action for strengthening blood banks in the Region of the Americas and on international recommendations [133, 134]. During 2004, a detailed analysis of the local situation allowed the development of pertinent strategies to convert all the hospital blood banks into transfusion services and to gradually reduce their participation in blood collection. In 2005, a 5-year 5.9-million Euro grant was obtained from the Grand Duchy of Luxembourg to support the investments in infrastructure and training identified as necessary for the implementation of the new national blood system. The interventions were carried out under the authority of the Ministry of Health (MoH) which covered all the expenses for the operation of the blood system using national resources. At the beginning of the project, Nicaragua had 20 hospital-based blood banks managed by the MoH and 4 operated by the Nicaraguan Red Cross. The 24 centers collected 54,117 units of whole blood, 54% of them from individuals who were recruited by patients to deposit blood on their behalf, as a requisite for being admitted or treated by the hospitals.

Once the central and hospital authorities agreed on the plan and strategies for the conversion of the national blood system, training of personnel in establishing VBD programs, quality assurance, clinical use of blood, and management of blood services was the first intervention. Technical and training materials produced by PAHO were used to improve skills of administrative, medical, and technical staff and to educate the general public [135–140]. The distance learning courses were taken online at the Benemérita Universidad Autónoma de Puebla, in Mexico, one of the three Ibero-American academic centers supported by PAHO in Ibero-America to establish the corresponding diploma courses. Three physicians were awarded Master's degrees in immunohematology and transfusion at the Universidad de Rosario, in Argentina, as part of program which trained 92 professionals from Ibero-America, supported by the Belgian Red Cross in which PAHO participated by proposing candidates. In late 2008, the decision was made to end coerced, replacement donation by 1 March 2009, a year when all hospital-based blood banks had been transformed into transfusion services and only three Red Cross centers remained in operation. Reducing the number of blood centers allowed the termination of replacement donation and the establishment of a comprehensive quality assurance program, which eventually lead to the accreditation of the National Blood Service in 2012. Associated with the reduction of operating blood banks and with universal VBD, in 2017 only 8.8% of prospective donors were deferred (Table 12.5). Additionally, of those individuals who donated, 0.54% were reactive for viral markers, and 0.25% had anti-$T\ cruzi$ antibodies, figures that represent 71% and 58% reductions, respectively, compared to those found in 2008 (Table 12.5).

One of the central considerations for the termination of hospital-based blood collection and processing was the timely delivery of sufficient blood components to those hospitals. The Regional Plan of Action [30], which Nicaragua adopted, called for the estimation of each blood component need at each patient care facility, as a first and necessary step to define centralized blood collection goals and the procedures required for the opportune distribution of blood components. To attain that purpose, PAHO requested the contribution of an expert from Argentina, the Director of the Transfusion Service at the Garrahan Hospital, to coordinate the development of the appropriate methodology to assess the medical practice of transfusion medicine and the associated clinical requirements of patients. In coordination with the

Table 12.5 Impact of voluntary, altruistic donation on indicators of blood safety

Indicator	Nicaragua 2008	Nicaragua 2017	Garrahan hospital 2010	Garrahan hospital 2017	Chihuahua state center 2010	Chihuahua state center 2017
Donor recruitment						
Voluntary, altruistic (%)	40	100	35	100	29	61
Interviewed (N)	60,769	92,952	13,324	19,176	10,893	13,460
Deferred (%)	13.1	8.8	20.5	21.6	25.9	22.2
Effective	52,829	84,765	10,583	15,026	8071	10,463
TTI markers (%)						
HIV reactive	0.49	0.08	0.24	0.09	0.11	0.13
Confirmed HIV positive			0.06	0.02		
HBsAg reactive	0.48	0.21	0.10	0.11	0.62	0.42
Confirmed HBsAg positive			0.08	0.006		
HCV reactive	0.92	0.25	1.09	0.35	0.57	0.49
Confirmed HCV positive			0.12	0.006		
Anti-*T. cruzi* reactive	0.59	0.25	1.16	0.31	0.21	0.13
Anti-*T. cruzi* confirmed positive			1.10	0.19		

Data from routine records of each service

Technical Officer of the Luxembourg project, a former PAHO blood services employee, arrangements were made with the Bureau of Education and Research of the Nicaraguan Ministry of Health to field-validate the proposed method in seven of its hospitals [138]. During the exercise, the Argentinian expert had the opportunity to learn the Nicaraguan strategy to terminate replacement donation and decided to adapt it to her center in Buenos Aires. 14 June 2011, when Buenos Aires was the venue for the global celebration of World Blood Donor Day, was chosen as the date to attain 100% VDA at the Garrahan Hospital [141], a goal that was achieved and has been sustained over the years. As shown in Table 12.5, employing the same laboratory methodology, the prevalence rates of viral infections among blood donors were reduced by 88% from 2010 to 2017, when only one donor was found to be positive for either HBsAg or HCV, and three were found to be infected with HIV. Four of the five individuals with positive tests in 2017 were first-time donors. During the post-test counseling sessions, the only repeat positive donor reported engaging in risky behaviors that were concealed during the pre-donation interview. The positivity rate for *T. cruzi* was reduced by 83% during the same period. It is important to note that the prevalence of *T. cruzi* infection among pregnant women in the Province of Buenos Aires, where the Garrahan hospital is located, was reported to be six times higher, 1.6% [54], and that the rate of viral TTI markers among all blood donors in Argentina was 1.06 in 2015, when the country had 45.7% VBD (Table 12.1). The continuous improvement in blood safety indicators cannot, however, be attributed only to repeat VBD, since the Garrahan Blood Bank implemented a comprehensive quality assurance program which includes personnel training and standardized operating procedures and is accredited by the AABB since 2013. Confirmatory testing allows a more precise estimation of the safety of the blood components prepared by the center and acts as a proxy indicator of the quality of laboratory screening of TTI.

An additional PAHO collaborative effort to improve blood safety through training of personnel in issues pertaining to VBD was initiated in 2003 by the United Blood Services (UBS) Blood Bank, in El Paso, Texas [142]. During a 3-year period, professionals from all the Ibero-American countries, except Cuba and Peru, spent 1 month in El Paso for hands-on training on donor recruitment, community involvement, volunteer coordinator development, blood collection processes, and media relations. A Mexico-focused approach was developed in 2006, with the involvement of the PAHO US/Mexico Border Field Office, to support the six Mexican states that border the United States. In 2007, Baja California, Nuevo Leon, Sonora, Tamaulipas, Coahuila, and Chihuahua had 0%, 3%, 6%, 16%, 22%, and 30% VBD, respectively [143]. The corresponding figures for 2015 were 4%, 29%, 8%, 15%, 21%, and 48% (Fig. 12.1 [144]), after the Chihuahua State Transfusion Center (CSTC) continued its efforts with support from UBS and the Global Blood Fund [142]. Table 12.5 shows that, in 2017, voluntary blood donation reached 61% at CSTC and that viral markers were detected in 1.04% of the donors, a 20% reduction from 2010. The proportion of donations found to be reactive for *T. cruzi* was 0.13%, which is one third of the national prevalence reported by Mexico in 2015, 0.37%, when the country had 3.8% VBD (Table 12.1) and incomplete coverage of screening for the parasite [37].

The results of these three experiences demonstrate that the safety of the blood supply is determined by the manner in which the health services, especially those involved in donor recruitment and blood collection, operate. The factors that are common to the three success cases presented above are the commitment of the higher authorities—national, state, or institutional—pertinent, evidence-based technical leadership; and involvement of the community. These facilitators are also very

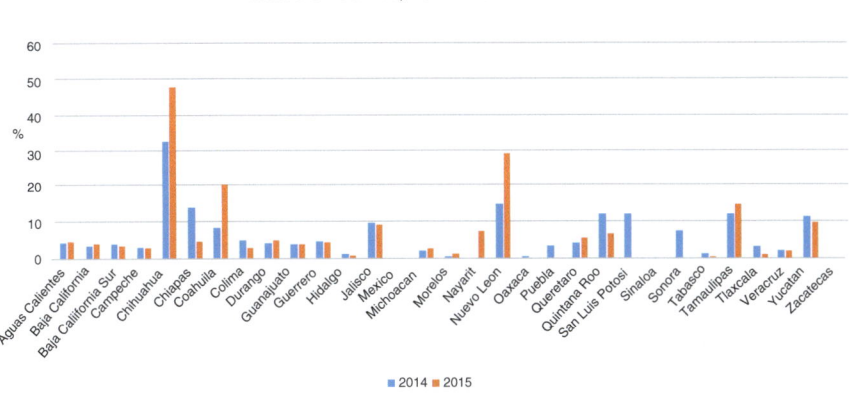

Fig. 12.1 Proportion of voluntary donors in the states of Mexico, 2014–2015. (Based on data from Rojo [144])

likely to attract external collaborators, financial resources, and media attention which, in turn, allow implementing extramural blood collections, enhance the confidence of both the medical and civil societies, and result in better blood donor services. The challenge is to invigorate all the countries and all the blood banks to move in the proper direction at the acceptable speed in order to achieve and protect the highest possible level of blood safety.

Approaches for International Collaboration

We believe that it is necessary to combine surveillance, training, research, oversight, governance, and collaboration among stakeholders in order to improve the selection of safe donors, laboratory screening, and preparation of blood components. International collaboration plays a vital role in the continuous improvement of blood safety and in the monitoring and response to microbial threats. Integration of the Ibero-American blood services into international initiatives to promote global health will undoubtedly contribute to improving blood safety locally and globally.

Table 12.6 has been constructed to represent the stages that we consider appropriate for productive implementation of international collaboration intended to monitor and respond to microbial threats to global blood safety, as defined in the introduction of this chapter.

With the basic understanding that the first and most efficient line of defense is a strong public health system [145], we suggest that international collaboration be initiated during non-emergencies. This approach will not only reduce the potential of emerging threats but will also result in conditions conductive to efficient collaboration when one is identified. In addition to brokering the commitment of local authorities, it is important to work with local individuals who are in positions to provide pertinent technical leadership and to facilitate community involvement. International public health surveillance and research should be carried out in strict adherence to the four Beauchamp and Childress principles: respect of autonomy, non-maleficence, beneficence, and justice [146, 147]. It is necessary to ensure that local authorities, health professionals, blood donors, patients, and their relatives understand the ramifications of research and its potential benefits to their communities and to individuals living elsewhere [148]. Special attention to social and moral values is required when communities are involved and should be viewed as vital to understand that blood donors and patients are not passive subjects who only provide biological material and information for either surveillance or research but active participants of the processes [149].

Other issue to be taken into consideration when conducting international research on global blood safety is the general applicability of the potential innovative technologies developed [150]. Intellectual property of health innovations and its financial and ethical implications must be clear before embarking in collaborative investigation [151–153].

Table 12.6 Strategies for collaboration to improve global blood safety and to monitor and respond to microbial threats in Ibero-America

Goal	Regional challenges	International collaboration
Continuously improve blood safety	Identify and implement the best approach to educate, recruit, select, and retain the safest donors Define and implement pertinent laboratory testing strategies Define the usefulness of pathogen inactivation technology Determine the impact of transfusions on clinical outcome of patients Improve communication and information pathways Report all transfusion-transmissible infections Ensure appropriate regulatory oversight of blood services Ensure appropriate financial resources for adequate blood service operation	Implement/strengthen permanent international working partnerships Develop/provide tools for epidemiological studies to assess efficacy of blood donor deferral criteria and of laboratory testing strategies Provide pertinent support to enhance efficiency of blood collection and processing Support training and infrastructure to improve production and use of clinical records in hospital Support the implementation of a regional system for accreditation of blood services Support the implementation of a regional system for training and certification of personnel Support the implementation of a regional system for blood transfusion technology assessment
Monitor new threats	Integrate blood services into surveillance systems Include blood donors as sentinel population Define and implement surveillance protocols Define and implement research protocols Implement an alert system for rapid dissemination of information on potential new threats to blood safety Adjust government policies and regulations	Develop/provide tools for multicenter research to assess the local microbial threats to blood safety Provide training on ethical issues on research among blood donors and in blood services Provide access to international surveillance and information systems Provide training and access to innovative testing technology
Respond to threats	Integrate blood services into emergency response system Develop preparedness and response plans Ensure adequate financial resources	Support preparedness and response capacity Provide access to innovative containment and control technologies

We believe that international collaboration is vital for attaining the safest possible blood for all patients in all nations and that it can promote establishing universal VBD, pertinent and precise laboratory blood testing, and appropriate preparation of components. International collaboration can be instrumental in surveillance, training, and research and may strengthen oversight of blood services and governance of health systems. We hope the content of this chapter contributes to fostering efficacious international collaboration and global blood safety.

References

1. Seeff LB, Wright EC, Zimmerman HJ, McCollum RW. VA Cooperative study of post transfusion hepatitis, 1969–1974: Incidence and characteristics of hepatitis and responsible risk factors. Am J Med Sci. 1975;270(2):355–62.
2. Johnston DG. Blood transfusion: use and abuse of blood components. West J Med. 1978;128:390–8.
3. Curran JW, Lawrence DN, Jaffe H, Kaplan JE, Zyla LD, Chamberland M, Weinstein R, Lui KJ, et al. Acquired Immunodeficiency syndrome (AID) associated with transfusions. N Engl J Med. 1984;310(2):69–75.
4. Schmunis GA. Chagas' disease and blood transfusion. Prog Clin Biol Res. 1985;182:127–45.
5. Alter HJ, Holland PV, Purcell RH, Lander JJ, Feinstone SM, Morrow AG, Schmidt PL. Posttranfusion hepatitis after exclusion of commercial and hepatitis-B antigen-positive donors. Ann Intern Med. 1972;77(5):691–8.
6. Comptroller General of the United States. Report to the Congress. Hepatitis from Blood Transfusions: Evaluation of Methods to Reduce the Problem. Department of Health, Education and Welfare; 1976.
7. Hsu HH, Gonzalez M, Foung SK, Feinstone SM, Greenberg HB. Antibodies to hepatitis C virus in low-risk blood donors: Implications for counseling positive donors. Gastroenterology. 1991;101:1724–7.
8. Allain JP, Stramer SL, Carneiro-Proietti AB, Martins ML, Lopes da Silva SN, Ribeiro M, Proietti FA, Reesink HW. Transfusion-transmitted infectious diseases. Biologics. 2009;37(2):71–7.
9. Remesar MC, Gamba C, Colaianni IF, Puppo M, Sartor PA, et al. Estimation of sensitivity and specificity of several Trypanosoma cruzi antibody assays in blood donors in Argentina. Transfusion. 2009;49(11):2352–8.
10. Chiqurupati P, Murphy KS. Automated nucleic acid amplification testing in blood banks: An additional layer of blood safety. Asian J Transfus Sci. 2015;9(1):9–11.
11. Simmons G, Bres V, Lu K, Liss NM, Ryff KR, et al. High incidence of Chikungunya virus and frequency of viremic blood donations during epidemic, Puerto Rico, USA, 2014. EID J. 2016;22(7):1221–8.
12. Kuenhert MJ, Basavaraju SV, Moseley RR, Pate LL, Galei SA, Williamson PC, et al. Screening blood donations for Zika virus infection – Puerto Rico, April 3- June 11, 2016. MMWR. 2016;65(24)
13. World Health Organization. Screening donated blood for transfusion-transmissible infections. Recommendations. Geneva; 2010.
14. Ministerio de Sanidad y Politica Social de España. Chagas disease and blood donation. Madrid; 2009. In http://www.msssi.gob.es/profesionales/saludPublica/medicinaTransfusional/publicaciones/docs/InformeChagasInglesJul09.pdf.
15. Center for Biologics Evaluation and Research. Guidance for Industry: Use of serological tests to reduce the risk of transmission of Trypanosoma cruzi infection in whole blood and blood components intended for transfusion. US Department of Health and Human Services. In https://www.fda.gov/biologicsbloodvaccines/guidancecomplianceregulatoryinformation/guidances/blood/ucm235855.htm.
16. O'Brian SF, Scalia V, Goldman M, Fan W, YI QL, et al. Selective testing for Trypanosoma cruzi: the first year after implementation at Canadian Blood Services. Transfusion. 2013;53(8):1706–13.
17. Shimian Z, Fang C, Schonberger LB. Transfusion transmission of human prion diseases. Transfus Med Rev. 2008;22(1):58–69.
18. Stramer SL. Current perspectives in transfusion-transmitted infectious diseases: emerging and re-emerging infections. ISBT Sci Series. 2014;9:30–6.
19. Leiby DA. Transfusion-transmitted Babesia spp: bull's eye on Babesia microti. Clin Microbiol Rev. 2011;24(1):14–8.

20. Glynn SA, Busch MP, Dodd RY, Katz LM, Stramer SL, Klein HG, et al. Emerging infectious agents and the nation's blood supply: responding to potential threats in the 21st century. Transfusion. 2013;53(2):438–54.
21. Bloch EM, Vermeulen M, Murphy E. Blood transfusion safety in Africa: a literature review of infectious disease and organizational challenges. Transfus Med Rev. 2012;26(2):164–80.
22. Caliendo AM, Gilbert DN, Ginocchio CC, Hanson KE, May L, et al. Better tests, better care: improved diagnostics of infectious diseases. Clin Infec Dis. 2013;57(Suppl 3):S139–70.
23. Remis RS, Delage G, RWH P. Risk of HIV infection from blood transfusion in Montreal. CMAJ. 1997;157:375–82.
24. Glynn SA, Kleinman SH, Wright DJ, Busch MP. NHLBI Retrovirus Epidemiology Donor Study. International Application of the incidence rate/window period model. Transfusion. 2002;42:966–72.
25. Schmunis GA, Zicker F, Pinheiro F, Brandling-Bennett D. Risk of transfusion-transmitted infectious diseases in Central and South America. Emerg Infect Dis. 1998;4(1):5–11.
26. World Health Organization. Blood Safety. Aide-Memoire for National Health Programmes. Geneva, 1999.
27. Debeir J, Noel L, Aullen JP, Frette C, Sari F. The French haemovigilance system. Vox Sang. 1999;77(2):77–81.
28. Strong M, Whitaker B, Kuehnert MJ, Holmberg JA. Biovigilance in the Unites States. Chapter 19. In: RRP DV, Faber J-C, editors. Hemovigilance. An effective tool for improving transfusion safety: Wiley-Blackwell. Hoboken, NJ. USA; 2012.
29. Faber JC. Hemovigilance: definition and overview of current hemovigilance systems. Transf Alt Transf Med. 2003;5(1):237–45.
30. Pan American Health Organization. Improving blood availability and transfusion safety in the Americas. Document CD48/11. 48th Directing Council, Washington, DC; 2008.
31. Institute of Medicine (US) Committee on the US Commitment to Global Health. The US Commitment to global health: Recommendations for the public and private sectors. pp18. Washington, DC: National Academy Press; 2009.
32. Organización de Estados Iberoamericanos. What is OEI? In http://www.oei.es/historico/isoei.htm.
33. Pan American Health Organization. Basic Indicators 2015. Washington, DC; 2016.
34. United Nations Development Programme. Human Development Report 2016. Human Development for Everyone. New York; 2016.
35. Central Intelligence Agency. Population below Poverty Line. The World Fact Book; 2016.
36. United Nations Development Program.Human Development Report 2014. Sustaining Human Progress: Reducing Vulnerabilities and Building Resilience. Washington, DC; 2014.
37. Organización Panamericana de la Salud. Suministro de sangre para transfusiones en los países de Latinoamérica y del Caribe, 2014 y 2015. Washington, DC; 2017.
38. Programa de Naciones Unidas para el Desarrollo. Informe Nacional sobre Desarrollo Humano 2013. Argentina en un mundo incierto: Asegurar el desarrollo humano en el siglo XXI. Buenos Aires; 2013.
39. Programa de Naciones Unidos para el Desarrollo. Informe sobre el Desarrollo Humano 2013. El Salvador. Imaginar un nuevo país. Hacerlo posible. Diagnóstico y Propuesta. La Libertad; 2013.
40. Chi-Square Goodness of Fit Test. In http://vassarstats.net/csfit.html.
41. Spearman Rank-Order Correlation Coefficient. In http://vassarstats.net/corr_rank.html.
42. Joint United Nations Programme on HIV/AIDS (UNAIDS). Global Summary of the AIDS Epidemic 2015. Geneva; 2016.
43. Joint United Nations Programme on HIV/AIDS (UNAIDS). The Gap Report. Latin America. Geneva; 2014.
44. About the Pan American Health Organization (PAHO). http://www.paho.org/hq/index.php?option=com_content&view=article&id=91%3Aabout-paho&lang=en.

45. Pan American Health Organization. Plan of action for the prevention and control of viral hepatitis. 54th Directing Council. 67th Session of the Regional Committee for the Americas. Document CD54/13 Rev.1. Washington, DC; 2015.
46. Pan American Health Organization. Hepatitis B and C in the Spotlight. A public health response in the Americas 2016. Washington, DC; 2016.
47. Ott JJ, Stevens GA, Groeger J, Wiersma ST. Global epidemiology of hepatitis B virus infection: New estimates of age-specific HBsAg seroprevalence and endemicity. Vaccine. 2012;30:2212–9.
48. Tanaka J. Hepatitis B epidemiology in Latin America. Vaccine. 2000;18(Suppl 1):S17–9.
49. Petruzziello A, Mariagliano A, Loquercio G, Cozzolino A, Cacciapuoti C. Global epidemiology of hepatitis C virus infection: An up-date of the distribution and circulation of hepatitis C virus genotypes. World J Gastroenterol. 2016;22(34):7824–40.
50. Hanafiah KM, Groeger J, Flaxman AD, Wiersma ST. Global epidemiology of hepatitis C virus infection: new estimates of age-specific antibody to HCV seroprevalence. Hepatology. 2013;57:1333–42.
51. Alonso M, Gutzman A, Mazin R, Pinzon CE, Reveiz L, Ghidinelli M. Hepatitis C in key populations in Latin America and the Caribbean: systematic review and meta-analysis. Int J Public Health. 2015;60:789–98.
52. World Health Organization. Chagas disease in Latin America: an epidemiological update based on 2010 estimates. Wkly Epidemiol Rec. 90;(6):33–43.
53. Sasawaga E, Guevara de Aguilar AV, Hernandez de Ramirez MA, Romero Chavez JE, Nakagawa J, et al. Prevalence of Trypanosoma cruzi infection in blood donors in El Salvador between 2001 and 2011. J Infect Dev Ctries. 2014;8(8):1029–36.
54. Chuit R, Segura EL. El control de la enfermedad de Chagas en Argentina. Sus resultados. Rev Fed Arg Cardiol. 2012;41(3):151–5.
55. Carter K, Singh P, Mujica O, Escalada RP, Ade MP, Castellanos LG, Espinal MA. Malaria in the Americas from 1959 to 2011. Am J Trop Med Hyg. 2015;92(2):302–16.
56. Pan American Health Organization. Report on the situation of malaria in the Americas 2014. Washington, DC; 2016.
57. Pan American Health Organization/World Health Organization. Epidemiological Alert: Increase in cases of malaria. 15 February, Washington, DC; 2017.
58. Patterson J, Sammon M, Garg M. Dengue, Zika and Chikungunya: Emerging Arbovirus in the New World. West J Emerg Med. 2016;17(6):671–9.
59. Pan American Health Organization/World Health Organization. Number of Reported Cases of Dengue and Severe Dengue (SD) in the Americas, by Country. Figures for 2016. Epidemiological week/EW/52. Updated 6 Feb 2017.
60. Pan American Health Organization/World Health Organization. Number of Reported Cases of Chikungunya Fever in the Americas, by Country or Territory 2016 (to week noted). Cumulative cases. Updated as of 27 Jan 2017.
61. Campos GS, Bandeira S, Sardi I. Zika Virus Outbreak, Bahia, Brazil. EID. 2015;21(10):1885–6.
62. Kinzer K, Morrison K, Brownstein JS, Marinho F, Santos AF, Nsoesie EO. Reconstruction of Zika Virus Introduction in Brazil. EID. 2017;23(1):92–4.
63. Schuler-Faccini L, Ribeiro EM, Feitosa IM, et al. Possible Association between Zika Virus Infection and Microcephaly –Brazil. MMWR Morb Mortal Wkly Rep. 2016;65(3):59–62.
64. Pan American Health Organization/World Health Organization. Zika cases and congenital syndrome associated with Zika virus reported by countries and territories in the Americas 2015–2017. Cumulative cases. Data as of 4 May 2017 2:00pm EST. Washington, DC; 2017.
65. Easterbrook PJ, Roberts T, Sands A, Peeling R. Diagnosis of viral hepatitis. Curr Opin HIV AIDS. 2017;12(3):302–14.
66. Schmidt M, Geilenkeuser W-J, Sireis W, Seifried E, Hourfar K. Emerging Pathogens – How safe is blood. Transf Med Hemother. 2014;41:1–17.
67. Arizona Department of Health Services. Arizona Arboviral Handbook for Chikungunya, Dengue, & Zika Viruses. Phoenix; 2016.

68. Murray KO, Gorchavkov R, Carlson AR, Berry R, Lai L, Natrajan M, et al. Prolonged Detection of Zika Virus in Vaginal Secretions and Whole Blood. EID. 2017;23(1):99–101.
69. Andrade DV, Gollob KJ, Dutra WO. Acute Chagas disease: new global challenges for an old neglected disease. PLoS Negl Trop Dis. 2014;8(7):1–10.
70. Denniston MM, Klevens RM, McQuillan GM, Jiles RB. Awareness of infection, knowledge of hepatitis C, and medical follow-up among individuals testing positive for hepatitis C: national health and nutrition examination survey 2001–2008. Hepatology. 2012;55(6):1652–61.
71. Sanchez DR, Traina M, Hernandez S, Smer AM, Khamag H, Meymandi SK. Chagas disease awareness among Latin American immigrants living in Los Angeles, California. Am J Trop Med. 2014;91(5):915–9.
72. Hoen AG, Hladish TJ, Eggo RM, Lenczner M, Brownstein JS, Meyers LA. Epidemic wave dynamics attributable to urban community structure: a theoretical characterization of disease transmission in a large network. J Med Inter Res. 2015;17(7):1–12.
73. Castillo-Chavez C, Bichara D, Morin BR. Perspectives on the role of mobility, behavior, and time scales in the spread of disease. PNAS. 2016;113(51):14582–8.
74. World Tourism Organization. Yearbook of Tourism Statistics. Compendium of Tourism Statistics and Data Files, 2015. Madrid; 2016 in http://data.worldbank.org/indicator/ST.INT.DPRT.
75. Pan American Health Organization. Eligibility for blood donation: recommendations for education and selection of prospective blood donors. Washington, DC; 2009.
76. Organización Panamericana de la Salud/Organización Mundial de la Salud. Documento de Trabajo. Recomendaciones preliminares para los servicios de sangre frente a la epidemia del virus del Zika: su potencial impacto en de diseminación de la infección y en la disponibilidad y seguridad de la sangre y componentes sanguíneos. Washington, DC; 2016.
77. Bellis MA, Hughes K, Bennett A, Thomson R. The role of an international nightlife resort in the proliferations of recreational drugs. Addiction. 2003;98(12):1713–21.
78. Vivancos R, Abubakar I, Hunter PR. Foreign travel, casual sex, and sexually transmitted infections: a systematic review and meta-analysis. Int J Infect Dis. 2010;14(10):e842–51.
79. Croughs M, Remmen R, Van den Ende J. The effect of pre-travel advice on sexual risk behavior abroad: a systematic review. J Travel Med. 2014;21(1):45–51.
80. World Tourism Organization. International tourist arrivals. UNWTO Tourism Highlights 2016 Edition. Madrid; 2017. In http://data.worldbank.org/indicators/ST.INT.ARVL.
81. Kariyawasam R, Lau R, Eshaghi A, Patel SN, Sider D, Gubbay JB, Boggild AK. Spectrum of viral pathogens in blood of malaria-free Ill travelers returning to Canada. IED. 2016;22(5):854–61.
82. Anez G, Heisey DAR, Chancey C, Fares RCG, Espina LM, Souza KPR, et al. Distribution of dengue virus types 1 and 4 in blood components from infected blood donors from Puerto Rico. PLOS Negl Infect Dis. 2016;10(2):e0004445. https://doi.org/10.1371/journal.pntd.0004445. In http://journals.plos.org/plosntds/article/file?id=10.1371/journal.pntd.0004445&type=printable
83. Patients Beyond Borders. Medical tourism statistics and facts. In http://www.patientsbeyondborders.com/medical-tourism-statistics-facts.
84. Organización Panamericana de la Salud. Salud Materno Infantil en Bolivia. Análisis de la Respuesta del Sistema de Salud. Washington, DC; 2011.
85. Statistics Canada. National household survey. NHS Profile, Canada 2011. Ethic origin. In http://www12.statcan.gc.ca/nhs-enm/2011/dp-pd/prof/details/page.cfm?Lang=E&Geo1=PR&Code1=01&Data=Count&SearchText=canada&SearchType=Begins&SearchPR=01&A1=Ethnic%20origin&B1=All&Custom=&TABID=1.
86. Padilla B, Peixoto J. Latin American Migration to Southern Europe. Migration Information Source. Migration Policy Institute 2007. In http://www.migrationpolicy.org/article/latin-american-immigration-southern-europe.
87. Migration Policy Institute. United States Immigrant Population by Country of Birth, 2000-Present. In http://www.migrationpolicy.org/programs/data-hub/us-immigration-trends#source.

88. Migration Policy Institute. LAC immigrants in Europe. A statistical analysis 2007. In http://www.migrationpolicy.org/article/latin-american-immigration-southern-europe.
89. Martínez Pizarro J, Cano Christiany V, Contrucci MS. Tendencias y patrones de la migración latinoamericana y caribeña hacia 2010 y desafíos para una agenda regional. Centro Latinoamericano y Caribeno de Demografía, Comisión Económica para América Latina y el Caribe. Santiago de Chile; 2014.
90. Klein N, Hurwitz I, Durvasula R. Globalization of Chagas disease: a growing concern in noendemic countries. Epidemiol Res Internal 2012: 13 pages. https://doi.org/10.1155/2012/136793.
91. Jackson Y, Getax L, Wolff H, Holst M, Mauris A, Tardin A, et al. Prevalence, clinical staging and risk for blood-borne transmission of Chagas disease among Latin American migrants in Geneva, Switzerland. PLOS Neglected Trop Dis. 2010;4(2):e592.
92. Hotez PJ, Dumontell E, Betancourt Cravioto M, Botazzi ME, Tapia-Conyer R, et al. An unfolding tragedy of Chagas disease in North America. Editorial PLOS Neglected Infect Dis. 2013;7(10):e2300.
93. Gabrielli S, Girelli G, Vaia F, Santonicola M, Fakeri A, Cancrini G. Surveillance of Chagas disease among at-risk blood donors in Italy: preliminary results from Umberto I Polyclinic in Rome. Blood Transf. 2013;11:558–62.
94. Steele WR, Hewitt EH, Kaldun AM, Krysztof DE, Dodd RY, Stramer SL. Donors deferred for self-reported Chagas disease history: does it reduce risk? Transfusion. 2014;54(8):2092–7.
95. Murillo J, Bofill LM, Bolivar H, Torres-Viera C, Urbina JA, et al. Congenital Chagas' disease transmission in the United States: Diagnosis in adulthood. ID Cases. 2016;5:72–5.
96. Centers for Disease Control and Prevention. Congenital transmission of Chagas disease – Virginia, 2010. MMWR. 2012;61(26):477–9.
97. Ries J, Komarek A, Gottschalk J, Brand B, Amsler L, Jutzi M, Frey BM. A case of possible Chagas transmission by blood transfusion in Switzerland. Transf Med Hemother. 2016;43(6):415–7.
98. Centers for Disease Control and Prvention. Chagas disease after organ transplantation-United States, 2001. MMWR. 2002;51(10):210–2.
99. Requena-Mendez A, Albajar-Vinas P, Angheben A, Chiodini P, Goscon J, Munoz J, Chagas Disease COHEMI Working Group. Health policies to control Chagas disease transmission in European countries. PLOS Neglected Trop Dis. 2014;8(10):e3245.
100. US Food & Drug Administration. Guidance for Industry: Use of Serological Tests to Reduce the Risk of Transmission of Trypanosoma cruzi infection in Whole Blood and Blood Components Intended for Transfusion. US Department of Health and Human Services, Washington, DC; 2010.
101. Canadian Blood Services. Donor selection, transmissible disease testing and pathogen reduction. Professional Education; 2017.
102. da Silveira Baldy JL, Takaoka L, Pereira JD, Calizto AA, Duarte EF. Prevalencia da infeccao por Trypanosoma cruzi, em 1975, em dois bancos de sangue de Londrina, Parana, Brazil. Rev Saude publ, S Paulo. 1978;12:409–16.
103. Freitas JLP, Amato Neto V, Sonntag R, Biancalana A, Nussenzweig V, Barreto JG. Primeiras verificacoes de transmissao acidental da molestis de Chagas ao homem por transfusao de sangue. Rev Paul Med. 1952;40:36–40.
104. Organización Panamericana de la Salud/Organización Mundial de la Salud. Enfermedad de Chagas. Condiciones de salud en las Américas. Publicación Científica No. 524. 1990;1:171–3. http://www.paho.org/salud-en-las-americas-2012/dmdocuments/condiciones-salud-americas-1985-1988-vol1.pdf
105. Organización Panamericana de la Salud/Organización Mundial de la Salud. Síndrome de inmunodeficiencia adquirida (SIDA). Condiciones de salud en las Américas. Publicación Científica No. 524. 1990;(1):180–5. http://www.paho.org/salud-en-las-americas-2012/dmdocuments/condiciones-salud-americas-1985-1988-vol1.pdf
106. Organización Panamericana de la Salud. Situación de los bancos de sangre en la Región de las Américas, 1994-1995. Boletín Epidemiológico. 1997;18(1):11–2.

107. Organización Panamericana de la Salud. Situación de seguridad en los bancos de sangre de las Américas. Seguridad en los bancos de sangre: cuadros actualizados de países de América Latina. Boletín Epidemiológico. 1999;20(2):8–9.
108. Organización Panamericana de la Salud. II Conferencia Latinoamericana de Bancos de Sangre. Dra. Lorena Carboni Aguiluz (In Memoriam). Cartagena de Indias, Colombia. 31 de Mayo – 2 de Junio 1999. Documento OPS/HSP/HSE-LAB/06.99, Washington, DC; 1999.
109. Cruz JR, Perez-Rosales MD. Availability, safety and quality of blood for transfusion in the Americas. Pan Am J Public Health. 13(2/3):103–10.
110. Schmunis GA, Cruz JR. Safety of the blood supply in Latin America. Clin Microbiol Rev. 2005;18(1):12–29.
111. Saez-Alquezar A, Otani MA, Sabino EC, Salles NA, Chamone DF. Programas de control externo de la calidad en serología desarrollados en América Latina con el apoyo de OPS entre 1997 y 2000. Pan Am J Public Health. 2003;13(2/3):91–102.
112. Beltrán Duran M, Ayala Guzmán M. Evaluación externa de los resultados serológicos en los bancos de sangre de Colombia. Pan Am J Public Health. 2003;13(2/3):138–48.
113. Grijalva MJ, Chiriboga RF, Vanhassel H, Arcos-Teran L. Improving the safety of the blood supply in Ecuador through external performance evaluation of serological screening of blood donors. J Clin Virol. 2005;34(Suppl 2):S47–52.
114. Remesar M, Gamba C, Kuperman S, Marcos SA, Miguez G, et al. Antibodies to hepatitis C and other viral markers in multi-transfused patients from Argentina. J Clin Virol. 2005;34(Suppl 2):S20–6.
115. de Paula EV, Goncales NS, Xueref S, Addas-Carballo M, Gilli SC, et al. Transfusion-transmitted infections among multi-transfused patients in Brazil. J Clin Virol. 2005;34(Suppl 2):S27–S3.
116. Beltrán M, Navas MC, De la Hoz F, Muñoz MT, Jaramillo S, et al. Hepatitis C virus seroprevalence in multi-transfused patients in Colombia. J Clin Virol. 2005;34(Suppl 2):S33–8.
117. Ballester JM, Rivero RA, Villaescusa R, Merlin JC, Arce AA, et al. Hepatitis C virus antibodies and other markers of blood-transfusion transmitted infection in multi-transfused Cuban patients. J Clin Virol. 2005;34(Suppl 2):S39–46.
118. Vinelli E, Lorenzana I. Transfusion-transmitted infections in multi-transfused patients in Honduras. J Clin Virol. 2005;34(Suppl 2):S53–60.
119. Laguna-Torres VA, Perez-Bao J, Chauca G, Sovero M, Blichtein D, et al. Epidemiology of transfusion-transmitted infections among multi-transfused patients in seven hospitals in Peru. J Clin Virol. 2005;34(Suppl 2):S61–8.
120. Lopez L, Lopez P, Arago A, Rodriguez I, Lopez J, et al. Risk factors for hepatitis B and C in multi-transfused patients in Uruguay. J Clin Virol. 2005;34(Suppl 2):S69–74.
121. Calderon GM, Gonzalez Velazquez, Novelo Garza B. Risk factors and prevalence of HCV, HBV and HIV in multiple transfusion recipients in Mexico. Report submitted to PAHO; 2005.
122. Berrios R, Jiménez EV. Prevalencia de Hepatitis C y otras infecciones transmitidas por transfusión en pacientes multitransfundidos en Nicaragua. Informe final enviado a OPS; 2005.
123. Cruz JR. El estudio EPISANGRE. Una experiencia multipaís encaminada a mejorar la seguridad sanguínea. Boletín del Grupo Cooperativo Iberoamericano de Medicina Transfusional, GCIAMT. 2006;20:5–8.
124. Organizacion Panamericana de la Salud. Suministro de sangre para transfusiones en los países de Latinoamerica y del Caribe 2012 y 2013. Washington, DC; 2015.
125. Fundacao Pro-Sangue Hemocentro de Sao Paulo/Organización Panamericana de la Salud. Programa de Evaluación Externa de Desempeño en Serología. América Latina 2013. Sao Paulo; 2014.
126. Torres OW, León de González G. Haemovigilance in Latin America. Blood Transfus. 2014;12(Suppl 2):s430–1.
127. Agencia Nacional de Vigilancia Sanitaria. Hemovigilancia No Brasil. Relatorio Consolidado 2007–2015. Brasilia; 2016.

128. Instituto Nacional de Salud. Dirección Redes en Salud Pública. Coordinación Red Nacional de Bancos de Sangre y Servicios de Transfusión. Informe nacional de indicadores de red nacional bancos de sangre y servicios de transfusión. 1 de enero a 31 de diciembre de 2015. Bogotá; 2016.
129. Chi-square Goodness of Fit test. In http://vassarstats.net/csfit.html.
130. Cruz JR. Implementación de la donación voluntaria de sangre a nivel nacional: papel del Estado. Capítulo 12. In: Cortes A, Roig Oltra R, Cabezas Belalcalzar AL, Garcia-Castro Gutierrez M, Urcelay Uranga S, editors. Promoción de la Donación Voluntaria de Sangre. Colombia: Grupo Cooperativo Iberoamericano de Medicina Transfusional; 2017. p. 94–101.
131. Berrios R, Gonzalez A, Cruz JR. Achieving self-sufficiency of red blood cells based on universal voluntary blood donation in Latin America. The case of Nicaragua. Transf Aphe Sci. 2013;49:387–96.
132. Cruz JR. Introduction of programs for voluntary blood donation in Central America. ISBT Science Series. 2012;7(1):188–91.
133. Pan American Health Organization. Strengthening blood banks in the Region of the Americas. Document CD41/13. 41st Directing Council, San Juan (Puerto Rico). PAHO; 1999.
134. Cruz JR. Basic components of a national blood system. Pan Am J Pub Health. 2003;13(2/3):79–84.
135. Organización Panamericana de la Salud. Guía para la estimación de costos de la regionalización de los bancos de sangre. Washington, DC; 2005.
136. Organización Panamericana de la Salud. Estándares de Trabajo para Servicios de Sangre. Segunda Edición. Washington, DC; 2005.
137. Organización Mundial de la Salud. Sangre y Componentes Seguros. Edición Revisada. Ginebra; 2002.
138. Pan American Health Organization. Recommendations for Estimating the need for blood and blood components. Washington, DC; 2010.
139. International Federation of Red Cross and Red Crescent Societies. Making a difference: recruiting voluntary, non-remunerated blood donors. Geneva; 2008.
140. Pan American Health Organization. Eligibility for blood donation. Recommendations for education and selection of prospective blood donors. Washington, DC; 2009.
141. del Pozo A. Captación, selección y colecta de donantes de sangre. In: Cortes A, León G, Muñoz M, Jaramillo S, editors. Aplicaciones y Practica de la Medicina Transfusional. Santiago de Cali: Grupo Cooperativo Iberoamericano de Medicina Transfusional; 2012. p. 1289–312.
142. Villalobos P. Experiencia del United Blood Services para Latinoamérica. 1er Congreso Internacional de Donación Voluntaria Altruista de Sangre. Ciudad Juárez, Chihuahua; 2016.
143. Cruz JR. *Cambiemos la* Donación de Sangre en las Américas. Foro de Donación Voluntaria de Sangre. Monterrey; 2008.
144. Rojo J. ¿A dónde vamos? Panorama de DVA en México. 1er Congreso Internacional de Donación Voluntaria Altruista de Sangre. Ciudad Juárez, Chihuahua; 2016.
145. Commission on a Global Health Risk Framework for the Future. Strengthening public health as the foundation of the health system and first line of defense. In the neglected dimension of global security. A framework to counter infectious disease crises. US National Academy of Medicine; 2016.
146. Beauchamp TL, Childress JF. Principles of biomedical ethics. 5th ed. New York: Oxford University Press; 2001.
147. Klingler C, Silva DS, Schuermann C, Reis AA, Saxena A, Strech D. Ethical issues in public health surveillance: a systematic qualitative review. BMC Public Health. 2017;17:295.
148. Patino RM. Moving research to patient applications through commercialization: understanding and evaluating the role of intellectual property. J Am Assoc Lab Ani Sci. 2010;49(2):147–54.
149. Bromley E, Mikesell L, Jones F, Khodyakov D. From subject to participant: ethics and the evolving role of community in health research. Am J Pub Health. 2015;105(5):900–8.
150. Masum H, Lackman R, Bartleson K. Developing global health technology standards: what can other industries teach us? Glob Health. 2013;9:49.

151. Lysdahl KB, Oortwijn W, van der Wilt GJ, Refolo P, Sacchini D, Mozygemba K, Hofmann B. Ethical analysis in HTA of complex health interventions. BMC Med Ethics. 2016;17:16. https://doi.org/10.1186/s12910-016-0099-z.
152. Taubman A. A typology of intellectual property management for public health innovation and access: design considerations for policymakers. Open AIDS J. 2010:4–24.
153. Meslin EM, Were E, Ayuku D. Taking stock of the ethical foundations of international health research: pragmatic lessons from the IU–Moi Academic Research Ethics Partnership. J Gen Intern Med. 2013;28(Suppl 3):639–45.

Index

A
Abnormal prion protein, 151
Abnormal PrP, 150, 151
Acquired immune deficiency syndrome (AIDS), 3, 126–129
    See also Human immunodeficiency virus (HIV) infections
Acute parvovirus B19 (B19V) infection, 30
Aedes
    A. aegypti, 167
    mosquitoes, 5
Alanine aminotransferase (ALT), 10, 56
Alliance of Blood Operators (ABO) RBDM Framework, 44, 46, 48
Amoxicillin, 213
Anaplasma phagocytophilum, 208
    biology and epidemiology, 209
    clinical features/diagnosis/treatment, 209, 210
    mitigating risk, strategies for, 211
    seroprevalence and incidence, 210
    transfusion transmission/survival in blood, 210, 211
Anti-HBc, 131
Antihemophilic factor (AHF), 129
Anti-Zika IgM antibodies, 172
Arboviruses, 3, 160, 168
Assessing blood safety threats, 37–39, 41–47
    ABO RBDM Framework, 36
    consultation, 36
    fairness, 36
    risk communication
        applications, 41, 43–45
        goals of, 41
        principles, 41
        process, 42–43
    risk perception, 39
        blood safety (*see* Blood safety)
        collective risk judgement processes, 38, 39
        dynamics, 37, 38
        qualitative risk factors, 37
        trust in risk management, 39
    risk tolerability, 48–50
    stakeholder engagement, 44
        discovery, 46
        opportunities, 47
    transparency, 36

B
Babesia, 65–67
    B. microti, 66, 72
Babesiosis, 67
Biggerstaff-Petersen (BP) model, 90, 91, 96–98, 105
Blood bank community, 129
Blood components, 17, 18, 143, 144, 146, 151, 153
Blood donor screening, 137
Blood Product Advisory Committee (BPAC), 127, 131
Blood safety, 7–13, 40, 41, 53–57, 84, 107, 143, 160, 181
    donor suitability, 7
        donor information-based strategies, 7
        medical history, 8
        risk behaviors, 9
        risk exposure, 8, 9
    emerging infectious diseases, 4, 5
    global implications for, 14
    health economics in

Blood safety (*Cont.*)
   analysis study designs and methods,
      54–57 (*see also* Health economics,
      blood safety)
   healthcare policy decision-makers, 54
   principles, 53
  horizon scanning, 5, 6
  pathogen inactivation, 13
  prediction, 6, 7
  risk perception
   blood donors and donation, 40, 41
   blood products, 40
  RPV (*see* Ross River virus (RRV),
     Australia)
  testing, 9
   direct testing method, 11
   nucleic acid testing, 13
   pathogens, 10, 11
   rapid tests, 12–13
   serologic testing, 11, 12
   surrogate testing, 9, 10
Borrelia burgdorferi, 208
Borrelia microti, 208
Borrelia miyamotoi, 207
  biology and epidemiology, 212
  clinical features/diagnosis/treatment,
     212, 213
  mitigating risk, strategies for, 214
  seroprevalence and incidence, 213
  transfusion transmission/survival in blood,
     213, 214
Bovine spongiform encephalopathy (BSE),
     4, 143, 192
Budget impact analysis (BIA), 55, 57

C

Ceftriaxone, 213
Centers for Disease Control and Prevention
     (CDC), 125, 128, 129, 131, 171
Chemiluminescence, 12
Chikungunya, 26, 168, 169, 176, 194–196
  fever, 98
  virus, 6
CJD Incidents Panel, 147
Congenital neurological disease, 171
Congenital Zika Syndrome (CZS), 166,
     170–172
Consolidated Health Economic Evaluation
     Reporting Standards (CHEERS), 62
Cost-benefit analysis (CBA), 55, 56
Cost-effectiveness (CE)
  plane, 58, 61
  thresholds, 56, 59, 60, 62, 64

Cost-effectiveness acceptability curve
     (CEACs), 61, 62
Cost-effectiveness analysis (CEA), 55
Cost-effectiveness ratio (CER), 56
Cost-effectiveness/utility analysis, 57
Cost-minimization analysis (CMA), 55, 56
Cost of illness (COI), 55
Cost-utility analysis (CUA), 55, 56
Creutzfeldt-Jakob disease (CJD), 143, 144,
     146, 148, 151
"Current good manufacturing practices"
     (cGMP), 190

D

Deer tick virus (DTV), 215
Dengue, 168, 169, 194–196
Dengue virus (DENV), 87
  in Cains, Australia, 100, 101
  in Singapore, 100, 101
Deterministic sensitivity analysis, 61
Direct costs, 57
Direct testing method, 11
Disability-adjusted life years averted
     (DALYs), 56
DNA/RNA of pathogen, 28–30
Donor deferral strategies, 200
Donor information-based strategies, 7
Donor screening, 18, 26–28, 32

E

Ebola Virus, 193, 194
Emerging infection, 26, 27
Emerging infectious diseases (EIDs), 4, 5, 83,
     84, 86–103
  interpreting risk assessments
   local context, 102
   quantitatively estimating TT risk, 103
   threat to blood safety, 103
  qualitative assessment
   agent and competent vector(s), 86
   asymtomatic blood phase, 86, 87
   clinically apparent disease, associated
     with, 88, 89
   humans and spread within human
     populations, 86
   survive, ability to, 88
   transfusion-transmissible, 87, 88
  quantitative assessment
   Biggerstaff-Petersen models,
     90–91, 96–98
   DENV, 100, 101
   EUFRAT, 90–91, 98, 99

Index

HEV in Australia, 100, 102
IgM detection and incident infections in donors, 100, 101
risk modelling, 90, 92–95
risk assessment, 84
Enzyme-linked immunosorbent assay (ELISA), 133, 212
Epidemic polyarthritis, 105
European Center for Disease Control (ECDC), 5, 98
European Centre for Disease Prevention and Control (ECDC), 98
European Up-Front Risk Assessment Tool (EUFRAT) models, 26–28, 90–91, 98, 99, 105

F

Flaviviruses, 169, 194, 217
"4H disease", 126, 127
Fresh frozen plasma (FFP), 28, 70, 149

G

Gay-related immunodeficiency (GRID), 126
Global blood safety, international cooperation, 229–239
    approaches, 240, 241
    definition, 226
    Ibero-America, 226–229, 232, 233
        altruistic donation on indicators, 237, 238
        blood safety indicators, 235, 236
        hospital-based blood collection, 237
        impact of voluntary, 237, 238
        potential implications, 231–234
        T. cruzi, 234, 238
        TTI, 229–231
        VBD, 235, 237
        voluntary donors in states of Mexico, 239
GlpQ-Luminex assay, 213
G'lycerophosphodiester phosphodiesterase (GlpQ) antigen, 212
Gross domestic product (GDP), 60
Gross national income (GNI), 60
Guillain-Barré Syndrome (GBS), 89, 164, 166, 172, 173

H

Haematological and biochemical blood tests, 151
Health economics, blood safety, 55–69
    analysis study designs and methods, 54–57
    BIA, 55
    budget impact, 57
    CBA, 56
    CEA, 56
    CEACs, 61, 62
    CE plane, 58
    CMA, 56
    conducting and reporting analyses, 62
    cost-effectiveness thresholds, 59, 60
    cost-effectiveness/utility analysis, 57
    DALYs, 56
    discounting, 58
    ICERs, 57
    perspective, 57–58
    posttransfusion survival, 62
    QALYs, 56
    residual risk calculations, 63
    uncertainty and sensitivity, 60, 61
    healthcare policy decision-makers, 54
    implications for, 72, 73
    pathogen reduction/inactivation technologies, 70, 71
    principles, 53
    ZIKV, 63, 64
    Babesia, 65–67
    HIV, HBV and HCV, 67–69
    HTLV, 64, 65
HealthMap, 5
Health technology assessments, 54
Hendra viruses, 198–200
Henipaviruses, 198
Hepatitis A virus (HAV), 160
Hepatitis B core antibody (anti-HBc), 10, 128
Hepatitis B virus (HBV), 12, 67–69
Hepatitis C virus (HCV), 12, 67–69, 230
Heterosexual intercourse, 126
Human immunodeficiency virus (HIV)
    infections, 12, 13, 27–29, 67–69, 229
    in Australia, 100, 102
    discovery of, 132
    "4H disease", 126, 127
    funding and politics, 135–137
    history of, 125, 126
    screening test, 133, 134
    serologic testing, 12
    statements and **r**ecommendations, 128–130
    surrogate screening tests, 130, 131
    transfusion-transmissible disease, 127, 128
    transmission data, 134
Homosexuality, 126
Horizon scanning, 5, 6
Human Development Index (HDI), 226–228

Human Health Index (HHI), 227–229
Human pegivirus (HPgV), 89
Human T-cell lymphotropic virus (HTLV), 12, 64, 65
Human T-lymphotropic retrovirus types I/II (HTLVs), 189
Human-to-human transmission, 4, 199

I
Immunoglobulin M (IgM), 102
Immunohistochemical techniques, 170
Incremental cost-effectiveness ratio (ICER), 56, 58
Indirect costs, 57
Individual-donation (ID) nucleic acid testing (NAT) screening, 63, 68, 72
International Society for Blood Transfusion (ISBT), 67
International Society for Pharmaceutical Outcomes Research (ISPOR), 54
Investigational new drug (IND), 158, 180
IV drug, 126
Ixodes scapularis, 208, 209

L
Leucodepleted red cells, 148, 153
Leucodepletion, 143
Leukoreduced red cell, 211, 214
Lumbar puncture, 146
Lyme disease, 213
Lymphadenopathy-associated virus (LAV), 132

M
Mendrone, 179
Metagenomics, 190, 202
Microcephalic babies, 171
Microcephalic newborns, 170
Microcephaly, 164, 168, 170, 171
Middle East Respiratory Syndrome Coronavirus (MERS-CoV), 196–198
Mini-mental state examination (MMSE), 150
Minipool (MP) NAT screening, 68
Monte Carlo simulation, 61, 99, 177, 179
Morbidity and Mortality Weekly Report (MMWR), 125
Morulae, 210
Myelopathy, 190

N
Nucleic acid testing (NAT), 13, 67, 68, 133, 134, 160, 175, 177
National CJD Research & Surveillance Unit (NCJDRSU), 143, 144, 146
National Hemophilia Foundation (NHF), 129
Nipah viruses, 198–200
Non-leucodepleted red cells, 148–150, 214
Normal human flora, 202
Nucleic acid testing, 159

O
Occult HBV infection (OBI), 12
Ophthalmic lesions, 172
Ophthalmologic lesions, 170
Opportunistic infections, 126

P
Pan American Health Organization (PAHO), 5, 169, 196, 229, 234, 237–239
Parameter uncertainty, 60
Pathogen inactivation (PI), 13, 70, 71, 181, 190, 211
Pathogen reduction, 13, 70, 71, 190
Post-donation information (PDI), 8
Posttransfusion hepatitis, 10
Posttransfusion survival, 62
Powassan virus (POWV)
  biology and epidemiology, 215
  clinical features/diagnosis/treatment, 216
  mitigating risk, strategies for, 217
  seroprevalence and incidence, 216
  transfusion transmission/survival in blood, 217
Prion-protein typing, 146
Probabilistic sensitivity analysis, 61
ProMed-mail, 5
Protease-resistant prion protein (PrP^{res}), 148
Pteropus (flying foxes), 199
Public health, 18–29
  DNA/RNA of pathogen, 28–30
  Dutch blood transfusion service, 17
  mitigating interventions, 17
  outbreak, 17
  structured approach
    collect facts and uncertainties, 18
    report and conclude, 18–25
  TTI
    advanced quantitative assessment, 27–29
    tools for quantitative assessment, 25–27
  vCJD, impacts of, 30, 31

Index 255

Public trust, 40
Pulvinar sign, 145, 150

Q
Q-fever, 26
Quality-adjusted life year (QALY), 27, 56, 59, 60, 63, 65, 73

R
Residual risk calculations, 63
Retrovirus Epidemiology Donor Study (REDS), 176
Retroviruses, 12
Riboflavin, 198
Risk-based decision-making (RBDM), 35, 54, 84
Risk modelling, 90, 92–95, 100
Risk tolerability, 48–50
Ross River virus (RRV), Australia, 97
  Alphavirus genus, 104
  evidence-based decision-making, 106, 107
  threat to blood safety, 104, 105
  transmission cycle, 104
  TT risk, 105, 106

S
Safety measure, 27, 30, 31
Second-order uncertainty, 60
Serologic testing, 11, 12
Severe acute respiratory syndrome (SARS), 7, 197
Severe acute respiratory syndrome coronavirus (SARS-CoV), 191, 193
Sexual transmission, 173, 174
Simian immunodeficiency virus (SIV), 125
Stakeholder identification tool, 47
Surrogate testing, 9, 10, 189

T
T-cell growth factor (TCGF), 132
Teratogenic syndrome, 171
Tick-borne agents, 217
Tick-borne infections, 209–217
  Anaplasma phagocytophilum
    biology and epidemiology, 209
    clinical feayures/diagnosis/treatment, 209, 210
    mitigating risk, strategies for, 211
    seroprevalence and incidence, 210
    transfusion transmission/survival in blood, 210, 211

  B. burgdorferi, 208
  B. microti, 208
  B. miyamotoi, 207
    biology and epidemiology, 212
    clinical features/diagnosis/treatment, 212, 213
    mitigating risk, strategies for, 214
    seroprevalence and incidence, 213
    transfusion transmission/survival in blood, 213, 214
  blood safety threats, 208
  I. scapularis, 208
  phagocytophilum, 208
  POWV
    biology and epidemiology, 215
    clinical features/diagnosis/treatment, 216
    mitigating risk, strategies for, 217
    seroprevalence and incidence, 216
    transfusion transmission/survival in blood, 217
  tick-borne agents, 207, 217
Tortoises, 207
Transcription-mediated amplification (TMA) multiplex assay, 176
Transfusion medicine, 191
  ZIKV, 178–181
  zoonotic pathogens (*see* Zoonotic pathogens)
Transfusion Medicine Epidemiology Review (TMER) study, 144–146, 148, 149, 151–153
Transfusion-transmission (TT) risk, 87, 88, 90–91, 96–99, 101, 102, 127, 128
  definition, 85
  efficiency, 87
  EID agent, 103
    BP model, 90–91, 96–98
    DENV in Singapore, 101
    EUFRAT models, 90–91, 98, 99
    HEV in Australia, 102
    IgM detection and incident infections in donors, 102
    RRV in Australia, 105, 106
Transfusion-transmitted anaplasmosis (TTA), 209
Transfusion-transmitted infections (TTI), 17, 53, 63, 67, 68, 160, 189, 229–231, 234
  advanced quantitative assessment, 27–29
  tools for quantitative assessment, 25–27
Tropical arboviruses, 6
Trypanosoma cruzi, 234, 238

U

United Nations AIDS (UNAIDS) Program, 229
US Centers for Disease Control and Prevention (CDC), 5

V

Variant Creutzfeldt-Jakob disease (vCJD), 4, 8, 27, 144
  "at risk" donor, 151, 152
  after blood donation, 145, 146, 148, 149
  blood donors and recipients notification, 153, 154
  impacts of, 30, 31
  donors identification, 152, 153
  recipients received red cells from donor 1, 146, 147
  recipients received red cells from donor 2, 148
  recipients 3 received red cells from donor 3, 149–151
  TMER study, information flow in, 144, 145
  zoonotic pathogens, 192
VBD programs, 235, 237, 238

W

Wernicke's encephalopathy, 151
West Nile virus (WNV), 4, 6, 207
  BP model, 91, 96
  Flavivirus genus, 157
  incubation period, 157
  international reaction, 160
  minipool testing, 160
  RNA, 30
  severe neuroinvasive disease, 158
  symptoms, 157
  transfusion safety, 158, 159
  transmittion, 157
  in United Sates, 3
  zoonotic pathogens, 193
WNV neurologic disease (WNND), 96
World Health Organization (WHO), 5

Z

Zika virus (ZIKV), 6, 26, 64–69, 72, 159, 160, 166–178
  clinical manifestations
    chikungunya, 168, 169
    clinical characteristics of, 170
    CZS, 170–172
    dengue, 168, 169
    GBS, 172, 173
    PAHO, 169
  epidemiology, 166, 167
    in Brazil, 166, 167
    French Polynesian epidemic, 166
    microcephaly in Brazil, 168
    in USA, 168
    in Yap Island epidemic, 166
  health economics, blood safety, 63, 64
    Babesia, 65–67
    HIV, HBV and HCV, 67–69
    HTLV, 64, 65
  historical aspects, 163, 164
  minimize risk, approaches to, 178–181
  nonvector transmission
    by breast milk, 174
    laboratory contamination, 175
    by saliva, 173
    sexual transmission, 173–174
    ZIKV persistence in body fluids, 175
  single-donation testing, 159
  transfusion medicine, impacts on, 178–181
  transfusion-transmission
    in asymptomatic blood donors in Brazil, 176
    in Brazil, 176–178
    minipool testing, 177
    NAT tests, 177
    viremic and asymptomatic donors, 175
    worldwide Zika positive rates in blood donors, 178
  vectors of, 166
  virology, 165, 166
  zoonotic pathogens, 194
Zoonotic pathogens, 192–194, 202
  dengue and chikungunya viruses, 194–196
  emerging infections, 201
  emerging zoonotic agents, 190–192
  historical zoonoses
    Ebola virus, 193, 194
    SARS-CoV, 193
    vCJD, 192
    WNV, 193
    Zika virus, 194
  MERS-CoV, 196–198
  nipah and hendra viruses, 198–200

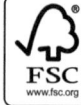

MIX
Papier aus verantwortungsvollen Quellen
Paper from responsible sources
FSC® C105338

If you have any concerns about our products,
you can contact us on
ProductSafety@springernature.com

In case Publisher is established outside the EU,
the EU authorized representative is:
**Springer Nature Customer Service Center GmbH
Europaplatz 3, 69115 Heidelberg, Germany**

Printed by Libri Plureos GmbH
in Hamburg, Germany